Management
of Healthcare
Organizations

Management of Healthcare Organizations

An Introduction

Peter C. Olden

THIRD EDITION

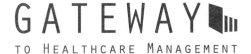

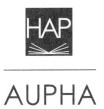

AUPHA

Health Administration Press, Chicago, Illinois
Association of University Programs in Health Administration, Washington, DC

Library of Congress Cataloging-in-Publication Data

Names: Olden, Peter C., author.
Title: Management of healthcare organizations : an introduction / Peter C. Olden,
    Gateway to Healthcare Management.
Description: Third edition. | Chicago, Illinois : Health Administration Press ;
    Washington, DC : Association of University Programs in Health Administration : ,
    [2019] | Includes bibliographical references and index.
Identifiers: LCCN 2018049642 | ISBN 9781640550438 (print : alk. paper) | ISBN
    9781640550452 (xml) | ISBN 9781640550469 (epub) | ISBN 9781640550476 (mobi)
Subjects: LCSH: Health services administration. | Health facilities—Administration. |
    Hospitals—Administration.
Classification: LCC RA971 .O415 2019 | DDC 362.1068—dc23 LC record available
    at https://lccn.loc.gov/2018049642

The paper used in this publication meets the minimum requirements of American National Standard for Information Sciences—Permanence of Paper for Printed Library Materials, ANSI Z39.48-1984. ∞™

Acquisitions editor: Jennette McClain; Manuscript editor: Sharon Sofinski; Project manager: Andrew Baumann; Cover designer: James Slate; Layout: PerfecType

Health Administration Press
A division of the Foundation of the American
    College of Healthcare Executives
300 S. Riverside Plaza, Suite 1900
Chicago, IL 60606-6698
(312) 424-2800

Association of University Programs
    in Health Administration
1730 M Street, NW
Suite 407
Washington, DC 20036
(202) 763-7283

*To the students
who will manage healthcare organizations
to help people live healthier lives.*

BRIEF CONTENTS

DETAILED CONTENTS

PREFACE

The healthcare field and the size of healthcare organizations (HCOs) continue to grow. So does the need for excellent management of these HCOs. Fortunately, many students and healthcare professionals aspire to management positions in HCOs. Management education for HCOs will help them succeed.

Having been a healthcare management student, healthcare manager, and healthcare management professor, I appreciate good books that help us learn management and how to apply it to HCOs. I studied management at the undergraduate, graduate, and doctoral levels. I worked in senior management at three hospitals during 14 years as a hospital executive. And for 25 years, I taught undergraduate and graduate courses in healthcare management and related subjects. All that has motivated and enabled me to write this book.

The purpose of this book is to help people learn the body of knowledge we call *management* and then apply it to HCOs. The primary intended audience is undergraduate students who are interested in managing HCOs but have no prior knowledge of the subject. This book will also be useful to students who are majoring in allied health professions and want to understand management of HCOs, and to current supervisors seeking to learn more about management. This book can help healthcare professionals prepare for advancement to management positions.

The content includes timeless fundamental principles as well as new concepts and current information. Both theory and practice are presented, along with terms, concepts, theories, principles, methods, and tools—and how to use them. A recurring theme in the book is that management is contingent and the "right" approach depends on changing factors. Students will learn that management problems are not multiple-choice questions with a single best answer. The book teaches the principles, theories, methods, and tools so students can assess situations and develop solutions. Students can practice skills using exercises and activities within and at the end of each chapter. Both the content and the writing style strive to engage students, keep them actively interested, provide a few laughs, and help them understand and remember what they read. I have used this approach to successfully teach management of HCOs to undergraduate and graduate students. The publication design further enhances learning by making the material visually appealing and easy to read and understand.

The book has 15 chapters on 15 interrelated subjects needed for management of HCOs. They are connected and organized into a cohesive body of knowledge. By the end of this book, students will understand management and how to apply it to HCOs. (Because this book is about management, it does not include some other disciplines found in healthcare management curricula, such as finance, law, and marketing.)

Each chapter opens with a relevant quote or saying, which is followed by Learning Objectives. Next is Here's What Happened—a real-world example that demonstrates concepts discussed in the chapter. Each Here's What Happened is drawn from the same complex, real-world case study that we follow through the book. In each chapter, headings and subheadings organize content and guide the reader. Key points are **bolded in a different font**. Important terms are defined in the page margins and included in the end-of-book glossary. Exhibits, bulleted lists, examples, activities, and exercises in each chapter keep students engaged and learning. There are sidebars and boxes called Check It Out Online; Try It, Apply It; and Using Chapter _ in the Real World. At the end of each chapter are One More Time (a chapter summary), For Your Toolbox, For Discussion, Case Study Questions, Riverbend Orthopedics Mini Case Study with questions, and References. The Riverbend mini case study and questions at the end of each chapter make up a practical hands-on exercise that is new in this edition. In each chapter, this mini case begins with a recurring paragraph (applicable to all chapters), which is followed by brief additional content and questions that are unique and relevant to that one chapter.

At the back of the book are appendices with more resources. The first is the lengthy, real-world management case study of Partners HealthCare (used to create the Here's What Happened in each chapter). The next appendix—Integrative Case Studies—has seven short (one- to two-page) case studies for which there are questions at the end of each chapter. The Real-World Applied Integrative Projects appendix suggests ten real-world applied projects that students can work on during the course using and integrating management tools from multiple chapters. All tools listed at the end of the chapters throughout the book are combined in the Your Management Toolbox appendix. All defined terms from throughout the book are repeated in the glossary, which is followed by an extensive detailed index.

Several features help students understand how chapters (and management methods) are interrelated. The book is arranged in a logical sequence of chapters that continually build on and connect with previous chapters. Chapter by chapter in the Here's What

Happened examples, students follow managers at Partners HealthCare who create and manage telehealth services to improve population health. When students read the example that begins each chapter, they may also look at the entire Partners HealthCare case in the appendix to appreciate how each chapter's opening case is interrelated with other chapters and management topics. Chapters are further interconnected by end-of-chapter case study questions, which all pertain to the same seven cases (three new to this edition) included in the appendix. Students will realize that fully solving a case study (i.e., management problem) requires them to use different kinds of management principles and tools (from different chapters) just like managers do in the real world. Also, when students try to explain how to address a project listed in the Real-World Applied Integrated Projects appendix, they will realize they must combine various tools and methods (from multiple chapters) like in the real world. This learning activity will develop their understanding of how chapters must be used together to solve real-world problems. In addition, the book sometimes states explicitly how specific chapters and concepts work together.

The purpose of each chapter, and the changes to each chapter in this new edition, are described below. This third edition is longer and has more depth, topics, and tools than prior editions. Prior content has been updated.

Chapter 1 provides the context and background for why HCOs exist and why HCO managers are needed. It introduces readers to health, healthcare, healthcare services, HCOs, and healthcare management jobs. This edition has more discussion of population health, with a newer health model and explanation of forces that determine health (emphasizing social determinants of health). The continuum of care is explained in more detail with a new exhibit. The types of healthcare services, types of HCOs, and current trends and developments are updated. The chapter now includes a section on stakeholders. The discussion and lists of healthcare management job titles, careers, specialty areas, and employment trends have been updated.

Chapter 2 teaches what management is and how it evolved as a body of knowledge, theory, and practice beginning more than a century ago. The chapter briefly explains important developments in the history of management theory. From this comes a framework for organizing and connecting the subsequent chapters and content. New in this edition is an explanation of organization development theory. The section on systems theory has been moved here from chapter 4 and expanded. The chapter has additional explanation of some concepts (e.g., authority) and updated examples.

In chapter 3, students learn how managers plan the purpose, goals, and work of their HCOs. The chapter's strategic planning section has been significantly revised and expanded, with new real-world methods, examples, content, and exhibits from a consulting company. Content for planning at lower levels (involving recent graduates in entry-level jobs) was revised. Tools and techniques for short-term planning are described.

After managers plan as described in chapter 3, they must organize to achieve those plans. We learn about organizing in chapters 4–6. In chapter 4, managers organize work into jobs and departments. This edition contains an expanded section on job design to explain more about tasks, jobs, delegation, and authority. The chapter includes an expanded description of mechanistic and organic structures and more detail about the informal organization. It explains how current trends (mentioned in chapter 1) are affecting how work is organized. In chapter 5, the text and exhibits describe how managers organize departments into larger organization structures seen in organization charts. Concepts are applied to organizing for clinical integration and the continuum of care. This edition includes a new section on horizontal structure, which is explained and illustrated in an exhibit. This chapter has an expanded section on coordination (previously split between chapters 4 and 5). Explanation of how a medical staff is organized has been updated to reflect current trends. Chapter 6 focuses on how managers organize groups and teams. In this edition, this chapter has revised definitions for *group*, *team*, and *committee*. Characteristics of groups and group membership are explained in more depth. This new edition explains huddles and self-managed work teams. The "Effective Groups and Teams" section now includes a discussion of virtual teams.

After organizing, managers must staff the positions, departments, and organizations. Chapter 7 explains how managers obtain staff. This new edition added two new sections and expanded one existing section to emphasize three special concerns for staffing: (1) staff diversity and inclusion; (2) centralized, decentralized, and outsourced staffing; and (3) laws and regulations that affect staffing. The explanation of hiring, recruiting, and selecting staff was expanded with more information and methods (e.g., realistic job previews) tied to macro trends. Real examples of how HCOs have increased staff diversity were added, and the chapter introduces a cultural competency assessment tool. Chapter 8 focuses on how managers retain staff. This edition includes substantial revisions to prior content. It emphasizes developing (rather than training) staff. The performance appraisal section describes the shift from traditional annual appraisals to the newer approach of frequent informal feedback. Compensation and incentives are connected to newer trends in healthcare, and the chapter further explains how pay is determined. There is additional discussion of cultural diversity, including the multigenerational workforce. New information about workplace violence and surveillance was added.

After managers staff the HCO, they must lead, direct, influence, and motivate the staff. This is explained in a trilogy of leadership chapters. Chapter 9 presents leadership theories and models. Compared to the prior edition, it reflects a slight shift from "leadership" to "leading" (i.e., what managers do). This edition has added a section on situational leadership theory and its practical application. The discussion of transformational and servant leadership theories has been expanded, and the chapter touches on authentic leadership and ethical leadership. It also has an important new section on leadership competency models for the twenty-first century. Chapter 10 teaches leading by motivating, influencing, and using power. It explains and applies motivation theories and methods. Exhibits for two theories were updated, and Hackman and Oldham's job characteristics model has been added for practical application of Herzberg's motivation theory. The exhibit detailing types of power was revised. This edition presents more discussion of political tactics and explanation of how leaders use hard power and soft power. Chapter 11 explains leading with culture and ethics. New in this edition are espoused (stated) and enacted (actual) organizational cultures. Explanation of organizational socialization is also new, as is nonmaleficence as a fourth ethical principle. Many short examples (to explain exhibits 11.1 and 11.2) were revised to connect with current HCO trends described in chapter 1.

After planning, organizing, staffing, and leading, managers must control performance. Chapter 12 teaches control and performance improvement. This edition provides more information about Six Sigma. It greatly expands the explanation of Lean management with value stream mapping (and an exhibit) along with root-cause analysis as a new tool. The topics of high-reliability organization and key performance indicators are both explained. New examples pertain to current priorities in healthcare, such as patient experience, value rather than volume, and patient safety. There is an expanded explanation of where managers obtain the data needed to measure and control performance.

After chapters 2 through 12 explain the five basic management functions (planning, organizing, staffing, leading, and controlling), the book presents three additional chapters that will help students to manage HCOs. Chapter 13 teaches how to make decisions needed to solve problems and resolve conflicts. This edition has updated definitions and expanded sections on intuition and evidence-based decisions. The previous edition's section on data for rational decisions has been expanded to address data for all types of decisions. That section was combined with more explanation of big data and analytics to form a new "Data for Decision Making" section that is applicable to all decision-making approaches. The "Who Makes Decisions" section was simplified. This edition describes the conflict resolution process required by The Joint Commission and presents such a process for HCOs.

Chapter 14 teaches how to manage change in organizations. The chapter has a new section on assessing organizational and individual readiness for change. A new exhibit and explanation of the force field analysis tool is also included. There is more detailed explanation of why and how people resist change. The chapter has a new section on organization learning and development, as well as a detailed example of primary care practices trying to implement change in work processes.

Because all the management work taught in chapters 1–14 should be done with professionalism, Chapter 15 explains professionalism for managers in HCOs. This includes sections on professionalism, emotional intelligence (EI), cultural competence, and communication. A new opening quote starts this chapter with relevant career advice. The new edition provides more context, explanation, and examples for EI, along with advice on how to improve EI for management. The chapter has added explanation of cultural competence and steps to improve it (personally and organizationally). The communication model exhibit was revised to better portray people communicating.

The content of this book contributes to numerous curriculum requirements for Association of University Programs in Health Administration (AUPHA) undergraduate certification. These include organization development, organization behavior, management of HCOs, operations assessment and improvement, management of human resources and professionals, governance, leadership, and strategy formulation and implementation.

Instructor resources for each chapter include PowerPoint slides, suggested answers to discussion questions, and a test bank. For access to these instructor resources, please e-mail hapbooks@ache.org.

When Enrico Fermi (who later won a Nobel Prize in physics) was a student, he once told a professor, "Before I came here I was confused about this subject. Having listened to your lecture I am still confused. But on a higher level." I hope that after reading this book, you will be less confused and on a higher level about the subject of management for HCOs. Please share with me your feedback about this book. Thank you.

Peter C. Olden, PhD, MHA, LFACHE
University of Scranton
peter.olden@scranton.edu

INSTRUCTOR RESOURCES

This book's Instructor Resources include PowerPoint slides for each chapter, suggested answers to discussion questions, and a test bank.

For the most up-to-date information about this book and its Instructor Resources, go to ache.org/HAP and search for the book's order code (2378).

This book's Instructor Resources are available to instructors who adopt this book for use in their course. For access information, please e-mail hapbooks@ache.org.

ACKNOWLEDGMENTS

This book and my work on it have benefited from many people. I gratefully acknowledge and deeply appreciate the support of the following, among others.

Many wonderful students at the University of Scranton inspired me to teach, write, and educate future students. Graduate teaching assistant Michaela Dolde helped with research, exhibit preparation, and other tasks. Colleagues at my university and elsewhere shared resources, advice, and feedback on my writing. Faculty and students who used the prior edition of this book gave positive feedback and suggestions.

Staff at Health Administration Press, especially Jennette McClain, Janet Davis, Andrew Baumann, Sharon Sofinski, and Michael Cunningham have helped in more ways than I can list. Health Administration Press kindly gave permission to use material from some of its books, including exhibits prepared by Rose T. Dunn, Daniel B. McLaughlin, John R. Olson, and Patrice Spath, as well as cases prepared by Deborah Bender, Jennifer Lynn Hefner, Ann Scheck McAlearney, and Susan Moffatt-Bruce. Veralon Partners Inc. graciously allowed use of several of its strategic-planning exhibits in this book. Brian Rinker of Highmark Blue Cross Blue Shield gave permission to modify and use a diagram. The Commonwealth Fund gave permission to use a case prepared by Andrew Broderick.

When I was a student, many professors helped me study and learn about managing healthcare organizations. During my management career, I worked with three hospital CEOs—Dana Bamford, Charlie Boone, and Kirby Smith—each of whom helped me develop practical management experience. What I learned from all of them has helped me write this book.

My wife, Debbie, and sons, Ryan and Alex, have been supportive and understanding of my professional work and the time and effort needed to write this book. They have also enriched my life in many ways for which I am especially grateful.

Finally, and yet before everyone noted above, my parents, Walter and Helen, instilled in me a passion for reading and learning.

Thank you, everyone. I appreciate your support and could not have written this book without you.

Peter C. Olden, PhD, MHA, LFACHE
University of Scranton

CHAPTER 1

HEALTH, HEALTHCARE, AND HEALTHCARE ORGANIZATIONS

Strike a balance between population health and individual health.

Howard R. Grant, CEO of Lahey Health

LEARNING OBJECTIVES

Studying this chapter will help you to

➤ explain what health and population health are,

➤ describe the major forces that determine the health of a population,

➤ identify types of health services in the continuum of care,

➤ identify types of healthcare organizations,

➤ explain the external environment and how it affects healthcare organizations,

➤ describe trends that will affect management of healthcare organizations in the future, and

➤ appreciate the variety of healthcare management jobs and careers.

HERE'S WHAT HAPPENED

Partners HealthCare is an integrated healthcare delivery system that owns and operates numerous healthcare organizations (HCOs), including community health centers, physician practices, hospitals, urgent care clinics, and home care businesses. Together, these HCOs provide the continuum of care from prenatal to end-of-life. Based in Boston, Partners is committed to its community, and it values innovation, technology, openness, and preparation. Its managers have watched developments in the external environment, such as demographic trends, the growth of social media, the emphasis on population health, and value-based payment for healthcare. They have been transforming Partners HealthCare to better fit the changing external environment in which it operates. For example, the managers have been forming patient-centered medical homes and are striving to keep the local population healthy through proactive preventive care (rather than reactive cure). Managers implemented a Connected Cardiac Care program that uses telehealth to connect with remote patients and help them care for their heart disease. People are living healthier lives because of what Partners HealthCare's executives, managers, supervisors, and staff have done.

A s the opening example shows, healthcare organizations need managers. We will follow managers at Partners HealthCare throughout this book as a management case study. A brief example from Partners HealthCare opens each chapter to demonstrate that chapter's subject. (These examples are based on a lengthy case study that is presented in "A Management Case Study: Partners HealthCare" later in this book.) This book will help you learn how to manage HCOs to help people live healthier lives, as managers at Partners do. You will be able to do important work (while earning a good paycheck).

This chapter explains health and population health and examines the main forces that determine them. It identifies health services in the continuum of care and the types of HCOs in the healthcare sector. The chapter then describes the external environment and important trends that are affecting HCOs, the healthcare industry, and the healthcare sector. The chapter ends with information about healthcare management jobs and careers, for which this book will prepare you. After reading this chapter, you will better understand why communities need HCOs—and why HCOs need people like you to manage them.

health
A state of complete physical, mental, and social well-being; not merely the absence of disease or infirmity.

HEALTH AND WHAT DETERMINES IT

What is health? In a classic definition still widely used today, the World Health Organization (WHO 1946, 100) states that **health** is "a state of complete physical, mental, and social well-being and not merely the absence of disease or infirmity." **Note that the definition of health is based on being well rather than just not having a health problem.**

An individual's health status may be measured by how well that person feels and functions physically, mentally, and socially. Health status can be evaluated through many measures, such as physical ability, emotions, socialization, blood pressure, and absence of pain. For a group or population, health status may be measured by birth rates, life expectancy, death rates, prevalence of diseases, and group averages for individual health measures.

In recent years, healthcare leaders, clinicians, policymakers, and others have become more concerned about **population health**. The well-established definition of this concept used by the Institute of Medicine (2018) and a population health book (Caron 2017) comes from Kindig and Stoddart (2003, 381): "the health outcomes of a group of individuals, including the distribution of outcomes within the group." A population can be a group of people identified by their shared community, occupation, ethnicity, geographic region, or other characteristic. Kindig (2017) emphasized that distribution of outcomes in a group is important because although a population can be healthy on average, some people may have bad outcomes. Population health has gained prominence because of population health provisions in the Affordable Care Act of 2010 and because it is one of the three goals in the Institute for Healthcare Improvement's (IHI 2018) widely accepted Triple Aim. The concept focuses on the health of a population or group rather than on the health of a patient or person.

Managers of HCOs historically focused on the health of their individual patients. Now they also are addressing the health of their local populations (Morrison 2017). Managers must strive to improve health at both the community population level and the individual person level. You will have to do the same when you are managing an HCO. The techniques presented in this book will help you manage programs, activities, and services to improve population health and individual health in your community. This chapter's opening quote reflects this approach to managing HCOs. As we learned in the opening Here's What Happened, Partners HealthCare's managers are using this approach.

population health
The health outcomes of a group of individuals, including the distribution of outcomes within the group.

DETERMINANTS OF HEALTH

Many forces determine (influence) the health status and health outcomes of populations and individuals. To understand these forces, consider the main determinants of health as described by various sources:

◆ Heredity, medical care services, lifestyles, and environment (fetal, physical, and sociocultural) (Blum 1983)

◆ Genetics, medical care, behavior, physical environment, and social circumstances (McGovern, Miller, and Hughes-Cromwick 2014)

◆ Social and economic environment, physical environment, individual characteristics and behaviors, and health services (WHO 2018)

◆ Policymaking (by governments), social factors (including physical environment), health services, biology (genetics), and individual behavior (HealthyPeople.gov 2018)

◆ Biology (genetics), individual behavior, social environment, physical environment, and health services (Centers for Disease Control and Prevention 2014)

◆ Healthcare, individual behavior, genetics, social environment, and physical environment (Kindig 2017)

Exhibit 1.1 shows Kindig's (2017) five determinants influencing the health outcomes of a person or population. Though not shown in the exhibit (to avoid too many arrows cluttering the exhibit), these determinants interact; they are not independent of each other. For example, the *social environment* in which someone lives affects that person's *individual behavior* and *healthcare*, and those three determinants all affect the person's health. Another point is that the five determinants do not all have an equally strong influence on health.

Genetics is the starting point of health. Genes and characteristics inherited from parents make a person more likely or less likely to develop certain health problems, such as heart disease or cystic fibrosis. Perhaps your parents have mentioned genetic traits and characteristics that run in your family. Although scientists in research laboratories can modify a gene to avoid a disease-causing mutation, genetics is not yet a practical approach

Exhibit 1.1
Five Determinants of Health Model

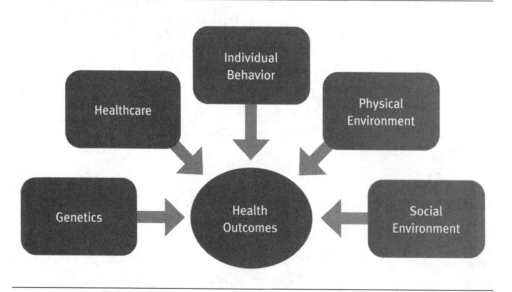

Source: Data from Kindig (2017).

to improving health. That might change in the future as science and ethics evolve (Reardon 2017). For now, managers have to modify the other four determinants to improve health.

Healthcare is "the maintaining and restoration of health by the treatment and prevention of disease [and injury] especially by trained and licensed professionals" (*Merriam-Webster Medical Dictionary* 2018). (The definition of *medical care* is similar but often limited to care performed by physicians.) Healthcare services exist for all ages and stages of life, from womb to tomb. Together, they form a continuum of care that is explained later in this chapter. Managers can improve people's health by helping to ensure people's appropriate use of quality healthcare. Most healthcare spending in the United States has been for diagnosis and treatment of health problems. However, other determinants, such as behavior and social environment, often have a larger effect on health (Caron 2017; McGovern, Miller, and Hughes-Cromwick 2014). Researchers, HCO managers, clinicians, policymakers, and others are realizing this. They are giving more attention and allocating more resources to the other three determinants of health: individual behavior, physical environment, and social environment.

Individual behaviors, such as smoking, seat belt use, diet, flossing, handwashing, and exercise, strongly affect health. For example, heart disease has been linked to behaviors that include smoking, eating unhealthy foods, and not exercising. Healthcare managers can improve people's health by helping them improve their lifestyle and behavior. Some HCOs offer smoking cessation programs, nutrition classes, and fitness walks.

Physical environment is the physical setting (natural and built) in which someone lives. Many elements of the physical environment affect health, such as sanitation, climate, parks, nighttime lighting, forests, safe roads, and air pollution. We can understand the importance of the physical environment by considering the health problems caused by floods and hurricanes. Healthcare managers can improve people's health by helping them improve their physical environment. For example, HCOs have helped their communities reduce air pollution, build parks, and remove garbage.

The social environment includes factors such as socioeconomic status, availability of fresh food, job opportunities, social interaction and support, discrimination, education, language, poverty, prevailing attitudes, and neighbors. Many of these factors vary based on location. Thus, a person's zip code is a stronger predictor of health than is his genetic code (Hinton and Artiga 2018). The effect of these factors on health has gained recognition in recent years. Healthcare managers can improve people's health by helping them improve their social circumstances. Healthcare providers are entering more of this information into patients' medical and health records to monitor and address it with patients (McCulloch 2017).

These determinants can lead to differences in the health of specific groups or subpopulations (e.g., those based on ethnicity, gender, and other characteristics). A **health disparity** is "a health difference that is closely linked with social, economic, or environmental disadvantage" (HealthyPeople.gov 2008). Health disparities are common among groups that face barriers based on their gender, race, ethnicity, disability,

healthcare
The maintaining and restoration of health by the treatment and prevention of disease and injury, especially by trained and licensed professionals.

health disparity
A health difference that is closely linked with social, economic, or environmental disadvantage.

✓ CHECK IT OUT ONLINE

The US Department of Health and Human Services develops health objectives for the country to pursue during each decade. The objectives are designed to help the country become a "society in which all people live long, healthy lives" (HealthyPeople. gov 2018). The 2020 health objectives are available at www. healthypeople.gov/2020/About-Healthy-People. These objectives pertain to dozens of health topics and aspects of health, some relevant to college students. Several new topics were added for 2010–2020, including adolescent health, dementia, genomics, global health, and sleep health. Information provided for each topic includes an overview, objectives, data, and resources. You can also see early work on developing objectives for the 2020–2030 decade. Check it out online and see what you discover.

location, and other factors. The US population is becoming more diverse, and many healthcare managers are striving to reduce disparities so that everyone can live healthy lives. You too will do that in your career.

How can healthcare managers use determinants of health to improve people's health? Realize that factors other than healthcare are important. For example, HCO managers in Wichita can improve people's health by improving their behavior, physical environment, and social environment. These three determinants can help prevent disease, illness, and injury from occurring in the first place. HCOs such as sports medicine clinics, hospitals, health insurers, physician practices, mental health clinics, and others have implemented many interesting approaches. Examples include offering wellness programs to seniors, helping children adopt healthy lifestyles, building walking trails and playgrounds, and using social media to guide behavioral change. Think about your community. What have HCOs done there (besides delivering medical care) to improve health?

HEALTHCARE AND HEALTH SERVICES

There are many different kinds of healthcare and health services. Which ones have you heard of? Some prevent problems, some diagnose problems, some treat problems, and some support people at the end of life. Some are short-term; others are long-term. The many

TRY IT, APPLY IT

Suppose you are asked to serve on a college task force whose mandate is to recommend what the college should do to help students improve their health. Using what you have learned in this chapter about the determinants of health, suggest how students' individual health and population health can be improved. Discuss your ideas with other students.

kinds of healthcare and health services can be grouped into categories, such as preventive, diagnostic, curative, rehabilitative, and so on. Exhibit 1.2 lists several types of healthcare and services. (It is beyond the purpose and scope of this book to explain all these services. If necessary, you can research any unfamiliar services online.) Some types of care, such as hospital care, take place in one kind of HCO. Yet most types of care occur in more than one kind of HCO. For example, diagnostic care occurs in freestanding diagnostic centers, outpatient clinics, physician practices, hospitals, urgent care centers, and other HCOs.

EXHIBIT 1.2
Types of Healthcare Services

Acute care	Health promotion	Preventive care
Adult day care	Home care	Primary care
Ambulatory care	Hospice/palliative care	Public health services
Assisted living	Hospital care	Rehabilitative care
Behavioral health care	Inpatient services	Respite care
Chiropractic care	Long-term care	Self-care
Chronic care	Mental health care	Skilled nursing care
Community health services	Office-based care	Specialty care
Complementary care	Outpatient services	Sports medicine
Dental care	Personal lifestyle care	Subacute care
Diagnostic care	Physician care	Urgent care
Emergency care	Post-acute care	Virtual care

Healthcare and health services together can be thought of as a **continuum of care** (CoC) or care continuum with a range of services needed to care for a person or population (Buell 2017). A comprehensive "womb-to-tomb" CoC begins with prenatal care, ends with palliative end-of-life care, and includes all other health services in between that people might use during their lifetime. Some HCOs extend the CoC into the community and call it a "health continuum" to more fully improve the population health (not merely patient health) of their communities. The health continuum extends beyond direct healthcare services to include housing, food support, employment, and other social determinants of health that come from outside the usual healthcare system (Buell 2018).

Exhibit 1.3 shows an example of a general CoC with a comprehensive sequence of services that many patients might follow. It begins with prenatal and preventive care, followed by primary care, specialty care, diagnostic care, acute care (outpatient and inpatient),

continuum of care
A range of services needed to care for a person or population.

EXHIBIT 1.3

Continuum of Care

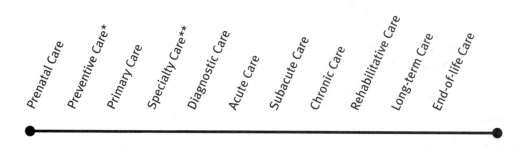

Source: Adapted from Barton (2010) and Shi and Singh (2015).

*Preventive Care occurs at many stages of the continuum to prevent occurrence and reoccurrence of disease, illness, and injury.

**Specialty Care occurs at many stages of the continuum.

subacute care, chronic care, rehabilitative care, long-term care, and end-of-life care (Barton 2010; Shi and Singh 2015). Preventive care and specialty care occur at multiple stages of the continuum.

The continuum can be considered a person's journey through the healthcare system and related community services that are needed to care for that individual (Buell 2017). The complete continuum provides physical health services and mental and behavioral health services throughout the individual's life. Smaller CoCs exist for particular kinds of patients or stages of life, such as CoCs for obstetrics, HIV (human immunodeficiency virus), rehabilitation, or behavioral health. For example, the University of Pittsburgh Medical Center Rehabilitation Institute uses a rehabilitation CoC that includes inpatient, outpatient, and community services. A CoC shows in a typical sequence the types of care and services needed for a specific patient population. Health professionals use CoC models as tools to plan how to meet the healthcare needs of a person or population in the most cost-effective way (Buell 2017). All services in a CoC should be seamlessly coordinated to work together. Thus, managers of HCOs must consider their place in their patients' CoCs and form effective links with other services and organizations in those CoCs.

Recent changes in how providers are paid have been driving HCOs, particularly hospitals and post-acute care HCOs, to use a CoC approach with their patients (Buell 2017; Van Dyke 2017). These changes include value-based payment for care, incentives to keep patients out of hospitals, requirements for discharge planning, bundled payments for episodes of care, and plans for unified post-acute payment. Driven by these new payment methods, hospitals are trying to avoid patient admission and readmission to the hospital. Their approaches include providing preventive, primary, specialty, and diagnostic care early in the continuum to prevent admission, and then subacute, chronic, rehabilitative, and long-term care later in the continuum to prevent readmission. Managers are trying to more closely connect mental and behavioral healthcare with physical healthcare in the continuum.

Besides payment changes, stakeholder demands for population health and coordinated, integrated (rather than fragmented) care are driving HCOs to develop optimal CoCs for patients and communities. This goes beyond the services that HCOs provide. HCOs must focus on social determinants of health (discussed earlier in this chapter) and the patient's role in self-care to keep people healthy and avoid expensive healthcare (Bosko and Gulotta 2016; Buell 2018). Thus, some HCOs are trying to gather data about patients' housing, food security, education, income stability, and other social factors that strongly affect health.

HEALTHCARE ORGANIZATIONS

The Here's What Happened at the beginning of the chapter introduced Partners HealthCare—a large, complex HCO (made up of smaller HCOs) that we will follow throughout the book. What HCOs have you heard of, worked at, or volunteered at? Some HCOs, such as large general hospitals, provide a wide range of services spanning many parts of the CoC. Other HCOs, such as hospices, specialize and provide only a narrow range of services in one part of the continuum. Hospitals may also specialize, such as hospitals for only psychiatric care or for only rehabilitation services.

Ambulatory HCOs provide healthcare services to people who obtain care but do not stay overnight. Medical group practices and physician offices provide many ambulatory medical services in specialties such as cardiology, pulmonology, and neurology. They might offer diagnostic testing, on-site therapy services, outpatient surgery, and other services. Outpatient diagnostic centers perform lab tests, medical imaging, and other services to diagnose health problems. Other outpatient HCOs are ambulatory surgery centers, urgent care facilities, mental health clinics, public health agencies, sports medicine businesses, dental practices, and counseling offices. Some retail stores operated by large companies (e.g., Walmart, Target, CVS, Kroger) offer basic urgent care. Home care organizations provide an array of nursing care, therapy, and health services in people's homes. Telehealth and virtual care methods have expanded the range of health services delivered in people's residences. Some organizations—such as skilled nursing facilities, personal care homes, and assisted living communities—provide services for people (not all of whom are elderly) who need care for an extended period of time.

In addition to HCOs that provide hands-on healthcare services to patients, other types of HCOs are essential for improving individual health and population health. Organizations such as the American Cancer Society and the American Lung Association improve people's health by funding research, developing educational programs, reducing risk factors, and assisting people who need treatment. Medical supply firms and pharmaceutical companies such as Johnson & Johnson produce and distribute supplies, drugs, and equipment that other HCOs use for their healthcare. Companies such as General Electric and Philips make complex medical equipment. Some companies make catheters, intravenous solutions, antibiotics, bandages, and many other daily supplies. Health insurance companies, such as Blue Cross, are another type of HCO. These businesses assist in the financing of and payment for healthcare services. Trade organizations (e.g., the Medical Group Management Association) and professional associations (e.g., the American College of Healthcare Executives) are other types of HCOs. Colleges and universities educate people to work in dozens of types of healthcare jobs. Professional and governmental organizations such as The Joint Commission and the Ohio Department of Health accredit, license, and regulate HCOs. Philanthropic organizations such as The Commonwealth Fund and the Kaiser Family Foundation provide research, education, and financial grants to improve health.

The list of HCOs could go on and on. Try to think of other kinds of HCOs. There is no distinct boundary between HCOs and non-HCOs. For example, Amazon, Apple, and Uber have announced their intentions to get involved with healthcare (Michelson 2018). Managers of HCOs should realize that their organizations must interact with many others to produce a CoC and healthcare services for their population.

THE EXTERNAL ENVIRONMENT OF HEALTHCARE ORGANIZATIONS

An HCO exists in an external environment of people, organizations, industries, trends, forces, events, and developments that are outside of the HCO. Most of these external elements are beyond the HCO's control. The external environment of a specific HCO includes all the other HCOs along with citizens, schools, colleges, banks, information technology (IT) companies, labor unions, competitors, stock markets, governments, venture capitalists, and more. This environment includes economic, demographic, technological, cultural, legal, social, and other kinds of developments in society. For example, in the opening Here's What Happened, the external environment of Partners HealthCare includes the invention of new devices for mobile technology.

Let's analyze the external environment of a home care business in Baltimore. The other home care businesses around the city are part of the environment. They exist in the healthcare realm, which also includes public health agencies, subacute care facilities, health insurers, and all the other HCOs in and around Baltimore. The larger society, including government, banking, transportation, education, housing, and many other elements, are all part of that home care business's external environment. In addition, that environment includes potential customers, volunteers, employees, student interns, donors, and suppliers. We can also think of this environment in terms of forces and influences, such as cultural diversity, local employment trends, 24/7 mobile communication, and opioid addiction rates, that affect the home care business.

These other organizations, forces, and people affect HCOs in many ways. For example, the home care business depends on people to use its services, but those clients may want more weekend services and social media interaction. They can use a different home care business if their preferences are not met. The government could force the business to make changes to maintain its license and stay open. The home care business depends on other businesses to provide services and supplies, so it will have to contract with an internet service provider and medical supply vendors.

An HCO exists in, and is influenced by, a larger world. The HCO must be open to its external environment and interact effectively with it. To paraphrase an old saying, no HCO is an island unto itself. An HCO depends on people and organizations in its environment just as a person does. When you are a manager, pay attention to your external environment!

If we just think of "the environment," we are likely to overlook parts of it. The environment is so big (and somewhat vague) that we might not fully realize what it includes. To better understand the external environment outside of and beyond our own HCO, we can divide it into 11 sectors (Daft 2016, 143). Thinking about each of these sectors helps managers analyze their external environment and more fully comprehend how it affects their HCO.

1. *Industry sector*—related businesses and competitors that offer products and services similar to what your organization offers

2. *Raw materials sector*—suppliers, manufacturers, and service providers, from which your organization obtains needed supplies, equipment, and services

3. *Human resources sector*—employees, labor unions, schools, colleges, employment agencies, and labor markets, from which your organization obtains human resources (employees)

4. *Financial resources sector*—banks, lenders, stock markets, and investors, from which your organization obtains loans, credit, and other financial resources (not customers and insurers who pay your organization for products and services)

5. *Market sector*—actual and potential customers, clients, and users of your organization's products and services

6. *Technology sector*—science and technological methods of producing products and services, some of which your organization uses

7. *Economic conditions sector*—levels and rates of employment, inflation, growth, investment, and other economic circumstances in which your organization exists (not financial resources or money for your specific organization)

8. *Government sector*—laws, regulations, court rulings, political systems, and governments at the local, state, and federal levels, some of which affect your organization

9. *Natural sector*—natural resources, the green movement, and forces for sustainability

10. *Sociocultural sector*—characteristics of the society and culture (e.g., education, values, attitudes) in which your organization exists

11. *International sector*—globalization, and other countries and their customs, industries, businesses, and people, some of which might affect your organization

When you think about an HCO, think about its external environment, too, because that strongly affects the HCO. The full Partners HealthCare case study at the end of this book explains how sectors of the external environment affected that HCO. Managers must develop good relationships between their HCO and the external environment, as explained further in this book's chapters on planning and organizing. For example, HCO managers use Facebook to interact with customers and suppliers in the environment.

HEALTHCARE TRENDS AND FUTURE DEVELOPMENTS

Healthcare is always changing—you have probably noticed that. Many powerful trends and developments affect health, healthcare, and healthcare organizations. Managers can use the methods, tools, principles, and techniques in this book to help their HCOs monitor and adjust to these changes. However, trends sometimes unexpectedly stop, change, turn around, or start anew, making it hard to accurately predict the future. Thus, managers should know "how to create a healthcare organization that can succeed in an unpredictable future" (Olden and Haynos 2013, 193). This book will help you learn how to do that.

The following list includes important trends and developments in US healthcare and its environment. These trends are interrelated and thus affect each other as well as HCOs. Watch for the Using Chapter _ in the Real World sidebar feature in each chapter of this book. The sidebars provide real-world examples of how managers use the concepts in each chapter to address such trends and developments.

◆   *Demographics.* What will the US population be like during your career? Here are estimates based on the last US census in 2010 and the subsequent US Census Bureau's 2014 National Projections (Colby and Ortman 2015, 1):

Between 2014 and 2060, the U.S. population is projected to increase from 319 million to 417 million, reaching 400 million in 2051. The U.S.

population is projected to grow more slowly in future decades than in the recent past, as these projections assume that fertility rates will continue to decline and that there will be a modest decline in the overall rate of net international migration. By 2030, one in five Americans is projected to be 65 and over; by 2044, more than half of all Americans are projected to belong to a minority group (any group other than non-Hispanic White alone); and by 2060, nearly one in five of the nation's total population is projected to be foreign born.

◆ *Workforce.* Many HCOs are striving to develop a diverse workforce that better matches the diversity of the population they serve. The workforce comprises up to five generations of very diverse workers with very different expectations. Managers are more concerned about workers' engagement, safety, joy, human interaction, and overall work experience. Employers are striving to reduce employees' fatigue, stress, burnout, and turnover while improving work flexibility, rewards, development, work space, well-being, feedback, and support. HCOs continue to use a mix of permanent and "gig economy" arrangements—full-time, part-time, freelance, on call, per diem, contractual, on-site, online, and others. Continual training, upskilling, and development of workers are essential. Shortages of nurses, pharmacists, and primary care professionals continue to challenge HCOs. Larger HCOs are creating management positions for innovation, transformation, process improvement, clinical integration, diversity and inclusion, strategy, population health, patient experience, and analytics. More physicians are working in senior management and leadership positions (Bisognano 2017; Dye 2017; Noe et al. 2016; Schawbel 2016, 2017; Spitzer 2018).

◆ *Payment.* Though still common, fee-for-service payment is on the decline. Healthcare payment is increasingly based on value of care rather than volume of care. Payments are being tied to performance as measured by benchmarks and standards for quality, patient experience, clinical outcomes, and best practices. Payment may be based on bundles of services for episodes of care, or on care that is accountable for keeping people healthy. Thus, HCOs are redesigning healthcare processes, monitoring care more closely, and using more detailed and sophisticated cost accounting. More payment is population based, where "providers typically receive a target budget to care for a defined population over a specified period, generally a year. Healthcare organizations are responsible for all services their patients use during the specified period" (Chernew 2017, 12). Thus, HCOs are strengthening how they manage patients through the CoC, especially before and after inpatient care.

◆ *Connectedness.* People and organizations are becoming more connected locally, regionally, nationally, and globally. Healthcare is investing in more communications technology and IT. HCOs are expanding their use of social media to share blogs, infographics, videos, and stories and to enable two-way conversations, feedback, and engagement with patients, employees, and other stakeholders. There are more e-health providers, and HCOs are delivering more telehealth, mobile health, and virtual health.

◆ *Patient experience.* Healthcare consumers are becoming more knowledgeable about their own health and more demanding of HCOs. People are more engaged in their health and healthcare including their wellness, health literacy, decision making, and self-management. They want to obtain and consume healthcare on their terms, not providers' paternalistic terms (Dowling 2017). Thus, HCOs are striving to improve the **patient experience**—all that a patient experiences and perceives while interacting with the healthcare system, HCOs, and healthcare workers (Radick 2016). The patient experience emphasizes the total experience of the CoC (not just medical care), including empathy, convenience, respect, trust, fulfillment of expectations, responsiveness, and individual attention. Care is becoming more patient centered and less provider centered to better meet the needs of patients, family members, consumers, and communities. Personalized medicine is becoming more common to address each patient's unique wants, needs, and life situation.

◆ *Population health.* The healthcare system and HCOs are giving more attention to population health and healthy communities through increased use of epidemiology and public health services to address risk factors (Caron 2017). HCOs are becoming more involved in health promotion, disease prevention, primary care, and wellness that require improving the upstream social, economic, behavioral, environmental, and educational factors that affect health. Stakeholders are focusing more on communities and not just one patient at a time. Care continues to shift from inpatient to outpatient settings and to many nontraditional points of service in retail stores, kiosks, and cyberspace. Mental and behavioral health are receiving more attention. Healthcare providers are collaborating with communities to improve social determinants of health. The CoC continues to expand beyond healthcare.

◆ *Consolidation.* HCOs continue to consolidate into a variety of larger organization forms (Dowling 2017; Kaufman 2017; Keckley 2018; Michelson 2018). Hospitals, medical groups, insurers, ambulatory clinics, long-term

patient experience
All that a patient experiences and perceives while interacting with the healthcare system, healthcare organizations, and healthcare workers.

care businesses, community agencies, and other HCOs are forming mergers, alliances, networks, vertically integrated delivery systems, accountable care organizations, and other collaborative structures. There are fewer HCOs, yet they are bigger and more complex. These structures are expected to improve coordination through the CoC, reduce fragmentation of services, share scarce resources, gain economies of scale, increase power, and improve quality. Their size and complexity may create challenges for patients and other stakeholders. Extremely large businesses (both inside and outside healthcare) are taking on bigger—and disruptive—roles in the US healthcare system.

◆ *Health science and technology.* Continual advances in science and technology enable new approaches to health prevention, diagnosis, and treatment. This evolution will continue in the future with developments in telehealth, robotics, genetics, bionic limbs, artificial organs, 3-D printing of body parts, IT and connectivity, virtual reality, artificial intelligence, voice activation, molecular imaging, implantable chips, personal health monitoring, e-health, customized medicines, gene therapy, regenerative medicine, and smart devices with medical attachments (Diamandis 2017; Harris 2018; Michelson 2018; Moore 2017). Artificial intelligence is gaining momentum and is expected to improve population health, chronic disease management, and clinical decision making. These developments require increased cybersecurity and raise many ethical, legal, financial, and social questions.

◆ *Big data and predictive analytics.* Clinicians and managers are developing systems to use big data from all aspects of people's lives to predict future health problems of individuals and populations. Some health data are obtained from people's wearables, mobile devices, and personal health monitors or trackers (Ebadollahi 2017). Healthcare is becoming more proactive. Besides population health and clinical care, analysis of big data is being used for management decisions, strategic planning, human resources, financial management, and many other aspects of managing HCOs.

Some of these trends and developments are included in the Triple Aim that many HCOs have been working toward. The Institute for Healthcare Improvement (2018) advocates

◆ improving the patient's experience of care (including quality and satisfaction),

◆ improving the health of populations, and

◆ reducing the per capita cost of healthcare.

STAKEHOLDERS AND EXPECTATIONS OF HEALTHCARE ORGANIZATIONS

As discussed earlier, HCO managers can better understand what is expected of them and their HCO by examining the external environment and the trends and future developments in healthcare. To further understand expectations, managers can analyze stakeholders. For a designated organization, **stakeholders** are people or groups of people (inside and outside the organization) and other organizations (outside the designated organization) that have a stake (interest) in the designated organization. To do this analysis for an HCO, a manager first lists the stakeholders of the HCO. Then the manager identifies the stake (i.e., interest, demand, expectation) of each stakeholder. The manager can also judge how much each stakeholder could affect the HCO (favorably or unfavorably) if the stakeholder's expectation is not met. Examples of an HCO's stakeholders are employees, the media, financial lenders, business coalitions, patients, other HCOs, governments, special interest groups, accreditors,

stakeholders
For a designated organization, people and other organizations who have a stake (interest) in what the organization does.

🌐 USING CHAPTER 1 IN THE REAL WORLD

Sven Gierlinger, chief experience officer at Northwell Health in New Hyde Park, New York, thinks healthcare is gradually catching up with the consumerism movement. Northwell is improving the patient experience by means of four approaches. *Culture change* sets expectations (backed by mandatory training) for how employees communicate with patients. *Innovation* changes work processes to provide better service to patients and families. The *environment* that patients experience is being made more welcoming, visually appealing, and focused on healing. *Accountability* of all employees for patient experience is achieved via standards, metrics, and data (Radick 2016).

Mosaic Life Care in Missouri is emphasizing population health. Mark Laney, CEO of the integrated delivery system, said, "We decided to . . . shift to what we call 'life care,' a patient-centered population health model that places greater focus on keeping people healthy than on treating acute illness" (Van Dyke 2016, 21). This health system is moving more care from the hospital to the home. For example, IT enables virtual house calls and ongoing two-way patient–provider communication via a portal. Patients access their electronic health records and discuss concerns with their physicians. These approaches are improving the health of the local population.

and labor unions. Exhibit 1.4 shows common stakeholders and what they typically expect of HCOs. Which other stakeholders can you think of in healthcare?

Stakeholder	Stakes in (Expectations of) HCOs
Employees	Job satisfaction, good compensation, safe work conditions
Patients, clients	Quality care, compassion, convenience, affordable prices
Media and press	Prompt, candid replies to questions; access to top managers
Creditors	Repayment as scheduled
Physicians	Superb patient care, new equipment, convenient scheduling
Businesses	Affordable healthcare, low insurance premiums and prices
Other HCOs	Cooperation for patients' transfers and transitions
Governments	Compliance with laws and regulations
Special interest groups	Support for their interests (e.g., hiring minorities, caring for people with diabetes)
Accreditation commissions	Compliance with accreditation standards
Vendors and suppliers	Prompt payment
Neighbors	Respect for their property and neighborhood

EXHIBIT 1.4
Stakeholders and Their Stakes in HCOs

Now and in the future, managers and their HCOs must strive to adapt to the trends and developments described earlier. They also must address stakeholders' expectations, which include the following:

◆ Reduce disparities in healthcare.

◆ Increase the efficiency of healthcare with lower cost and less variation.

◆ Improve the inclusiveness and diversity of the workforce based on age, gender, ethnicity, race, profession, education, skill, view, scope of practice, and other characteristics.

◆ Create high-performing employees, teams, and HCOs while helping workers deal with burnout and stress.

◆ Adjust work and the workforce to adapt to changes in healthcare.

◆ Expand the use of newer technologies (e.g., robotics, nanotechnology, artificial intelligence, genomics) to improve medicine, healthcare, and customer service.

◆ Provide excellent personalized healthcare to individual patients while also providing excellent population-based services to populations served.

HEALTHCARE MANAGEMENT JOBS AND CAREERS

Earlier, this chapter mentioned the many services and organizations that make up our healthcare system. Within them, many kinds of healthcare management jobs exist. According to the US Bureau of Labor Statistics (2018), there were 352,200 jobs in health services management in 2016; by 2026, this number is expected to grow by 20 percent (much faster than the average for all jobs). New graduates should expect to begin their careers in entry-level jobs. From there, promotions can lead to middle-management and then upper-management positions. After gaining some experience, you will be able to move between different types of HCOs, such as from a hospital to a health insurance company or a primary care network. There are many opportunities for students to develop exciting, rewarding healthcare management careers, as shown in exhibits 1.5 and 1.6. Although this book was written to help you prepare to enter this profession, its lessons, principles, tools, and methods will be useful throughout your career.

People who are preparing for a healthcare management job (or who already have one) can choose from a wide variety of potential jobs and career tracks. Yet demand and supply differ among jobs and careers, so students should follow hiring trends and be alert for new opportunities. For example, the number of management jobs in ambulatory care and long-term care is likely to increase more than the number of management jobs in inpatient hospital care. Healthcare management jobs that focus on quality, process improvement, social media, and population

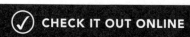

CHECK IT OUT ONLINE

Interested in the future of healthcare and healthcare jobs? You can access trends and data at the US Bureau of Labor Statistics healthcare occupations website (www.bls.gov/ooh/healthcare/home.htm). Trends and data for management jobs are at www.bls.gov/ooh/management/. Check it out online and see what you discover—now and throughout your career.

EXHIBIT 1.5

Types of Healthcare Organizations and Jobs

Managers may work in these and other HCOs:

- Accountable care organizations
- Ambulatory clinics
- Community health alliances
- Consulting firms
- Diagnostic centers
- Healthcare associations
- Health insurance organizations
- Health insurance organizations
- Health-related charities, foundations, advocacy groups, and voluntary organizations
- Home care businesses
- Hospitals
- Integrated health care systems
- Medical supply companies
- Mental health organizations
- Outpatient surgery centers
- Personal care homes
- Pharmaceutical businesses
- Physician practices
- Public health departments
- Rehabilitation centers
- Research institutions
- Respite care facilities

Managers may work in these and other specialized areas:

- Business development
- Clinical integration
- Community relations
- Diversity and inclusion
- Facilities management
- Finance
- Government relations
- Human resources
- Information systems
- Innovation
- Logistics for supplies and equipment
- Marketing and public affairs
- Medical affairs
- Patient access
- Patient experience
- Population health
- Professional services
- Strategic planning
- Transformation

health are likely to increase more than the average for all healthcare management jobs. Further, healthcare evolves so rapidly that new kinds of management jobs will emerge in the coming years. An exciting variety of jobs will be available, so healthcare managers need not be stuck in a dead-end job if they prepare for a job change.

Exhibit 1.6
Examples of
Healthcare
Management
Job Titles

Account manager	Director of human resources	Patient experience coordinator
Administrator	Director of marketing	Physician recruitment specialist
Billing manager	Director of materials management	Population health manager
Budget analyst		
Business intelligence specialist	Director of patient access	Product manager
Chief executive officer	Director of physician relations	Program manager
Chief information officer	Director of safety	Project manager
Chief quality officer	Director of utilization management	Provider network supervisor
Chief strategy officer		Public health program manager
Community health center director	Education and training director	Quality analyst
Community resource adviser	Emergency management coordinator	Quality assurance coordinator
Compliance officer	Health systems specialist	Regional director of operations
Contracts administration supervisor	Human resources compensation specialist	Research analyst
Credentialing coordinator	Informatics lead	Risk manager
Director of business development	Information management specialist	Sales representative
Director of environmental services	Insurance coordinator	Vice president of women's services
Director of finance	Managed care coordinator	Volunteer services coordinator
Director of government affairs	Management engineer	
	Marketing associate	

Sources: Friedman and Kovner (2013); Monster (2018).

ONE MORE TIME

Health is more than the absence of disease. It includes complete well-being—physical, mental, and social. People's health is determined by five broad forces: genetics, healthcare, individual behavior, physical environment, and social environment. Although healthcare managers can't improve heredity, they can improve all the other forces to boost a population's health. Healthcare services range from prenatal care to end-of-life palliative care, and they form a womb-to-tomb continuum of care. Many kinds of healthcare organizations exist to provide these services. Some directly provide health services in the CoC. Others (e.g., suppliers, insurers) do not directly provide health services but perform other essential services, such as manufacturing healthcare supplies and financing healthcare. HCOs interact with each other and with many other elements in their external environment. All HCOs depend on many other organizations and their environment. When the external environment changes, those changes often affect HCOs. Thus, HCOs must monitor and adapt to changes in their environment. Healthcare managers work in a wide variety of jobs and HCOs throughout the CoC and health sector.

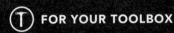

(T) FOR YOUR TOOLBOX

- Five determinants of health model
- Continuum of care
- External environment divided into sectors

FOR DISCUSSION

1. Based on what you learned in this chapter, discuss the determinants that affect health and well-being in the community where your college is located. Give an example of each determinant. Which determinants do you think healthcare managers can change the most to improve population health?

2. What are disparities in health? Give examples. Why must healthcare managers understand these disparities?

3. Why is the external environment so important to healthcare organizations? Which sectors of the environment do you think are most important for HCOs? Give examples.

4. Discuss several trends and issues presented in this chapter. Which of these trends and issues do you think are the most challenging for specific types of HCOs?

5. After students graduate with degrees in healthcare management, what are some HCOs and jobs that they could work in? Which of these are you interested in?

CASE STUDY QUESTIONS

These questions refer to the Integrative Case Studies at the back of this book.

1. All cases: Which healthcare services and HCOs are evident in these cases?

2. All cases: Which sectors of the external environment are evident in these cases?

3. All cases: Which healthcare management jobs are evident in these cases?

4. Disparities in Care at Southern Regional Health System case: How is the population health approach evident in this case?

5. How Can an ACO Improve the Health of Its Population? case: What problems with care coordination and the continuum of care are evident in this case? How could Ms. Dillow fix those problems to better manage population health?

 RIVERBEND ORTHOPEDICS MINI CASE STUDY

Riverbend Orthopedics is a busy group practice with expanded services for orthopedic care. It has seven physicians and a podiatrist, plus about 70 other employees. At its big, new clinic building, Riverbend provides extensive orthopedic care. Several technicians provide diagnostic medical imaging, from basic X-rays to magnetic resonance images. The physicians perform surgery in their own outpatient surgery center with Riverbend's own operating nurses and technicians. Therapy is provided by three physical therapists and one part-time contracted occupational therapist. In addition to staff providing actual patient care, the clinic has staff for financial management, medical records, human resources, information systems/technology, building maintenance, and other

(continued)

RIVERBEND ORTHOPEDICS MINI CASE STUDY *(continued)*

administrative matters. Occasional marketing work is done by an advertising company. Legal work is outsourced to a law firm. Riverbend is managed by a new president, Ms. Garcia. She and Riverbend have set a goal of achieving "Excellent" ratings for patient experience from at least 90 percent of Riverbend's patients this year.

Riverbend's physicians are not fully aware of the external environment and how it affects their group practice. Dr. Chen wonders how he can analyze the external environment to understand how it might affect Riverbend. Dr. Barr wonders what population health and continuum of care are and how they matter to Riverbend.

MINI CASE STUDY QUESTIONS

1. Using information from this book, how would you answer Dr. Chen?

2. Using information from this book, how would you answer Dr. Barr?

REFERENCES

Barton, P. L. 2010. *Understanding the US Health Services System*, 4th ed. Chicago: Health Administration Press.

Bisognano, M. 2017. "New Ways to Lead the Workforce of the Future." In *Futurescan 2017: Healthcare Trends and Implications 2017–2022*, edited by I. Morrison, 27–31. Chicago: Society for Healthcare Strategy & Market Development and Health Administration Press.

Blum, H. L. 1983. *Planning for Health*. New York: Human Sciences Press.

Bosko, T., and B. Gulotta. 2016. "Improving Care Across the Continuum." *Journal of Healthcare Management* 61 (2): 90–93.

Buell, J. M. 2018. "The Health Continuum: Leveraging IT to Optimize Care." *Healthcare Executive* 33 (1): 10–18.

———. 2017. "The Care Continuum Universe: Delivering on the Promise." *Healthcare Executive* 32 (1): 10–17.

Caron, R. M. 2017. *Population Health: Principles and Applications for Management*. Chicago: Health Administration Press.

Centers for Disease Control and Prevention. 2014. "Definitions." Accessed September 23, 2017. www.cdc.gov/nchhstp/socialdeterminants/definitions.html.

Chernew, M. E. 2017. "Two Payment Models Will Dominate the Move to Value-Based Care." In *Futurescan 2017: Healthcare Trends and Implications 2017–2022*, edited by I. Morrison, 12–16. Chicago: Society for Healthcare Strategy & Market Development and Health Administration Press.

Colby, S. L., and J. M. Ortman. 2015. *Projections of the Size and Composition of the U.S. Population: 2014 to 2060*. US Census Bureau Current Population Report P25-1143. Published March. www.census.gov/content/dam/Census/library/publications/2015/demo/p25-1143.pdf.

Daft, R. L. 2016. *Organization Theory and Design*, 12th ed. Mason, OH: South-Western Cengage.

Diamandis, P. H. 2017. "Exponential Change in Today's Healthcare System." In *Futurescan 2017: Healthcare Trends and Implications 2017–2022*, edited by I. Morrison, 42–47. Chicago: Society for Healthcare Strategy & Market Development and Health Administration Press.

Dowling, M. J. 2017. "4 Most Important Healthcare Trends in 2018." *Becker's Hospital Review*. Published December 18. www.beckershospitalreview.com/hospital-management-administration/michael-dowling-4-most-important-healthcare-trends-in-2018.html.

Dye, C. F. 2017. *Leadership in Healthcare*, 3rd ed. Chicago: Health Administration Press.

Ebadollahi, S. 2017. "The Power of Advanced Technologies to Transform Hospitals and Health Systems." In *Futurescan 2017: Healthcare Trends and Implications 2017–2022*, edited by I. Morrison, 17–21. Chicago: Society for Healthcare Strategy & Market Development and Health Administration Press.

Friedman, L. H., and A. R. Kovner. 2013. *101 Careers in Healthcare Management*. New York: Springer.

Harris, J. M. (ed.). 2018. *Healthcare Strategic Planning*, 4th ed. Chicago: Health Administration Press.

HealthyPeople.gov. 2018. "Determinants of Health." Accessed July 22. www.healthypeople. gov/2020/about/foundation-health-measures/Determinants-of-Health.

———. 2008. "Minutes: Sixth Meeting: October 15, 2008." Accessed August 6, 2017. www. healthypeople.gov/2020/minutes-sixth-meeting-october-15-2008/page/0/1.

Hinton, E., and S. Artiga. 2018. "Beyond Health Care: The Role of Social Determinants in Promoting Health and Health Equity." Kaiser Family Foundation. Published May 10. www. kff.org/disparities-policy/issue-brief/beyond-health-care-the-role-of-social-determinants-in-promoting-health-and-health-equity/.

Institute for Healthcare Improvement (IHI). 2018. "The IHI Triple Aim." Accessed July 24. www.ihi.org/engage/initiatives/TripleAim/Pages/default.aspx.

Institute of Medicine (IOM). 2018. "Working Definition of Population Health." Accessed July 27. http://nationalacademies.org/hmd/~/media/Files/Activity%20Files/PublicHealth/PopulationHealthImprovementRT/Pop%20Health%20RT%20Population%20Health%20Working%20Definition.pdf.

Kaufman, K. 2017. "The New Role of Healthcare Integration." In *Futurescan 2017: Healthcare Trends and Implications 2017–2022*, edited by I. Morrison, 2–6. Chicago: Society for Healthcare Strategy & Market Development and Health Administration Press.

Keckley, P. 2018. "Hospital Consolidation: The Third Wave." *Healthcare Executive* 33 (2): 60–63.

Kindig, D. A. 2017. "What Is Population Health?" *Improving Population Health* (blog). Accessed September 23. www.improvingpopulationhealth.org/blog/what-is-population-health.html.

Kindig, D. A., and G. Stoddart. 2003. "What Is Population Health?" *American Journal of Public Health* 93 (3): 380–83.

McCulloch, A. R. 2017. "Connecting Our Community to the Care It Needs." *Healthcare Executive* 32 (5): 52–55.

McGovern, L., G. Miller, and P. Hughes-Cromwick. 2014. "Health Policy Brief: The Relative Contribution of Multiple Determinants to Health Outcomes." *Health Affairs.* Published August 21. www.healthaffairs.org/do/10.1377/hpb20140821.404487/full/.

Merriam-Webster Medical Dictionary. 2018. "Health Care." Accessed July 22. www.merriam-webster.com/dictionary/health%20care#medicalDictionary.

Michelson, D. 2018. "The No. 1 Takeaway from HIMSS 2018: 'Amazon and Apple and Uber, Oh My!'" *Becker's Hospital Review*. Published March 9. www.beckershospitalreview.com/healthcare-information-technology/the-no-1-takeaway-from-himss-2018-amazon-and-apple-and-uber-oh-my.html.

Monster. 2018. "Healthcare Jobs." Accessed February 11. www.monster.com/jobs/browse/q-healthcare-jobs.aspx.

Moore, R. S. 2017. "Changing the Face of Medicine Through Virtual Care." In *Futurescan 2017: Healthcare Trends and Implications 2017–2022*, edited by I. Morrison, 36–41. Chicago: Society for Healthcare Strategy & Market Development and Health Administration Press.

Morrison, I. 2017. "The Building Blocks of Transformation." In *Futurescan 2017: Healthcare Trends and Implications 2017–2022*, edited by I. Morrison, 2–6. Chicago: Society for Healthcare Strategy & Market Development and Health Administration Press.

Noe, R., J. Hollenbeck, B. Gerhart, and P. Wright. 2016. *Human Resource Management: Gaining a Competitive Advantage*, 10th ed. Chicago: McGraw-Hill Higher Education.

Olden, P. C., and J. Haynos. 2013. "How to Create a Health Care Organization That Can Succeed in an Unpredictable Future." *Health Care Manager* 32 (2): 193–200.

Radick, L. E. 2016. "Improving the Patient Experience." *Healthcare Executive* 3 (6): 32–38.

Reardon, S. 2017. "US Science Advisers Outline Path to Genetically Modified Babies." *Nature*. Published February 14. www.nature.com/news/us-science-advisers-outline-path-to-genetically-modified-babies-1.21474.

Schawbel, D. 2017. "Workplace Trends You'll See in 2018." *Forbes*. Published November 1. www.forbes.com/sites/danschawbel/2017/11/01/10-workplace-trends-youll-see-in-2018/#300c33e24bf2.

———. 2016. "Workplace Trends You'll See in 2017." *Forbes*. Published November 1. www. forbes.com/sites/danschawbel/2016/11/01/workplace-trends-2017/#1cefa2dd56bd.

Shi, L., and D. A. Singh. 2015. *Delivering Health Care in America: A Systems Approach*, 6th ed. Burlington, MA: Jones & Bartlett Learning.

Spitzer, J. 2018. "5 New Executive Roles, Coming to a Hospital Near You." *Becker's Hospital Review*. Published May 4. www.beckershospitalreview.com/hospital-management -administration/5-new-executive-roles-coming-to-a-hospital-near-you.html.

US Bureau of Labor Statistics. 2018. "Medical and Health Services Managers." Accessed July 22. www.bls.gov/ooh/management/medical-and-health-services-managers.htm.

Van Dyke, M. 2017. "Strengthening Post-Acute Care Partnerships: 8 Factors for Success." *Healthcare Executive* 32 (1): 18–26.

———. 2016. "Leading in an Era of Value: 3 Key Strategies for Success." *Healthcare Executive* 31 (6): 20–28.

World Health Organization (WHO). 2018. "The Determinants of Health." Accessed July 22. www.who.int/hia/evidence/doh/en/.

———. 1946. *Preamble to the Constitution of the World Health Organization as Adopted by the International Health Conference, New York, 19–22 June, 1946; Signed on 22 July 1946 by the Representatives of 61 States (Official Records of the World Health Organization, No. 2, p. 100) and Entered into Force on 7 April 1948*. Geneva, Switzerland: WHO.

CHAPTER 2

MANAGEMENT

The worker is not the problem. The problem is at the top! Management!

W. Edwards Deming, quality expert,
business consultant, and writer

LEARNING OBJECTIVES

Studying this chapter will help you to

➤ define and explain management;

➤ describe how management has evolved as a field of knowledge, theory, and practice;

➤ explain major theories of management;

➤ identify important roles, functions, activities, and competencies of healthcare managers; and

➤ explain how management theory is used to manage healthcare organizations.

HERE'S WHAT HAPPENED

Partners HealthCare's management team planned, organized, staffed, led, and controlled the healthcare organization (HCO) and its work. Managers planned new initiatives for accountable care and population health. To accomplish plans, managers organized tasks, division of work, and jobs. They redesigned care processes for diabetes, heart attacks, and colorectal cancer. Specific tasks, responsibilities, and authority were assigned to specific jobs such as health coach, cardiologist, and nurse. A Connected Cardiac Care team coordinated diverse jobs toward the shared goal of improving cardiac care for remote patients. Managers staffed new jobs by hiring nurses and training them for telehealth responsibilities. When leading employees, managers overcame resistance from some nurses who disliked technology replacing their human touch. Managers led physicians by using financial incentives to motivate them. Performance of the telehealth program was controlled by monitoring enrollment, hospital readmissions, emergency room use, patient satisfaction, and cost savings. When data analytics showed that patient enrollment was below target, managers redesigned the enrollment process to increase the number of enrollees. All this planning, organizing, staffing, leading, and controlling by Partners HealthCare's managers—including new, entry-level managers—enabled the managers and HCO to serve their community and improve population health.

Chapter 1 introduced us to HCOs that provide healthcare services. As shown by Partners HealthCare, these HCOs must be managed. In this chapter's Here's What Happened, managers demonstrated five essential management functions—they planned, organized, staffed, led, and controlled. Managers at all career stages and organization levels use these management actions. This chapter introduces us to the management knowledge, theory, and practice used to manage HCOs. Management has evolved as a profession, and this chapter reviews how management has developed from the early twentieth century to today. We learn how managers today use classic management approaches in conjunction with more recent approaches. Chapter 2 introduces the work, skills, functions, roles, and competencies of managers; later chapters will review them in more depth and explain how to apply them to HCOs. You will learn about tools to include in your healthcare management toolbox and use throughout your career.

This chapter is important because it provides the foundation on which subsequent chapters will build. It explains many management terms, concepts, and principles that are used throughout the book—and in HCO management jobs and careers. The chapter opening quote suggests that problems in HCOs sometimes are caused by managers. Problems occur when managers do not properly use management principles and methods. Managers, including young professionals on their first day at work, can use this chapter to help them manage HCOs wisely. With a proper foundation in management principles, you can make a good start in your career and then build on it.

WHAT IS MANAGEMENT?

What comes to mind when you see the word *management*? Consider a manager you know. What does she do? What makes him a manager? Perhaps we have different ideas about what management means, what managers do, and who does management work. This book defines **management** as "the process of getting things done through and with people" (Dunn 2016, 14). **Always remember that management involves people—usually lots of them!** Managers can work at all levels of an organization.

People who perform management work (for much or all of their job) might have job titles such as *manager, executive, administrator, supervisor, coordinator*, or *lead*. However, people who only occasionally perform management work might also have job titles that imply they are managers. To determine whether someone really is a manager, we should consider how much of the work described in this chapter that person does.

management
The process of getting things done through and with people.

THE HISTORY AND EVOLUTION OF MANAGEMENT THEORY

As a field of study, management is younger than some (e.g., biology, mathematics, psychology) but older than others (e.g., computer science, aerospace engineering). Although management techniques surely were used before recorded history, writing about management as a body of knowledge is a more recent practice. This section draws from book chapters on both classical theories of organization (Olden and Diana 2019) and modern theories of organization (Diana and Olden 2019), plus other cited authors, to discuss theoretical approaches that created the foundation of management theory. As you read this section, think about how management has evolved by expanding on existing ideas, building on past ideas, and creating entirely new ideas that guide managers today. Also note that some management scholars studied work tasks, some studied work processes, others studied the structure of organizations, and still others studied the workers. Although some management theories are from long ago, they are still used today (just as theories of Sir Isaac Newton and Sigmund Freud are still used today in physics and psychology).

scientific management
A type of management that uses standardization, specialization, and scientific experiments to design jobs for greater efficiency and production.

TAYLOR AND SCIENTIFIC MANAGEMENT

Management began to develop as a body of knowledge more than a century ago with the **scientific management** work of Frederick W. Taylor (Olden and Diana 2019). He told factory managers they could increase productivity and output not by finding bigger, stronger workers to shovel coal and lift iron but instead by designing the workers' repetitive work for ease and efficiency. He analyzed factory workers' physical motions, postures, steps, actions, task completion times, and production. Based on the analysis, Taylor made changes that led to large improvements. For example, standing or sitting a certain way could help someone work with less strain on the body, similar to practicing good posture when working at a computer workstation today. Taylor also designed tools that enabled laborers to work with less effort yet accomplish more. (Does this remind you of the saying "Work smarter, not harder"?) Taylor developed detailed instructions, methods, rules, techniques, training, and time allowances for each job. Thus, work was based on objective scientific analysis rather than subjective personal preferences.

Taylor tested his ideas with the scientific method and detailed research in factories. He believed there was "one best way" to perform each repetitive job, and he set out to discover it. Factory managers then taught workers the one best way to do their job rather than let workers do their job however they wanted to (with varying results). Factory production and workers' pay increased. Managers' early efforts to redesign physical work led to redesigning their own management work. Managers now had to identify work tasks, set standards, and plan schedules for workers. Thus, managers' work also became more objective and less subjective.

Taylor's ideas became known as *Taylorism* and *scientific management*. This approach to management was further developed by Frank and Lillian Gilbreth (1917) and Henry L. Gantt (1919). The Gilbreths' work included studies of surgeons, which led to creating the surgical nurse job to assist the surgeon and the use of a tray to hold instruments (Langabeer and Helton 2017). Followers of Taylorism later realized that the best way to perform a job depended on a worker's experience, the work situation, and other factors. Nonetheless, principles of scientific management were useful back then and are still used today in many organizations, including HCOs.

Today we use terms such as *ergonomics* and *human engineering* to refer to how jobs, tools, work, postures, and workstations are designed to maximize productivity and minimize injury. When HCO managers design jobs such as nurse anesthetist, data analyst, and intake coordinator, they apply ideas that evolved from scientific management. We will learn more about this approach in later chapters.

administrative theory
An integrated set of ideas to organize work, positions, departments, supervisor–subordinate relationships, hierarchy, and span of control to design an organization.

FAYOL AND ADMINISTRATIVE THEORY

Early in the twentieth century, Henri Fayol was a pioneer in developing **administrative theory** to improve organizations (rather than improve individual jobs as Taylor did). His ideas were top-down, for top managers to apply to lower levels of the organization (Olden and Diana 2019). Fayol believed his principles were flexible and applicable to any kind of organization. Although history has shown that his principles work better in some types of organizations than in others, the principles have contributed much to the foundation of theory for managing people and organizations. His work helped develop administrative principles that are still widely used today. In the Partners HealthCare example in the opening Here's What Happened, we read how managers used some of these principles.

Have you seen an organization chart for a medical group practice, health website design company, pharmaceutical firm, or community health alliance? A typical organization chart (exhibit 2.1) reflects much administrative theory.

Division of work is how work is separated into smaller, more specialized tasks and activities. For example, building maintenance work is divided into plumbing, carpentry, painting, masonry, air-conditioning, and other types of specialized work to maintain buildings.

Specialization refers to the width of the range of tasks done by an employee or department. A maintenance worker who does only painting is more specialized than a maintenance worker who does painting, carpentry, and plumbing. A surgical nursing department is more specialized than a nursing department.

Coordination is connecting individual tasks, activities, jobs, departments, and people to work together toward a common purpose. It forms linkages and interrelationships to overcome the division of work caused by specialization. In a hospital, nursing is coordinated with laboratory, pharmacy, environmental services, patient access, and other specialized departments so they all work toward the common purpose of patient care.

Authority is power formally given to a job position (not to the person hired for a position) to make decisions and take actions, such as allocating resources and directing subordinates. The director position of a college wellness clinic has authority to allocate the clinic's resources and assign work to the director's subordinates. Whoever is hired as the director can use the director's authority to do the job. For example, Nicole was hired as the clinic director and used the authority of that position to perform her job. When she later transferred to a different job, Nicole no longer was able to use the authority of the

division of work
How work is separated into smaller, more specialized tasks and activities.

specialization
The width of the range of tasks and work done by an employee or department.

coordination
Connecting individual tasks, activities, jobs, departments, and people to work together toward a common purpose.

authority
Power formally given to a job position to make decisions, take actions, and direct and expect obedience from subordinates.

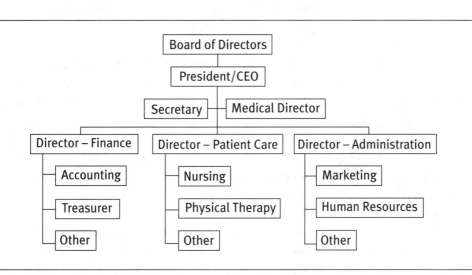

Exhibit 2.1
Organization Chart

clinic director job. This authority is sometimes referred to as *rational-legal authority* (Daft 2016) or *line authority* (Dunn 2016). It is based on the line of authority discussed later.

Some writers describe other kinds of authority. *Staff authority* and *functional authority* may be held by staff experts in specialties (e.g., accounting or marketing) who advise line managers (Dunn 2016). *Charismatic authority* may exist for some people based on their admirable personal character and charisma that inspire others (Daft 2016). These types of authority are based on the expertise or charisma of the person in a position (rather than on the position itself). To learn more about these kinds of authority, see chapter 10, which explains types of power.

Line of authority refers to the vertical chain of command, authority, and formal communication up and down an organization. In a health insurance company, the president gives commands and delegates authority down to the vice president of financial affairs, who gives commands and delegates authority down to the accounting director, who in turn gives commands and delegates authority down to the accounts payable supervisor. In the line of authority, the accounts payable supervisor communicates up to the accounting director, who communicates up to the vice president and so forth.

Managers usually organize work into **line jobs** (and departments) and **staff jobs** (and departments). These types of jobs are based on two different kinds of work and contributions to the organization's goals. Line jobs (and departments) contribute directly to—and are accountable for—achieving the organization's goals (Dunn 2016). Alternatively, staff jobs (and departments) indirectly help achieve the organization's goals by providing specialized advice, expertise, and support to the line jobs and departments (Dunn 2016). In a sports medicine clinic, physical therapists perform line work that contributes directly to their clinic's patient care goals. A secretary performs staff work for the clinic, such as scheduling patients, to support therapists in achieving the patient care goals. In a rehabilitation hospital, the nursing department performs line work to achieve the hospital's patient care goals. The strategic planning department does staff work to advise the line managers and board of directors (who then decide the strategic direction of the hospital). Compared to line workers, staff workers have less authority. Staff workers are expected to advise and support the line workers who have the authority to make the decisions. Yet line workers depend on staff workers and could not as readily accomplish their line work without the help of the staff workers.

The separation of line work and staff work is not always clear. For example, legal work may be staff work in a medical group practice but be line work in a law firm. Also, people might disagree on which jobs directly contribute to an organization's main goals. As noted in chapter 1, HCOs have become more concerned with the entire patient experience, which includes all interactions a patient has with the HCO's employees. Thus, any employee who interacts with a patient—including an employee who schedules appointments—contributes to the patient experience and could be viewed as contributing directly to patient experience goals. Managers should clarify for workers the extent to which a job

line of authority
The vertical chain of command, authority, and formal communication up and down an organization.

line jobs
Jobs that contribute directly to achieving an organization's purpose and main goals.

staff jobs
Jobs that use specialized skills, abilities, and expertise to support line jobs and thereby indirectly contribute to the organization's main goals.

is line or staff. That will help workers know if they have authority to make decisions or if they instead just advise others who then make decisions.

Separation of line work and staff work also may be unclear for managers of departments that perform staff work. Confusion can arise because a staff department in an organization has a manager who does line work within that one department (Dunn 2016). Assume the strategic planning department mentioned earlier has a department manager plus two employees who both gather and analyze data, study the external environment, and prepare reports. The department does staff work to assist line decision makers. Yet within that staff department, the department manager does line work, that is, she decides how to allocate resources, assign tasks to the two subordinates, and manage the department.

Unity of command means a worker takes commands from and is responsible to only one boss. An example is a computer technician who takes commands from and is responsible to only the director of information technology in a large cardiology group practice.

Span of control is how many subordinate workers a manager is directly responsible for, that is, how many workers report up one level (in an organization chart) to that boss. Suppose Brian is a hospital patient access manager in Scranton. Six employees report directly to Brian, so his span of control is six. Span of control varies based on factors such as the ability of the manager, ability of the subordinates, the proximity of the manager and subordinates to each other (physically and online), frequency and kinds of interactions, extent to which work is usually consistent and standardized, and variety and complexity of subordinates' tasks (Dunn 2016).

Centralization (and decentralization) is how high (and low) in an organization the authority to make a decision exists. In a mental health alliance, purchasing decisions costing $20,000 or more are centralized at the board of directors level. The board decentralizes authority for purchasing decisions costing less than $20,000 to the alliance executive director. Then the executive director decentralizes authority for purchases costing less than $1,000 to the department manager level.

unity of command
Arrangement in which a worker takes commands from and is responsible to only one boss.

span of control
How many subordinate workers a manager is directly responsible for; how many workers report directly to that manager (sometimes called *span of supervision* or *span of management*).

centralization
How high or low in an organization the authority exists to make a decision.

➡ TRY IT, APPLY IT

Think about a job you've had, such as a summer job or a current part-time job. Try to apply this chapter's administrative theory concepts to describe your job and the organization. For example, how was work divided? Which departments were coordinated with your department? What, if any, authority did your job have? Share your analysis with classmates.

These ideas from administrative theory help managers determine supervisor–subordinate relationships, group workers into work units such as departments, design levels of hierarchy in an organization chart, arrange who reports to whom, and structure the organization. Most HCOs apply at least some of these administrative principles. In later chapters on organizing and staffing, we will learn how managers and supervisors use these principles in HCOs.

✓ CHECK IT OUT ONLINE

The research of Roethlisberger, Dickson, Mayo, and others at the Western Electric Hawthorne Plant led to the discovery of the Hawthorne effect: We are motivated to change our behavior (e.g., produce more) when we are being watched. However, these researchers discovered much more than that about human behavior in the workplace. The Hawthorne studies ran from 1924 to 1936. Their deep effect on organization development and management still strongly influences managers today. The studies also led to new approaches for conducting research about organizations and people. You can learn more about the Hawthorne studies and lessons for today's managers at www.library.hbs.edu/hc/hawthorne/07.html#seven. Check it out online and see what you discover.

MAYO AND HUMAN RELATIONS

In the 1920s and 1930s, a team of researchers led by Fritz Roethlisberger and W. J. Dickson studied workers at the Western Electric Hawthorne Plant outside of Chicago. The researchers conducted experiments in which they changed the physical working conditions, such as lighting, of the rooms where workers manually assembled telephone components. These experiments, combined with observations, were to help Western Electric managers understand factors affecting workers' productivity, morale, and other aspects of performance. The researchers were puzzled that productivity did not vary as expected. Sometimes productivity improved in the experiment room where lighting was increased, yet it also improved in the control room where the lighting was not changed.

norms
Behaviors and attitudes expected of people in a group, organization, or society.

human relations
A type of management based on psychology and sociology that considers employees' feelings and behaviors, especially in groups.

Eventually, Elton Mayo and other scientists in the Hawthorne studies determined that social and psychological factors were involved. The experiments affected the workers' cooperation, teamwork, feelings of importance, and recognition, which then influenced their morale, work effort, and productivity. The workers were not machines or robots; they were humans. They had thoughts, feelings, emotions, and personalities, which they brought to work. They were more complex than previously realized, and they were not always rational. Western Electric was not a machine either; it was a social organization with **norms**, peer pressure, informal leaders, interpersonal relations, and group behaviors that affected workers (Dunn 2016).

This work led to the **human relations** approach in management, which was further developed by Chester Barnard (1938), an executive who emphasized cooperation based on communication and both social and psychological motivators. Decades of study have focused greater attention on the human relations aspects of management, such as motivation, organization culture, group behavior, and job design. In recent years, new approaches to human relations have led to innovations in management. We will learn more about human relations in later chapters on staffing, leadership, and communication.

Gulick, Urwick, and Management Functions

In the 1930s, Luther Gulick and Lyndall Urwick studied what executives do (Olden and Diana 2019). Executives plan, organize, staff, direct, coordinate, report, and budget (sometimes referred to as POSDCORB). Gulick and Urwick, and Fayol before them, identified five fundamental management functions: planning, organizing, staffing, directing, and controlling. **Managers plan, organize, staff, direct, and control.** In more recent years, the words *lead*, *influence*, and *motivate* have been used in place of *direct*.

In **planning**, managers decide what to do and how to do it. Planning can involve establishing mission, vision, goals, objectives, strategies, and methods. Planning may be short-term, such as a single eight-hour shift in an emergency department, or long-term, such as the five-year strategic plan of a medical school. What kind of short-term and long-term planning have you done in your life?

In **organizing**, managers arrange work into jobs, teams, departments, and other work units; arrange supervisor–subordinate relationships; and assign responsibility, authority, and resources. Organizing involves designing an organization chart. For example, five investors build a new assisted-living retirement home and then organize the jobs, departments, and 87 employees as shown on a new organization chart.

In **staffing**, managers obtain and retain people to fill jobs and do the work. Managers also recruit, select, orient, train, compensate, evaluate, protect, and develop employees. For example, an outpatient diagnostic center manager hires an ultrasonographer and decides how much to pay her.

In **directing** (also called *influencing* or *leading*), managers assign work to employees and motivate them to do the work. For example, a chemotherapy supervisor assigns three nurses to 13 patients who are scheduled for chemotherapy on Monday.

In **controlling**, managers compare actual performance to preset standards and make corrective adjustments if needed to meet the standards (Dunn 2016). For example, managers use real-time data collection, analysis, and reports at their digital desktops to control expenses, overtime hours, schedules, and customer satisfaction.

It makes sense for managers to carry out these five functions in the sequence shown, and the functions should be thought of as a cycle rather than a straight line. After all steps are completed, the original plans have been fulfilled (or revised), so new plans must be created. New plans lead to new organizing, staffing, directing, and controlling. The cycle suggests that managers plan goals to pursue, organize tasks to accomplish planned goals, hire staff to perform organized tasks, direct and motivate staff to do the tasks, and then control what happens so that planned goals are achieved. Although managers generally

planning
Deciding what to do and how to do it.

organizing
Arranging work into jobs, teams, departments, and other work units; arranging supervisor–subordinate relationships; assigning responsibility, authority, and other resources.

staffing
Obtaining and retaining people to fill jobs and do work.

directing
Assigning work to workers and motivating them to do the work.

controlling
Comparing actual performance to preset standards and making corrective adjustments if needed to meet the standards.

follow this approach, sometimes they might have to back up and redo a prior step before proceeding. For example, when interviewing applicants for an ethics officer position at a healthcare system in Portland, the CEO might realize he is unable to clearly explain to applicants the job's authority and reporting relationships throughout the health system. The job and its design are too fuzzy and have not been structured well. The CEO may return to the organizing function and more clearly design how the ethics officer will fit into the health system. Then the CEO can interview applicants and hire someone for the job. The five functions are used constantly by HCO managers—as they were used at Partners HealthCare in the scenario at the beginning of this chapter.

WEBER AND BUREAUCRATIC THEORY

The word *bureaucracy* may elicit negative or cynical feelings because bureaucratic rules sometimes create obstacles and delays. However, wise use of bureaucratic principles contributes to effective management. These ideas were developed by economist, sociologist, and political scientist Max Weber in the 1940s. He used perspectives from his three areas of expertise to study organization management and recommend changes. Here are some of Weber's basic principles of bureaucracy (Olden and Diana 2019):

◆   Staff members are subject to organization authority only in their work for the organization, not in their personal lives.

◆   Employees work in a hierarchy (organization chart) of bureaus, with a higher bureau (office) controlling lower ones.

◆   Control is based on authority rather than on personal relationships.

◆   Each bureau has an established division of labor and duties.

◆   A bureau is managed according to written documents kept in files for continuity.

◆   Workers are hired to fill positions based on open selection rather than election.

◆   Staff members are selected based on qualifications and ability rather than personal relationships.

◆   Staff members are paid based on position and responsibilities in the hierarchy.

◆   A worker can be promoted in the hierarchy based on seniority and achievement.

◆   Employees do not own rights to the bureau where they work, nor do they own property, equipment, or other resources used for work production.

◆ Staff must follow a system of rules, standards, and discipline that controls their work.

◆ Staff must follow orders given by superiors in official positions.

As you might have realized, the bureaucratic approach makes work and organizations more efficient but less personal. This design was intentional because Weber thought work and organizations were based too much on personal connections, favoritism, family relationships, and office politics. In bureaucracy, rules and authority dominate, and human creativity and personal feelings are stifled. This approach has advantages and disadvantages, as do other management approaches. Bureaucracy makes organizations more predictable, efficient, and stable. However, as Weber realized, it also makes them less flexible and less innovative.

Would you want to work in a bureaucracy? Today, many organizations and HCOs follow bureaucratic principles, some more rigidly than others. Bureaucracy helps you be paid properly, deters your boss from directing you to mow her lawn, and lets you be promoted even though you're not the president's nephew. However, bureaucracy might also stifle your creative ideas and control you with many rules. We will learn more about these principles in later chapters on organizing and controlling performance.

BERTALANFFY, BOULDING, AND OPEN SYSTEMS THEORY

A **system** is a "set of interrelated parts that function as a whole to achieve a common purpose" (Daft 2013, 33). The study of systems theory began in the 1950s with Bertalanffy's general systems theory and Boulding's classification of systems into nine hierarchical levels of complexity (Olden and Diana 2019). Boulding's fourth level is open systems, which are "self-maintaining structures that utilize a throughput of resources from their environment" (Diana and Olden 2019, 37). An open system obtains materials from its environment, uses them to maintain itself, and discharges its own materials into the organization's environment. This approach led to open systems theory, which has been applied extensively to organizations from the 1960s to the present. The theory asserts that an organization—as an open system—must understand, be open to, and interact with its external environment to sustain itself. Previously, managers and researchers had viewed an organization mostly as a closed system; they focused on the organization without regard to its external environment. Scholars and managers have further developed this open systems theory since the 1960s (Katz and Kahn 1978; Scott 2003; Thompson 1967), and it is now used more frequently than the closed system view.

Modern theories of organizations are open system theories that help us understand how an organization's external environment greatly influences the organization (Diana and Olden 2019). As an open system, an organization is open to (i.e., affected by) its external environment. It cannot seal itself off from external forces such as economic conditions,

system
A set of interrelated parts that function as a whole to achieve a common purpose.

new technology, people's attitudes, and competitors' actions. An organization is affected by its environment because external forces and external stakeholders act on the organization; recall the current trends and developments discussed in chapter 1. The organization must recognize these forces and adapt to them (or else suffer).

Organizations are also open systems, so they can import resources from the environment and export products and services into the environment. An organization must import staff, supplies, equipment, information, technology, and other inputs from the environment. These inputs are brought into the organization and used to produce services and products. This production occurs in the organization's production subsystem, which transforms inputs into outputs by mixing, arranging, connecting, combining, and processing inputs in different ways to create different services and products. Then the organization must be open to the external environment to export its outputs to customers, clients, and people outside the organization. For example, a medical lab in Teaneck is open to its

 USING CHAPTER 2 IN THE REAL WORLD

St. Joseph Hoag Health, a health system in Orange County, California, demonstrates the open system approach for improving population health. Based on demand from consumers in Orange County, the system has opened "wellness corners" in six locations, including an apartment community, a fitness center, and an office complex. Hoag Health managers choose locations convenient to where people live, work, and play. These facilities offer medical, fitness, and wellness services. Hoag Health strives to span the continuum of care, including preventive care and wellness, by partnering with other organizations in its community (Hegwer 2016; Perkes 2017).

The Brain Injury Alliance of Utah uses the systems approach to help people with traumatic brain injuries. The alliance works with many other organizations to create a seamless system of holistic care for patients at all stages of the brain injury continuum. This continuum ranges from emergency care and critical care to community care when the patient is living at home. Patients and families can get medical, social, financial, and other kinds of services and resources. Such services might include emergency care, acute care, post-acute care, diagnostic testing, treatment, therapies (physical, occupational, speech), case management, caregiver support, coping strategies, services to enable living at home, and yoga. Services and support may last for years. The alliance also offers community-based preventive education (Radick 2018).

environment to acquire lab equipment, test reagents, lab technicians, waiting room chairs, technical advice, lab certification, paper clips, blood tubes, and other inputs. The lab is also open to its environment to sell its services and outputs to patients, businesses, and health insurance companies.

Organizations are generally viewed as one of two types of open systems. Open *rational* systems strive to improve efficiency and performance and view organizations as somewhat mechanistic. Open *natural* systems strive to improve workers' satisfaction and view organizations as more organic. Both perspectives help us understand HCOs, as we will see throughout this book. The Using Chapter 2 in the Real World sidebar provides interesting examples of HCOs as systems striving to serve patients through the continuum of care (system).

LEWIN AND ORGANIZATION DEVELOPMENT THEORY

Organization development (OD) is "a process that applies . . . behavioral science knowledge and practices to help organizations build their capability to change and to achieve greater effectiveness" (Cummings and Worley 2015, 1). OD strives to change the whole system rather than focus only on a project, department, or part of the system. This approach began to evolve in the 1950s based on work by Kurt Lewin and Wilfred Bion (Johnson and Rossow 2019), and it strives to change social systems and organization culture to change human behavior in the organization. OD goes beyond continuing education and training. It uses interventions, team building, interdepartment activities, employee participation, constructive conflict resolution, organization redesign, process redesign, culture change, group dynamics, respect, trust, autonomy, fairness, and empowerment of employees (Cummings and Worley 2015; Daft 2016; Johnson and Rossow 2019).

OD has much applicability in HCOs. For example, UnitedHealth, a large national health insurance company, used OD with thousands of its managers to change toxic, hostile behavior into civil cooperation (Daft 2016). Other outcomes of OD have included improved change, decisions, employee satisfaction, customer satisfaction, innovation, and service quality (Dunn 2016). Cummings and Worley (2015, 690) suggest that OD will be useful for HCOs as they try to

- ◆ develop emotionally intelligent leaders and teams;
- ◆ develop more collaborative team-based organization systems, structures, and cultures;
- ◆ develop comprehensive learning for customer service and performance improvement; and
- ◆ develop engaged employees who have pride, passion, connection, and identity in their work.

organization development
A process that applies behavioral science knowledge and practices to help organizations build their capability to change and achieve greater effectiveness.

WOODWARD AND CONTINGENCY THEORY

There is no one best way to organize the structure of an organization, as discovered by management pioneers Joan Woodward; Tom Burns and G. M. Stalker; and Paul R. Lawrence and J. W. Lorsch in the late 1950s and 1960s (Diana and Olden 2019). Instead, the best organization structure is contingent. According to **contingency theory**, the best structure depends on other factors, such as the organization's environment, purpose, plans, size, and work technology (Daft 2016). For example, one organization structure works best if the external environment is mostly stable and predictable, whereas a different organization structure is best if the external environment changes quickly and unpredictably. This statement is true not only for an entire organization but also for individual departments and work units in the organization. Different departments face different circumstances, uncertainties, and contingencies and thus should be organized with different centralization, specialization, division of work, vertical hierarchy, coordination, and so forth. **There is no single best way to organize; instead, "it all depends."**

Think back to the kinds of HCOs identified in chapter 1, such as a consulting firm, rehabilitation center, accountable care organization, and public health department. How should these HCOs be organized? Which specialization, division of work, and vertical chain of command would be best? It depends on the unique circumstances and characteristics of each HCO. In a biotech company, should the research department be organized differently than the accounting department? Probably, yet it depends on the unique circumstances and characteristics of each department.

contingency theory
Theory that there is no single best way to organize; the best way depends on factors that differ from one situation to another.

KATZ AND MANAGEMENT SKILLS

Robert Katz (1974) spent years examining the work of managers. He found that they use three basic kinds of skills—technical, human, and conceptual—to perform three kinds of work. Managers use technical skills to work with things. They use human skills to work with people. They use conceptual skills to work with ideas. Managers may use these skills together, such as using conceptual skills with technical skills.

In HCOs, a manager's *technical* work might be preparing a therapist's job description, a dental clinic budget, or an outpatient lab marketing plan. An HCO manager's *human* interpersonal work might include motivating bereavement counselors or forming cooperative work relationships between the counselors and nurses. A manager's *conceptual* work might include envisioning future population health goals or considering how relocation to a new building could affect patients' access to care.

MEYER AND ROWAN, DIMAGGIO AND POWELL, AND INSTITUTIONAL THEORY

Institutional theory was developed by John Meyer and Brian Rowan in the late 1970s and later expanded by Paul DiMaggio and Walter Powell (Diana and Olden 2019). They argued that organizations feel compelled to fulfill expected obligations of the external environment even though those expectations may cause less efficiency. The external environment creates laws, regulations, customs, beliefs, standards, ethics, norms, and values about what should (and should not) be done. Some of these become firmly institutionalized (i.e., established) in society. For example, companies should not divulge confidential information. A local not-for-profit charitable organization should act for the good of its community. Dozens of healthcare professions, such as occupational therapy, have their own code of ethics. These codes establish social expectations that become institutionalized as expected normal behavior. (Look ahead to chapter 11 on leadership to see a code of ethics for healthcare managers.) Laws, ethical codes, local customs, and other institutions can force an organization's employees to behave a certain way.

Organizations that follow and comply with society's institutions are viewed as more appropriate and legitimate than organizations that do not. If an organization's stakeholders view the organization as legitimate, they will support it in many ways. If an organization loses legitimacy, stakeholders may withdraw support including funding, sales, accreditation, and resources. Then the organization might not survive. Therefore, managers feel pressure to do what is viewed as right and proper even if that action does not seem to be efficient. Why would a health education company buy supplies from a local vendor when it could buy the supplies for a lower price on Amazon? The manager feels external institutional pressure to "buy local" and support the community's supplier even though that is costlier (and thus less efficient). Managers must judge the pros and cons of complying with institutional expectations.

MINTZBERG AND MANAGEMENT ROLES

Henry Mintzberg (1990) helped analyze management by identifying ten roles performed by managers. He grouped the roles into three broad groups: interpersonal roles, informational roles, and decisional roles. The roles are shown in exhibit 2.2. (Note that in Mintzberg's view, leadership is not the same as management, nor is it separate from management: Leadership is one part of management.)

Mintzberg emphasized that these roles are interrelated. Suppose Kaitlyn manages an ambulatory surgery center in Cincinnati. She receives complaints from patients, families, and employees about insufficient parking. She uses interpersonal roles to represent the HCO and connect it with groups of people to resolve the problem. Kaitlyn uses informational roles to monitor the situation, gather information about the problem and possible solutions, and speak to others on behalf of the HCO. As the manager, she uses decisional roles to handle the problem, negotiate a solution, and allocate resources for more parking. Kaitlyn performs multiple managerial roles shown in exhibit 2.2. Because managers often perform different roles simultaneously—and may handle several projects at the same time—they need a special skill: juggling. We will learn more about these management roles in the remaining chapters.

EXHIBIT 2.2
Mintzberg's Ten
Managerial Roles

Role	Type	Action	Healthcare Example
Figurehead	Interpersonal	Symbolically representing one's own organization (or work unit) at ceremonial and social events	Appearing at a ground-breaking ceremony for a new healthcare building
Leader	Interpersonal	Developing, motivating, overseeing, and leading subordinate employees to achieve goals	Telling employees that with more teamwork the cancer center could improve survival rates
Liaison	Interpersonal	Connecting one's own organization (or work unit) to other organizations and people outside one's own chain of command	Meeting monthly with the city's youth sports council
Monitor	Informational	Gathering and using information (internal and external) to know what is happening	Analyzing opioid addiction rates based on zip codes and ages
Disseminator	Informational	Sharing information with others in one's own organization (or work unit)	Posting names and job titles of new employees on the company's intranet
Spokesperson	Informational	Sharing information with others outside one's own organization (or work unit)	Speaking at a college job fair about plans to increase employment
Entrepreneur	Decisional	Changing, adapting, and improving the organization (or work unit)	In a personal fitness business, adding evening yoga classes
Disturbance handler	Decisional	Taking care of problems and unexpected events	Arranging extra staffing in the emergency department after a nearby bus accident
Resource allocator	Decisional	Distributing and assigning organizational resources	Budgeting funds to create virtual reality tours of the facility
Negotiator	Decisional	Working with others to reach agreements and settle disputes	Meeting with a labor union to agree on wages for next year

Source: Adapted from Mintzberg (1990).

TRY IT, APPLY IT

External pressures and demands are causing many HCOs to merge and become larger. Suppose you manage a social media consulting company for HCOs. You are going to merge with a similar business. Explain in detail how you could use at least five of Mintzberg's managerial roles to do that.

Do All Managers Manage the Same Way?

By now you should know what management is and the roles, activities, and functions that managers carry out. Perhaps you wonder if all managers perform their management work the same way. What do you think? Consider people in general: Do they perform the same role, activity, or function in the same way? You have probably noticed that professors do not all teach the same way. Students do not all study the same way. The same goes for managers: They do not all manage the same way. Managers differ in personalities, attitudes, worldviews, biases, styles, and preferences. They also work with different situations, problems, and goals. **Although managers perform similar roles and functions, they do not perform them in the same way.**

One More Time

Management began to develop as a body of knowledge with the efforts of Taylor and the scientific method to improve work. Fayol pioneered administrative theory to improve organization structure, levels of organization, and supervisor–subordinate relationships. Mayo studied how using psychology and sociology could help managers understand workers' behaviors, norms, feelings, and motivations. Gulick and Urwick identified specific management functions, including planning, organizing, staffing, directing/influencing, and controlling. Weber developed bureaucracy theory to manage organizations with formal structure, bureaus, hierarchy, authority, responsibility, accountability, and consistent rules (rather than personal favoritism). Bertalanffy and Boulding began systems theory that led to viewing organizations as open systems that must interact with their external environments. Lewin's work led to organization development, which strives to improve performance by changing social systems and organization culture. Woodward and others argued that the best way to organize is contingent on external factors. Katz asserted that managers use technical, human, and conceptual skills to perform technical, human, and conceptual work.

DiMaggio and Powell developed institutional theory to explain that organizations and managers sometimes take actions in order to be viewed as proper and legitimate—even though the actions may reduce organization efficiency. Mintzberg summarized the work of managers into ten interpersonal, informational, and decisional roles.

Management is a mix of art and science. A body of scientific research, theories, principles, knowledge, and practice is available to guide managers. Yet scientific methods cannot fully address the many people, situations, and nuances of management. The art of management is also needed, which comes from judgment and experience that you will develop in your career.

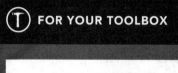

(T) FOR YOUR TOOLBOX

- Scientific management
- Administrative theory
- Human relations
- Management functions
- Bureaucratic theory
- Open systems theory

- Organization development
- Contingency theory
- Management skills
- Institutional theory
- Management roles

FOR DISCUSSION

1. How do you think Taylor's work has influenced present-day management of HCOs?

2. Why is Mayo's work important for present-day management of HCOs?

3. How do you feel about bureaucracy? What are the advantages and disadvantages of bureaucracy in HCOs?

4. What is a system? How is the open-system perspective useful for managing HCOs?

5. What does contingency theory tell us? How do you feel about this view of management?

6. Which of Mintzberg's ten managerial roles would come easily to you? Which of these roles would not come naturally to you and would require extra effort and practice?

CASE STUDY QUESTIONS

These questions refer to the Integrative Case Studies at the back of this book.

1. Disparities in Care at Southern Regional Health System case: Explain how Mr. Hank could use each of Gulick's five management functions to help his HCO reduce disparities in care.

2. Hospice Goes Hollywood case: Explain which of Mintzberg's management roles Ms. Thurmond should use to implement policies and procedures for accreditation.

3. Increasing the Focus on Patient Safety at First Medical Center case: Explain which management theories (tools) from this chapter you think Dr. Frame should use. (See the tools listed in the For Your Toolbox sidebar.)

4. Managing the Patient Experience case: Explain how Mr. Jackson could use each of Gulick's five management functions to implement his patient expectations program.

 RIVERBEND ORTHOPEDICS MINI CASE STUDY

Riverbend Orthopedics is a busy group practice with expanded services for orthopedic care. It has seven physicians and a podiatrist, plus about 70 other employees. At its big, new clinic building, Riverbend provides extensive orthopedic care. Several technicians provide diagnostic medical imaging, from basic X-rays to magnetic resonance images. The physicians perform surgery in their own outpatient surgery center with Riverbend's own operating nurses and technicians. Therapy is provided by three physical therapists and one part-time contracted occupational therapist. In addition to staff providing actual patient care, the clinic has staff for financial management, medical records, human resources, information systems/technology, building maintenance, and other administrative matters. Occasional marketing work is done by an advertising company. Legal work is outsourced to a law firm. Riverbend is managed by a new president, Ms. Garcia. She and Riverbend have set a goal of achieving "Excellent" ratings for patient experience from at least 90 percent of Riverbend's patients this year.

Ms. Garcia's expertise is in financial management, reimbursement, and contracting with insurers and payers. She did not study management in college but is now taking management courses at a local college.

(continued)

RIVERBEND ORTHOPEDICS MINI CASE STUDY *(continued)*

MINI CASE STUDY QUESTIONS

1. Ms. Garcia asks if bureaucracy could help Riverbend accomplish this goal. Using information from this book, how would you reply to Ms. Garcia? You may make reasonable assumptions and inferences.

2. Using information from this book, explain which of Mintzberg's management roles Ms. Garcia could use to help Riverbend achieve its goal.

REFERENCES

Barnard, C. 1938. *The Functions of the Executive.* Cambridge, MA: Harvard University Press.

Cummings, T. G., and C. G. Worley. 2015. *Organization Development and Change*, 10th ed. Stamford, CT: Cengage Learning.

Daft, R. L. 2016. *Organization Theory and Design*, 12th ed. Mason, OH: South-Western Cengage.

———. 2013. *Organization Theory and Design*, 11th ed. Mason, OH: South-Western Cengage.

Diana, M. L., and P. C. Olden. 2019. "Modern Theories of Organization." In *Health Organizations: Theory, Behavior, and Development*, 2nd ed., edited by J. A. Johnson and C. C. Rossow, 35–46. Burlington, MA: Jones & Bartlett Learning.

Dunn, R. 2016. *Dunn and Haimann's Healthcare Management*, 10th ed. Chicago: Health Administration Press.

Gantt, H. 1919. *Organizing for Work.* New York: Harcourt, Brace and Howe.

Gilbreth, F. B., and L. Gilbreth. 1917. *Applied Motion Study.* New York: Sturgis & Walton Company.

Hegwer, L. R. 2016. "6 Business Imperatives for Population Health Management." *Healthcare Executive* 31 (4): 10–20.

Johnson, J. A., and C. C. Rossow. 2019. *Health Organizations: Theory, Behavior, and Development*, 2nd ed. Burlington, MA: Jones & Bartlett Learning.

Katz, D. N., and R. L. Kahn. 1978. *The Social Psychology of Organizations*, 2nd ed. New York: John Wiley.

Katz, R. L. 1974. "Skills of an Effective Administrator." *Harvard Business Review* 52 (5): 90–102.

Langabeer II, J. R., and J. Helton. 2017. *Healthcare Operations Management*, 2nd ed. Burlington, MA: Jones & Bartlett Learning.

Mintzberg, H. 1990. "The Manager's Job: Folklore and Fact." *Harvard Business Review* 68 (2): 163–76.

Olden, P. C., and M. L. Diana. 2019. "Classical Theories of Organization." In *Health Organizations: Theory, Behavior, and Development*, 2nd ed., edited by J. A. Johnson and C. C. Rossow, 23–34. Burlington, MA: Jones & Bartlett Learning.

Perkes, C. 2017. "St. Joseph Hoag Health Opens Wellness Clinic Inside LA Fitness." *Orange County Register*. Published August 2. www.ocregister.com/2017/08/02/st-joseph-hoag-health-opens-wellness-clinic-inside-la-fitness/.

Radick, L. E. 2018. "Integrating Care Across the Continuum for Four Major Conditions." *Healthcare Executive* 33 (1): 20–30.

Scott, W. R. 2003. *Organizations: Rational, Natural, and Open Systems*, 5th ed. Upper Saddle River, NJ: Prentice Hall.

Thompson, J. D. 1967. *Organizations in Action: Social Science Bases of Administrative Theory*. New York: McGraw-Hill.

CHAPTER 3
PLANNING

People who fail to plan, plan to fail.

Business expression

LEARNING OBJECTIVES

Studying this chapter will help you to

➤ explain what planning is,

➤ compare and contrast planning at different levels,

➤ explain a model of strategic planning,

➤ examine types of strategies for HCOs,

➤ describe implementation of plans,

➤ explain project planning,

➤ identify sources of data and information for planning, and

➤ understand useful planning guidelines.

HERE'S WHAT HAPPENED

Managers at Partners HealthCare assessed their external environment and saw both opportunities (e.g., the continuum of care) and threats (e.g., reduced Medicare payments). They also considered Partners' strengths (e.g., extensive electronic health records system) and weaknesses (e.g., discharged hospital patients being readmitted for more care). Based on this and other information, top-level managers planned new strategic goals for Partners. One goal was to reduce the number of readmitted patients. Managers in the Center for Connected Health—a lower-level unit within Partners HealthCare—developed an implementation plan to achieve that goal. It involved using technology to connect Partners' staff with recently discharged patients at home. Managers planned which staff members would do which tasks in which sequence to accomplish the goal. They planned to use information technology, medical technology, and communications technology to coordinate care among several services in the continuum of care. They also planned to train discharged patients in self-care and to transmit their health data (blood pressure, weight, and pulse) to the center each day. Via telehealth, staff then could provide just-in-time care and education when needed. This complex project was successfully planned and implemented by managers and staff to achieve Partners' goal.

As demonstrated in the Here's What Happened, managers plan what their organizations and work units will do in the future and how to do it. Managers at all levels of a healthcare organization (HCO) must plan well. Many do so weekly and even daily. This chapter defines planning and explains how it varies at different levels of HCOs. Planning methods and real-world examples are presented for different levels of management and stages of planning. These methods include strategic planning, implementation planning, and project planning. This chapter provides useful planning tools to add to your healthcare management toolbox.

WHAT IS PLANNING?

In simple terms, planning is deciding what to do and how to do it. The planning activity is the first of the five fundamental management functions discussed in chapter 2. Planning should precede the other management functions because a manager cannot properly organize, staff, lead, or control an HCO without first planning. We can also relate planning to three of Mintzberg's ten management roles discussed in chapter 2: monitor, entrepreneur, and resource allocator.

Planning is, of course, future oriented. When planning, we anticipate and prepare for tomorrow. Students plan which courses to take next semester, where to do an internship next year, and what to do during spring break. Managers plan many aspects of HCOs. Can you think of some? Planning enables an HCO's manager to set a direction for the future that employees should pursue. **Managers plan a future direction and then plan how to go there.** We read about Partners HealthCare planning in the Here's What Happened. Good planning enables managers to be proactive rather than reactive. Being proactive is much more effective and fun than reactive crisis management.

Managers plan at all levels of the organization hierarchy. For example, the board of directors and high-level managers of a hospital in Grand Rapids plan for the organization as a whole using a broad perspective. They plan for the long-term future of the entire HCO. Their plans have enormous consequences for the HCO's survival and prosperity. At middle and lower levels of the organization hierarchy, managers plan for their individual smaller parts of the organization. They plan for shorter time periods. Their plans identify what different departments and smaller work units will do to achieve the bigger plans set by higher-level managers. Middle- and lower-level planning determines who will do what, when, where, and how with which resources to achieve the broad long-term plans. This type of planning is done by the department directors and unit supervisors within a department. For example, they plan their own department tasks, monthly work schedules, weekly inventory levels, daily staffing, and many activities. In larger HCOs that have specialized staff, a planning department, planner, decision support specialist, research analyst, or other staff may assist line managers with planning. Some health administration graduates choose planning jobs for their careers. Smaller HCOs have fewer staff specialists, so managers do more planning work themselves or hire planning consultants.

Many HCOs avoid pure top-down planning, in which top managers make the plans and determine the goals by themselves. Instead, the planning is partly bottom-up, meaning that lower-level work units and employees provide input to top managers for higher-level plans. This method provides important information and perspectives about the HCO's current and future needs, pros and cons of proposals, stakeholders' views, and whether proposed plans are realistic. Also, when lower-level workers participate in the planning process, they become more committed to implementing the final strategic plan and making it happen. They will not feel the plan was imposed on them without their input.

Planning should precede other management functions. It does not make sense for a community health alliance's manager to organize job positions, authority, responsibility, and the organization chart without first knowing what the alliance plans to do in the future. Nor does it make sense to hire staff yet. Only after knowing the alliance's future plans can the manager properly organize the work and jobs, staff the positions, direct the staff, and control their performance to achieve the plans. Let's learn how managers do high-level broad strategic planning. That will lead into how managers then do focused implementation planning.

STRATEGIC PLANNING

Strategic planning is an HCO's highest-level planning. It determines how the HCO can succeed in the future, often with an emphasis on beating competitors and satisfying customers. **Strategic planning** is a decision-making activity that defines where an organization is going, sets its future direction, and guides its future efforts to move the organization toward its intended future (Ginter, Duncan, and Swayne 2013, 21). This planning enables an organization to examine where it is now (point A), decide where it wants to be in the future (point B), and make decisions for how to get there (how to get from point A to point B). In the opening Here's What Happened, we saw strategic planning by Partners HealthCare.

Prior to doing actual strategic planning, the HCO must prepare for it (Harris 2018). The top management team must identify and communicate the planning process, the schedule, the participants, and the desired outcomes of strategic planning. In many HCOs, the CEO leads the process and may be assisted by a steering committee and a facilitator. The committee includes selected board members, top executives, and physician leaders if the HCO has a medical staff. Steering committee members choose the planning process, determine who should be involved in the process, and create the schedule for it. The committee also selects and works with a planning facilitator, who will manage the day-to-day planning process to ensure it stays on schedule. The facilitator might be an internal executive or an external consultant.

Individual participants, such as board members and other executives, also have key roles. Board members often represent key stakeholder groups, and they have to give final approval to the plan. In hospitals, the medical staff is an essential stakeholder that must participate in the process. However, each HCO has to decide who will be involved, to what extent, and in which parts of the planning process—from top managers and the governing body to middle- and lower-level managers. For example, at some stages of the process, lower-level managers will not participate in some planning meetings yet will offer essential input through surveys and interviews. Advisory groups may offer feedback on preliminary ideas that evolve during the planning process. The entire process may take about six months, although the time frame depends on the HCO's desire for expediency versus extensive stakeholder participation.

HCOs face many powerful trends and developments that are reshaping healthcare. Managers must make difficult decisions about how their HCO will adapt to changing demographics, value-based reimbursement, mobile health, patient experience, population health, mergers, scientific advances, workforce shortages, and other developments described in chapter 1. To guide decision making, strategic planning has many potential benefits for an HCO if it is done well (Harris 2018, 13–14). Strategic planning does the following:

◆ Gathers input for planning from all parts of the HCO

◆ Provides viable future direction and focus for the HCO

◆ Enables each part of the HCO to align its activities with the HCO's direction

strategic planning
A decision-making activity that defines where an organization is going, sets its future direction, and guides its future efforts to move the organization toward its intended future.

◆ Sets priorities to address crucial issues

◆ Allocates scarce resources to activities with the biggest potential payoff

◆ Establishes measures of success to gauge progress

◆ Generates commitment to implementation of the plan

◆ Coordinates and unifies the actions of diverse parts of the HCO

◆ Creates shared learning and shared context

However, these potential benefits will be realized only if managers avoid the following potential problems (Harris 2018, 11–13):

◆ Not involving the appropriate stakeholders (internal and external)

◆ Overanalyzing data and thereby delaying the planning process

◆ Avoiding difficult critical issues

◆ Not including financial planning in strategic planning

◆ Ignoring resistance to change

◆ Not developing consensus and enthusiasm for the plan

◆ Not transitioning effectively from planning to execution

We will next study a strategic planning approach developed by Veralon (a healthcare management consulting firm). Veralon has used this approach to assist many HCOs with strategic planning (Harris 2018). This approach and its four stages are shown in exhibit 3.1 and explained in the following sections.

STRATEGIC PLANNING STAGE 1: ENVIRONMENTAL ASSESSMENT

An HCO's managers must assess the organization's external environment and the HCO's current position in that environment. Thus, this stage actually includes both an external environmental assessment and an internal organizational assessment. This stage helps managers understand the following (Harris 2018):

◆ Assumptions about the external environment in the future

◆ The HCO's current and future positions relative to competitors, and pros and cons of those positions

◆ Important strategic issues that must be addressed

EXHIBIT 3.1
The Strategic
Planning Approach

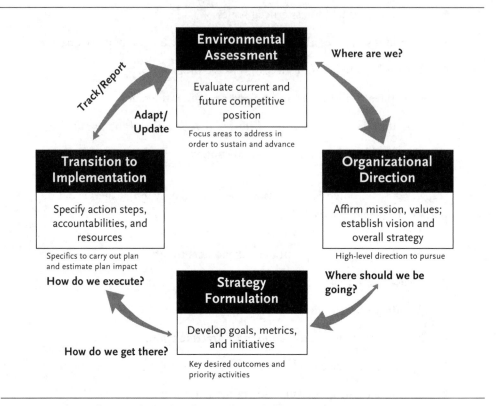

Source: Harris (2018, 8). Copyright Veralon Partners Inc. Used with permission.

With these three pieces of information, managers can judge how well the HCO will thrive and survive in the future. They can also identify factors that will strongly affect future advantage against competitors.

For the external assessment, planners should consider healthcare forces and trends (e.g., demographic, economic, social, financial, technological, and legal, as discussed in chapter 1) and how they affect—or could affect—the HCO. For the internal (organizational) assessment, planners should consider the HCO's mission, culture, image, facilities, equipment, quality, workforce, finances, competencies, management, and other characteristics. They should also examine services and programs, including distinctive features and key performance indicators (e.g., market share, utilization, profitability). Exhibit 3.2 is an example of an organizational assessment. Planners can then analyze the competitive market to prepare profiles of competitors (including newer, nontraditional competitors) and market forecasts. Exhibit 3.3 is an example of a competitor assessment. (A later section of this chapter describes sources of data for these assessments.)

Exhibit 3.2
Community Hospital's Organizational Assessment, 2017

Categories	Assessment Focus	Urgent Need for Medical Attention	Major Changes Required for Long-term Stability	On the Right Track; Needs Additional Development for Continued Success	Well-positioned for Long-term Success with Minor Gaps	Well-positioned for Current and Future Competitive Advantage
Scale/scope	– Relative size of operations – Mix and distribution of services and site – Care continuum coverage				★	
Financial position	– Current and historical financial performance, position, and access to capital			★		
Market position	– Current and historic market share performance and position			★		
Value position	– Quality and service outcomes relative to cost and price			★		
Integration	– Physician alignment – Coordination among services and sites within the system – Care continuum integration		★			

Source: Harris (2018, 115). Copyright Veralon Partners Inc. Used with permission.

The environmental assessment in stage 1 provides information regarding the HCO's

◆   internal strengths that it can build on,

◆   internal weaknesses that it can try to reduce,

◆   internal and external opportunities to pursue for competitive advantage, and

◆   external threats to protect against.

SWOTs
Strengths, weaknesses, opportunities, and threats.

With this information, managers can clearly see where their HCO stands relative to competitors in its market. In the Here's What Happened at the beginning of this chapter, managers identified strengths, weaknesses, opportunities, and threats, or **SWOTs**, of Partners HealthCare. (For another example, see exhibit 3.4.) In addition to SWOTs, strategic planners should identify critical issues that must be resolved. Examples of critical issues include the following:

Exhibit 3.3
Analysis of XYZ's Competitors' Strategies, 2017

Strategy	System A	System B	AMC A	AMC B	Comm. Hospital	Niche Provider
Value position	✪	O	O	O	●	●
Market capture	✪	●	●	✪	O	✪
Horizontal integration (w/ other health systems)	✪	●	●	✪	●	O
Vertical integration (w/ payers and physicians)	✪	O	O	✪	O	O
GME and research	O	O	✪	✪	O	O
Marketing and consumer preferences	✪	O	●	✪	O	●

Symbol	Description
✪	High risk to XYZ
●	Moderate risk to XYZ
O	Low risk to XYZ

System A and AMC B are XYZ's most significant competitors

Source: Harris (2018, 120). Copyright Veralon Partners Inc. Used with permission.

◆   Considering possible merger with a competitor

◆   Integrating the continuum of care to improve care coordination

◆   Partnering with community organizations to improve social determinants of health

◆   Using more horizontal organizational structure

◆   Implementing mobile health to improve health outcomes

By the end of this first stage of strategic planning, managers know the organization's advantages and disadvantages relative to its competitors, its SWOTs, the strategic issues it must resolve, and where the HCO is (point A). Next, managers must decide where the

Exhibit 3.4

An Integrated Health System's Strategic Profile and SWOTs

Strengths	Weaknesses
• Facilities (hospital campuses) • Scope of services • Variety of specialized services • Medical equipment and technology • Owned health plan • Primary care base • Quality outcomes relative to competitors	• Limited debt capacity • Siloed system components • Relationship with medical staff • Condition of post-acute and ambulatory facilities • Leadership in transition • Patient satisfaction
Opportunities	**Threats**
• Rural outreach • System integration • Competitor ownership transition • Shift to customer-focused culture • University affiliation • Insurance product advancement • Affiliations • Transition to value-based environment	• Local/regional economy • Declining or flat reimbursement • Specialist alignment to other systems • Competitor market share gains • Historical perspective of the organization as non-collaborative

Source: Harris (2018, 125). Copyright Veralon Partners Inc. Used with permission.

TRY IT, APPLY IT

Think about your college or university. Try to list three internal strengths, three internal weaknesses, three internal or external opportunities, and three external threats for that organization. Discuss your SWOTs with another student.

HCO should be going (point B). This task involves planning the HCO's future direction and forming a broad strategy to get from point A to point B.

STRATEGIC PLANNING STAGE 2: ORGANIZATIONAL DIRECTION

Managers plan their HCO's organizational direction as their desired future state (Harris 2018). To do this, they review and decide four things: their organizational **mission**, **vision**, **values**, and **strategy**. This process establishes the HCO's general direction, which will enable the HCO to fit and prosper in the future external environment conceived in stage 1. The mission, vision, values, and strategy should focus on the specific HCO rather than the health sector in general, and "sharp, tailored, directional statements are most useful" (Harris, 2018, 138). In large, complex HCOs (e.g., Partners HealthCare) comprising multiple smaller HCOs (e.g., physician practices, hospitals, clinics, home care businesses), strategic planning must develop a unified organizational direction pertinent for all entities. That will guide all parts of the HCO to move in the same direction.

 The HCO's mission statement should clearly and concisely tell stakeholders why the HCO exists—the HCO's purpose. The statement should be short enough that employees can easily memorize it (Harris 2018). Washington University Physicians in St. Louis has this mission statement: "Our mission is to improve the health of people through excellence in patient care and medical discovery" (Washington University Physicians 2018). Although it might seem that this mission statement did not take long to write, it is actually the result of a lot of thought, analysis, and discussion among strategic planning participants who considered assessments of the organization and its external environment. The same is true for vision, value, and strategy statements. Planning participants should decide on these only after much thoughtful discussion and consideration of assessments from stage 1.

 The vision should clearly and concisely tell stakeholders what the HCO aspires to be in the future—for example, in five to ten years. It should be a desirable future state that motivates the HCO's workers so that they become excited about and strive for the vision. Yet, the vision must be realistic and based on the assessments of stage 1. Amazon states,

mission
The purpose of an organization; why the organization exists.

vision
What the organization wants to be in the long-term future; what it aspires to become.

values
Deeply held beliefs, ideals, and standards of behavior.

strategy
An idea that guides an organization's decisions, actions, and behaviors in a consistent way to gain competitive advantage.

"Our vision is to be Earth's most customer centric company" (Harris 2018, 148).

Values portray the character and soul of the organization. Values are the core beliefs an organization is strongly committed to. They are usually enduring and should not change much or at all during strategic planning each year. These values are part of the organization's culture, which will be studied in chapter 11. The core values of Washington University Physicians in St. Louis are quality, respect, integrity, discovery, education, partnership, and professionalism (Washington University Physicians 2018). See the Check It Out Online box for the mission, vision, and values of the American College of Healthcare Executives. The Using Chapter 3 in the Real World sidebar provides other interesting examples.

Strategy is the primary means by which an organization intends to achieve its mission and vision (Harris 2018, 150). The strategy is an idea that guides an organization's decisions, actions, and behaviors in a consistent way to gain competitive advantage (Luke, Walston, and Plummer 2003). Managers may have to revise the strategy during each strategic planning cycle to ensure it fits the changing environment, competitors' strategies, and new threats and opportunities. Here are two examples of strategy statements (Harris 2018, 153):

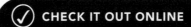

CHECK IT OUT ONLINE

Many organizations post their mission, vision, and values on their websites. They want stakeholders to know what they are about. The American College of Healthcare Executives (ACHE) is the leading professional association for healthcare leaders and has more than 40,000 members. The ACHE (2018) website lists its mission, vision, and values as follows:

- *Mission:* To advance our members and healthcare management excellence

- *Vision:* To be the preeminent professional society for leaders dedicated to improving health

- *Core Values:* Integrity, lifelong learning, leadership, and diversity and inclusion

The ACHE website also explains its strategic framework for setting organizational direction. Learn more about this HCO and its mission, vision, values, and strategic framework at www.ache.org/about-ache/strategy. Then research online the mission, vision, and values of other HCOs. Check it out online and see what you discover.

◆ Banner Health (a regional healthcare system based in Phoenix, Arizona): Develop a highly coordinated patient experience.

◆ Anthem (a national health insurer based in Indianapolis, Indiana): Capitalize on new opportunities to drive growth.

One well-known approach to strategy is based on two broad patterns of action (Porter 1985). A business may gain competitive advantage to succeed in its market by using either the *low-cost strategy* or the *differentiation strategy*. Using the low-cost strategy, an HCO would drive down its costs as low as possible. The HCO would not offer expensive features and upscale comforts. The HCO's facility would not be spacious and

USING CHAPTER 3 IN THE REAL WORLD

Grand View Health Urgent Care in Kulpsville, Pennsylvania

Mission: To provide prompt, customer-focused, quality urgent care services with convenient hours and shorter visit times to those with common illnesses and injuries

Vision: To improve the health of our community through convenient patient-centered urgent care services and partnerships with primary healthcare practitioners

Values:

Compassion—I act with kindness and empathy.

Integrity—I do the moral and ethical thing.

Respect—I treat others fairly and with dignity.

Collaboration—I value the contributions of others in building teams.

Leadership—I embrace these values and lead by example.

Excellence—I go above and beyond.

Service—I am passionate about meeting the needs of others.
Source: Grand View Urgent Care (2018).

Four Rivers Behavioral Health in Paducah, Kentucky

Mission: To provide comprehensive, integrated mental health, substance abuse, and mental retardation–developmental disability services that promote the health and quality of life of our community members.

Vision: To inspire confidence and respect as a provider of comprehensive behavioral health care. To be a valued partner in alliances that promote the health and quality of life for our community and its members.
Source: Four Rivers Behavioral Health (2018).

attractive, but its costs would be low. An HCO using a differentiation strategy would add features that make its products and services different in a way customers like. For example, the facility would be more spacious and attractive than other facilities (but its costs would be higher).

Each of Porter's two broad strategies can be applied to a wide or a narrow market. A business might use the low-cost strategy with a wide customer market (e.g., all people aged 18 or older) or with only a narrow customer market (e.g., only college students). Thus, there are four possible strategies:

Low-cost for a wide market	Differentiation for a wide market
Low-cost for a narrow market	Differentiation for a narrow market

Managers of HCOs should be careful when using the low-cost strategy. Although many people want lower costs and prices for healthcare, some people assume that low costs and prices mean low quality. An HCO with a low-cost strategy that advertises "We have the lowest-cost healthcare in town" might scare away some potential customers. When their health is involved, many people want the best, especially when insurance pays for it. The low-cost strategy can work for some healthcare services, but managers need to think carefully about how it will be perceived.

STRATEGIC PLANNING STAGE 3: STRATEGY FORMULATION

In stage 3 of strategic planning, the strategy formulation builds on the general organization direction (set in stage 2) to set specific goals, objectives, and major initiatives that can achieve the new organizational direction. Further, strategy formulation addresses the critical issues previously identified in stage 1 assessments, and it either reaffirms or revises them. These issues must be resolved for the HCO to achieve its vision and mission in the forecasted market and environment. Two examples of critical issues are (1) integration with partners in the continuum of care, and (2) cost reduction to thrive under value-based reimbursement. These issues are based on trends and developments (discussed in chapter 1), which many HCOs address in their strategic planning.

Planners and managers should choose a limited number of critical issues. A typical approach is to identify no more than ten potential issues for further consideration (Harris 2018). Who should choose the final issues to go in the strategic plan? That depends on the planning process. Top managers, board members, a board committee, a task force of selected stakeholders, or others might select the issues (Harris 2018). Diverse perspectives, a manageable number, and comprehensive representation of key stakeholders are useful. Participants can nominate issues and then prioritize them as essential, important, or useful. The most time and effort should then be devoted to the essential issues. For each issue, managers must set a measurable **goal** that, when achieved, will resolve the issue and enable

goal
A specific, measurable outcome that will help achieve the mission and vision.

the HCO to move toward its vision and mission. Exhibit 3.5 shows examples of critical issues and metrics to measure goal achievement for those issues.

The management team can now break down each goal into objectives (smaller pieces) that should be achieved in shorter time periods. At this point, the HCO has a clear idea of what is point B and a plan of how to get from the current point A to the future point B in the forecasted future. Goals take longer to achieve than the smaller objectives do. Managers should strive to establish SMART goals and objectives. The SMART acronym "stands for *specific, measurable, attainable, result oriented*, and *time limited* (or, alternatively, *specific, measurable, action oriented, realistic*, and *time limited*)" (Dunn 2016, 163).

STRATEGIC PLANNING STAGE 4: TRANSITION TO IMPLEMENTATION

In stage 4 of strategic planning, transition to implementation, managers add even more detail to the plans. They specify the actions, steps, tasks, and schedules to achieve the objectives to achieve the goals that resolve critical issues and achieve the organization's mission and vision. Managers allocate resources and assign responsibility to specific positions to achieve the objectives and goals. Work now shifts from the top managers to managers and staff at lower levels of the vertical hierarchy. Work also shifts from strategic planning to project planning and day-to-day operations. Specific projects are begun that will change work

EXHIBIT 3.5
Critical Issues and Metrics for Goals

Critical Issues	Key Metrics for Goals
Coordinate care to deliver value	• Top decile nationally in clinical quality • Top decile nationally in service excellence • Top decile in the state in lowest cost of care • Service area counties perform in the 90th percentile nationally for the majority of health-related indicators
Expand partnerships	• 80% of affiliated providers (e.g., physicians, care extenders) are accountable for performance measures • 25% more incremental providers and staff • "Employer of choice" in the market • 50% increase in annual philanthropic contributions
Grow across the full continuum of care	• Grow net revenue by 25%+ to ensure the appropriate scale to execute strategic initiatives • Increase market share by 5% (on average) across all services • Increase total covered lives by 30%

Source: Harris (2018, 168). Copyright Veralon Partners Inc. Used with permission.

structure, processes, methods, staff, actions, techniques, and other aspects of day-to-day operations. Lower-level planning by managers, departments, and individual work units results in implementation plans that are less abstract and have more concrete tasks and actions.

Detailed work plans may be prepared that outline who will do what, when, and using which resources. Exhibit 3.6 is an example of a detailed implementation plan. Partners HealthCare also developed (in this chapter's opening scenario) an implementation plan detailing what it must do to achieve its goal of reducing hospital readmissions. Top managers use a progress tracking system to monitor implementation progress on all parts of the strategic plan. Monitoring and controlling performance will be discussed in chapter 12.

The outcomes that follow implementation will answer managers' questions, such as: How well did our strategies enable us to resolve our critical issues and achieve our mission

EXHIBIT 3.6
Strategic Goal with Detailed Objectives and Year 1 Implementation Plan

Strategic Goal #1

Our health system successfully participates in alternative reimbursement models that emphasize coordinated and longitudinal care for patients

Objectives for Strategic Goal #1

	1-Year Target	5-Year Target
Reduction in inpatient stays for ambulatory sensitive conditions	–10%	–30%
Reduction in readmission rates	–10%	–40%
Reduction in per member cost of care for ACO attributed lives	–5%	–15%
Positive overall operating margin from risk-based reimbursement contracts	2%	5%
Growth in total net revenue attributed to risk-based reimbursement models	+10%	+60%

Major Initiatives for Strategic Goal #1

- Refine care models to focus on providing "Right care, Right time, Right place"
- Improve coordination and efficacy across care locations—within our system and with external partners
- Enhance operational capabilities to assume financial risk under alternative reimbursement models
- Seek out new and expanded opportunities to participate in alternative reimbursement models

(continued)

EXHIBIT 3.6
Strategic Goal
with Detailed
Objectives
and Year 1
Implementation
Plan *(continued)*

Projects and Tactics for Year 1	Time Frame	Lead	Resource Requirements[1]	Estimated Impact[2]
Implement three new care coordinator positions for primary care offices	Q1	JS	Medium	High
Implement nurse hotline service for ACO members	Q2	JS	Low	Medium
Utilize ACO data to identify opportunities to improve care delivery	Q1–Q4	GJ	Low	Medium
Institute Lean as a means for streamlining and improving care processes	Q1–Q4	SD	Medium	Medium
Improve continuity of patient care by providing community partners with an appropriate level of access to patient information	Q3	GJ	Low	Medium
Develop cost accounting system	Q3–Q4	BL	High	Medium
Pursue bundled payments for selected procedures	Q3–Q4	DD	Medium	Low
Explore opportunities for alternative reimbursement contracts with commercial payers	Q3–Q4	DD	Low	Low

Source: Harris (2018, 190–91). Copyright Veralon Partners Inc. Used with permission.

[1]Time and/or financial resources: Low=0.50 person days and/or <$250K during the year; Medium = 50–100 person days and/or $250K–$500K; High = 100+ person days and/or >$500K.

[2]Net impact from incremental revenue and/or decreased costs: Low = <$100K during the year; Medium = $100K–$500K; High = >$500K.

and vision? How well did we achieve our goals? How much did our hospital reduce its readmissions? How well are we addressing the Triple Aim? The answers to these questions will affect future planning and create a new "where we are now" (point A). With implementation, changes occur (internally and externally) that lead back to the beginning of the strategic planning cycle and influence future planning.

PLANNING AT LOWER LEVELS

Middle- and lower-level managers plan annual goals, projects, and work in their departments that, when accomplished, will help the HCO achieve its higher-level mission, vision, and goals. During the four stages of strategic planning, high-level managers set workload forecasts for departments in the HCO. These forecasts become the basis for plans in those departments. Department managers can then plan monthly and weekly workloads, such as student interns supervised, healthy lifestyle classes taught, language translation services used, or patient navigators hired. Based on planned workloads, managers forecast the resources needed to produce those workloads—staff, equipment, space, supplies, training, funds, and other resources. They prepare schedules and targets to show when staff will be hired, equipment will be bought, new services will be started, seasonal workloads will vary, and so forth. The cost of each resource is calculated and used to prepare annual and monthly budgets for the coming year. Department managers can get cost data from vendors, finance staff, human resources staff, and procurement staff. The department workload forecast, anticipated resource requirements, and budgets are plans that guide future action and provide targets to reach.

In each department, such as a medical lab, supervisors of smaller work units cooperate with department managers to plan for even smaller parts of the overall HCO. The supervisor of the lab's cytology section may create monthly work schedules for staff, weekly estimates of supplies needed, and daily task lists. The histology supervisor, microbiology supervisor, and hematology supervisor do the same. Shift supervisors plan how to divide the work of an eight-hour shift among the staff and may have to adjust plans if the work unit is short-staffed on a particular day.

Individual divisions, departments, and lower-level work units within the HCO prepare their own plans to support the higher-level plans and HCO mission. Managers of these divisions, departments, and units may follow a similar approach to that described previously for strategic planning, although planning at lower levels is more specific to each work unit and focused on implementation plans. For example, imagine a medical supply company in Las Cruces. The sales department, led by Fernando, is responsible for selling medical equipment and supplies. After the company makes its strategic plan, its sales department prepares annual sales plans for products and customer groups that must be achieved for the company to fulfill its strategic plan. As sales manager, Fernando plans by answering for his department the four key questions seen in exhibit 3.1: Where are we now? Where should we be going? How do we get there? How do we execute (implement)?

Fernando answers the first question by assessing the relevant external environment and his department's current situation and by analyzing the sales department's SWOTs. The answer to the second question will reflect the higher-level plan's mission, vision, values, and strategy. The sales department might also have a department mission, vision, and values that must be consistent with those of the overall organization. These can help guide the department and its employees. The third question may be answered by goals and targets set during the high-level strategic planning. That plan may call for a 4 percent increase in revenue from sales to hospitals, a 7 percent increase from sales to long-term care HCOs, a 5 percent increase from sales to medical groups, a 4 percent increase from sales to retail HCOs, and a 3 percent increase from sales to all other customers.

As sales manager, Fernando breaks these targets down into smaller targets—for example, dividing them up by geographic area. Breaking down the targets helps him plan how to assign his sales team so his department can achieve the target sales increases. This activity answers the fourth question: How do we execute (implement)? How do we increase sales to hospitals by 4 percent, to medical groups by 5 percent, and so on? The answer will be guided by the strategy developed during the company's strategic planning process, such as a strategy of superior customer service. At this focused level, planning identifies who will do what, when, and with which resources to achieve the target increases in sales. Fernando plans how to assign his sales staff for each month of the year, when to provide sales training, and how much to expect in sales for each potential customer group each month.

The main point is that lower-level work units plan implementation of higher-level goals set by top management's strategic planning. After higher-level plans are approved by upper management and the board of directors, they are shared with middle- and lower-level managers. These managers are responsible for departments that perform the day-to-day, hands-on work to produce and support the products and services. They prepare implementation plans that, when executed, bring to life the higher-level managers' plans for mission, vision, values, strategy, and goals. Lower-level department managers draft department implementation plans that identify in detail what their departments must do to help achieve the strategic plan and goals. They review their plans with higher-level managers and reach agreement on priorities, staff requirements, supplies and equipment needs, budgets, funds, and timelines. Sometimes, a higher-level or lower-level project manager and project team might develop the implementation plan, as explained later in this chapter.

Besides determining what their department must do to help achieve an organization's larger plans and goals, managers must plan for their own department. In Fernando's case, he and the sales department will identify the department's goals for next year. For example, one goal might be to devise a better summer vacation schedule for department staff.

PROJECT PLANNING AND PROJECT MANAGEMENT

project
A temporary endeavor undertaken to create a unique product, service, or result.

Managers often implement projects to achieve goals in an organization's strategic plan. According to the Project Management Institute (PMI 2017, 4), a "**project** is a temporary endeavor undertaken to create a unique product, service, or result." It is an organized effort with sequenced activities that are temporarily done to accomplish an outcome (Langabeer and Helton 2016). Unlike ongoing routine activity, a project is temporary. It has a start and a finish; the total time may range from hours to years. After the project is finished, the product, service, or result is absorbed into the organization's day-to-day operations.

Think of an HCO you know. What projects might have been done there? Perhaps its projects included establishing a patient portal to enhance customer engagement, creating an opioid addiction treatment service as part of the care continuum, or arranging better supply chain logistics.

A project does not just happen; someone has to plan and manage it to make it happen. This task can be simple or complex, depending on the project and organization. At a minimum, someone should plan the purpose of the project, identify specific outputs the project will deliver, list the tasks that must be done, schedule the tasks, assign people to do the tasks, and list the resources needed to carry out the plan. For complex projects, an HCO is likely to use project management, which is a more comprehensive approach. "**Project management** is the application of knowledge, skills, tools, and techniques to project activities to meet the project requirements" (PMI 2017, 10). Project management is essential for the implementation (execution) stage of strategic planning. Organizations—including HCOs—believe project management helps them achieve many benefits, including better control of resources, customer relations, development times, costs, quality, profit margins, productivity, coordination, worker morale, and reliability (Schwalbe and Furlong 2013, 3).

To start, a senior-level manager appoints a project manager. This individual may be someone other than the line managers shown in a vertical hierarchy. The project manager has responsibility and authority to initiate, plan, execute, monitor and control, and close the project. These processes are defined as follows (PMI 2017, 23):

◆ *Initiate.* Define a new project or new phase of an existing project by obtaining authorization to start the project or phase.

◆ *Plan.* Establish the scope of the project, refine the objectives, and define the course of action required to attain the objectives.

◆ *Execute.* Complete the work defined in the project management plan to satisfy the project requirements.

◆ *Monitor and control.* Track, review, and regulate the progress and performance of the project; identify any areas in which changes to the plan are required; and initiate the corresponding changes.

◆ *Close.* Formally complete or close the project, phase, or contract.

Innovative HCOs depend on project managers to bring the organization's goals and plans to life. Project managers work to ensure assigned projects are completed within established constraints of time, budget, risk, scope, quality, and available resources (PMI 2017; Schwalbe and Furlong 2013). This work involves much thought and action. Project managers analyze the organization's structure, culture, processes, and people, as well as the influence each might have on a project. They determine key individuals—stakeholders—who

project management
The application of knowledge, skills, tools, and techniques to project activities to meet the project requirements.

have interests in and expectations for the project. Some stakeholders might have conflicting interests (stakes) that must be resolved so the project is not pulled in different directions.

To accomplish this work, a project manager carefully forms a team of people for the project. The size, membership, and structure of the team will vary depending on the project, the organization, and other factors. Forming a project team requires wise thought and choices, as explained in chapter 6. The project manager and team use management skills (many of which are presented in this book), as well as project management tools, software, portals, and apps to plan and manage the following for the project (PMI 2017; Schwalbe and Furlong 2013):

◆ Scope (i.e., expected results and project boundaries)

◆ Schedule and timing of detailed tasks and activities required

◆ Resources needed

◆ Cost and budget

◆ Procurement of supplies, equipment, and services

◆ Risks involved

◆ Work needed from other people and stakeholders

Managers in HCOs may like the excitement, involvement, and achievement that come with project management. Some earn special certifications from the PMI, such as Certified Associate in Project Management (CAPM) or the more advanced Project Management Professional (PMP). Project management requires many of the same tools, methods, and competencies as general management, but it applies them to specific, time-limited projects. Recall, from chapter 2, Gulick's five management functions and Katz's three types of management skills. Project managers use all of them. Project managers create teams, coach, lead, motivate, make decisions, resolve conflicts, communicate with others, and so on (PMI 2017). You will learn many of these skills in later chapters of this book on team building, motivation, decision making, leading, and other management work. While you study this book, think about how you can apply what you learn to project management.

Project managers in HCOs should realize that healthcare is different from many other products and services. Healthcare projects may directly affect people's health and have life-and-death consequences. Healthcare is often personal and emotional, especially for patients. Finances may be complex, hard to measure, and difficult to assign within a project. Compared to outcomes in other industries, healthcare outcomes often are harder to measure, quantify, and link to a specific project, although outcome measurement has been improving. Thus, managing healthcare projects can involve unique challenges (Schwalbe and Furlong 2013).

Project management requires the breakdown of work activities into ever-smaller, increasingly detailed steps that enable more precise plans (Langabeer and Helton 2016). To do this well, the project manager must interview people who have relevant knowledge, observe relevant activities, and read relevant documents, taking detailed notes. With this information, the project manager can then prepare a **Gantt chart**. This project planning tool shows what must be done, when, and in which sequence to accomplish a project on time. Besides showing start and end points for each step, the chart may also name who is responsible for each step. Gantt charts have many variations; one example is shown in exhibit 3.7. Simple Gantt charts can be made in Microsoft Excel by inserting a bar chart. For more complex charts, managers use commercial software designed specifically for project planning and management.

A Gantt chart shows the tasks or activities needed to complete a project. A good practice is to state each task using a verb followed by a noun: for example, *identify* (verb) *employees* (noun). Each task can be broken down into smaller tasks; managers decide how much subtasking to include. Managers set anticipated start and end dates for each task, considering constraints, deadlines, work schedules, and other factors. When managers decide how tight to make the timeline, allowing some flexibility is usually a good idea. Tasks are generally listed vertically on the left side by start date, beginning with the first task at the top and continuing to the last task at the bottom. A horizontal bar beside each task shows its start and end points. Many variations are possible. Different shapes may indicate different tasks and activities; different colors may indicate importance, risk, or other characteristics. If more than one person will be responsible for a task, planners can label the task with initials, names, or job titles. Once the project begins, managers monitor progress and gradually darken each task bar to show progress on (or completion of) each task. All tasks in exhibit 3.7 have been completed except the last task (monitor training outcomes). Actual (versus planned) start and end dates may be added. Managers can revise the chart if necessary. We will return to Gantt charts in chapter 12.

Gantt chart
Graphic arrangement of tasks needed to complete a project, in sequence and with start and end dates for each task; may include other information, such as the person responsible and resources needed for each task.

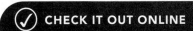

✓ CHECK IT OUT ONLINE

You can find many examples of Gantt charts online. Some are simple with just basic information, while others are complex with detailed layers of information. Some charts become so large that they are divided into subcharts that combine to portray an entire project. A search for *Gantt charts* will find many variations of this useful planning tool. Check it out online and see what you discover.

DATA AND INFORMATION FOR PLANNING

How do managers find data and information for planning? What sources can you think of? Some people believe they can find anything on the internet, and in fact the internet is very helpful to planners and managers. A lot of quantitative information for assessing the

EXHIBIT 3.7
Gantt Chart for Training Employees

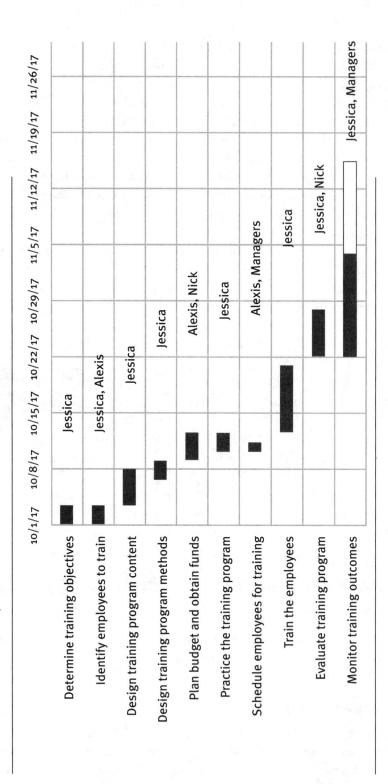

local and national external environments is available online. Resources include websites, government databases on hundreds of relevant topics, competitors' promotional materials, spokespersons' speeches, interviews with industry experts, and predictions of stakeholders such as vendors, professional associations, and community leaders.

Another source is your own HCO. It has printed and digital records, files, documents, reports, past plans, and archives. HCOs continually capture data about customers, supplies bought and used, quantities of products and services, staff hours worked, and much more. Some HCOs combine their data with data from hundreds of other sources and then perform data analytics to better understand their organization, customers, competitors, and external environments. Ask your HCO's chief information officer or other managers what types of data are available and how to access them.

People are another source of data and information, especially qualitative information. Talk with stakeholders (internal and external) to obtain their feelings and opinions. Gather their points of view about what might happen next year. Ask others what they think your main competitor will do. Be sure to talk to people who use your products and services and people you coordinate with. They can help you learn about the strengths and weaknesses of your HCO and its departments. Your manager will have valuable opinions, as will your department's workers. Talk with people outside your HCO, too—vendors and sales representatives, staff in relevant local government agencies, and employees of health organizations that your HCO works with. These sources will get you started. You will surely discover others during your career.

FINAL THOUGHTS ABOUT PLANNING

Managers should consider these guidelines when they plan:

- ◆ View planning as a continual process, not as a one-time event.

- ◆ Realize that planning is orderly yet messy, sequential yet circular.

- ◆ Allow for flexibility in the planning process and in the plan.

- ◆ Combine objective analysis with subjective judgment.

- ◆ Use—but don't overuse—historical records and data.

- ◆ Be open to new ideas, including "crazy" ideas.

- ◆ Look inward (at the organization) and look outward (at the external environment).

- ◆ Value both the plan and the process of planning.

Planning is deciding what to do and how to do it. Planning is future oriented, continual, and done at all levels of an HCO. Planning must be done well because it sets the stage for the other management functions—organizing, staffing, leading, and controlling. Managers at higher levels plan for the long term with a broad perspective of the HCO. At lower levels, managers plan for shorter periods and for smaller parts of the HCO. Higher-level planning is concerned with *what* to do, while lower-level planning is concerned with *how* to do it.

Strategic planning is essential for an HCO to prepare for its future. This type of planning enables an HCO to examine where it is now in its external competitive environment, where it wants to be in the future, how it will get there, and how it will execute (implement) the plan to get there. Strategic planning should include analysis of SWOTs, stakeholders, and critical issues. This analysis leads to creation of the HCO's mission, vision, values, strategy, goals, and objectives. An HCO then uses more detailed implementation plans and project plans to determine how to achieve its goals. Managers use project management methods and tools to plan and implement complex projects to achieve these goals. Quantitative and qualitative data and information for planning may come from many sources inside and outside of an HCO.

(T) **FOR YOUR TOOLBOX**

- Strategic planning approach
- Strategy
- Environmental assessment
- Organizational assessment
- SWOT analysis

- Porter's strategies
- Project management
- Gantt chart
- Planning guidelines

FOR DISCUSSION

1. Discuss what is planning and what is strategic planning.

2. Compare and contrast planning at higher levels of an HCO with planning at lower levels.

3. Referring to exhibit 3.1, discuss how strategic planning is done. Which part of the model do you think would be most challenging for you?

4. Discuss how project planning and project management are done. Which parts of project management do you think would be most challenging?

CASE STUDY QUESTIONS

These questions refer to the Integrative Case Studies at the back of this book.

1. Disparities in Care at Southern Regional Health System case: Apply the first stage of the strategic planning model (shown in exhibit 3.1). Use information from the case to describe "where we are now" for Southern Regional Health System (SRHS). Then write a proposed mission and vision to indicate "where we should be going" for SRHS.

2. Hospice Goes Hollywood case: Apply the first stage of the strategic planning model (shown in exhibit 3.1). Use information from the case to describe "where we are now" for Hollywood Hospice. Then write a proposed mission and vision to indicate "where we should be going" for the hospice.

3. How Can an ACO Improve the Health of Its Population? case: Assume Vandalia Medical Center (VMC) developed the Vandalia Care accountable care organization (ACO) as part of VMC's strategic planning. Which external opportunities and which external threats might have led VMC to start the ACO? Which critical issues do you think VMC is trying to resolve by developing the ACO?

4. Managing the Patient Experience case: Skim the case and then focus on the next-to-last paragraph that describes the development of the educational video. Prepare a Gantt chart to show a plan to implement Mr. Jackson's video project. Use information from the case and your imagination to decide which tasks to include in your Gantt chart.

5. The Rocky Road to Patient Satisfaction at Leonard-Griggs case: Prepare a Gantt chart to show a plan to implement the survey process at one of the physician practices. Use information from the case and your imagination to decide which tasks to include in your Gantt chart.

RIVERBEND ORTHOPEDICS MINI CASE STUDY

Riverbend Orthopedics is a busy group practice with expanded services for orthopedic care. It has seven physicians and a podiatrist, plus about 70 other employees. At its big, new clinic building, Riverbend provides extensive orthopedic care. Several technicians provide diagnostic medical imaging, from basic X-rays to magnetic resonance images. The physicians perform surgery in their own outpatient surgery center with Riverbend's own operating nurses and technicians. Therapy is provided by three physical therapists and one part-time contracted occupational therapist. In addition to staff providing actual patient care, the clinic has staff for financial management, medical records, human resources, information systems/technology, building maintenance, and other administrative matters. Occasional marketing work is done by an advertising company. Legal work is outsourced to a law firm. Riverbend is managed by a new president, Ms. Garcia. She and Riverbend have set a goal of achieving "Excellent" ratings for patient experience from at least 90 percent of Riverbend's patients this year.

The seven physicians and one podiatrist own Riverbend Orthopedics and together are the board of directors. Ms. Garcia is currently leading the board of directors in its strategic planning. They all feel the "Healthcare Trends and Future Developments" section of chapter 1 is relevant to Riverbend. They also note that only 57 percent of patients rated the ease of scheduling appointments as "Excellent" during the past year. All appointments are scheduled by telephone.

MINI CASE STUDY QUESTIONS

1. Ms. Garcia asks you to help identify five to seven critical planning issues for Riverbend based on the trends and developments in chapter 1. What issues do you suggest the planning should address? Rank the issues as high, medium, and low priorities. You may make reasonable assumptions and inferences.

2. Ms. Garcia asks you if project planning could be used to improve the scheduling of appointments. How would you answer her?

REFERENCES

American College of Healthcare Executives (ACHE). 2018. "2018–2020 Strategic Plan Overview." Accessed July 25. www.ache.org/about-ache/strategy.

Dunn, R. T. 2016. *Dunn and Haimann's Healthcare Management*, 10th ed. Chicago: Health Administration Press.

Four Rivers Behavioral Health. 2018. "Mission Statement." Accessed July 25. https://four-riversmirco.com/mainsite/about-us/.

Ginter, P. M., W. J. Duncan, and L. E. Swayne. 2013. *Strategic Management of Health Care Organizations*, 7th ed. San Francisco: Jossey-Bass.

Grand View Urgent Care. 2018. "Our Mission." Accessed July 25. www.gvhurgentcare.com/our-mission/.

Harris, J. M. (ed.). 2018. *Healthcare Strategic Planning*, 4th ed. Chicago: Health Administration Press.

Langabeer, J. R., and J. Helton. 2016. *Health Care Operations Management*, 2nd ed. Burlington, MA: Jones & Bartlett Learning.

Luke, R. D., S. L. Walston, and P. M. Plummer. 2003. *Healthcare Strategy: In Pursuit of Competitive Advantage*. Chicago: Health Administration Press.

Porter, M. E. 1985. *Competitive Advantage: Creating and Sustaining Superior Performance*. New York: Free Press.

Project Management Institute (PMI). 2017. *A Guide to the Project Management Body of Knowledge (PMBOK Guide)*, 6th ed. Newtown Square, PA: PMI.

Schwalbe, K., and D. Furlong. 2013. *Healthcare Project Management*. Minneapolis, MN: Schwalbe Publishing.

Washington University Physicians. 2018. "Mission, Clinical Vision and Core Values." Accessed July 25. https://wuphysicians.wustl.edu/about-us/mission-clinical-vision-and-core-values.

CHAPTER 4

ORGANIZING: JOBS, POSITIONS, AND DEPARTMENTS

For every minute spent organizing, an hour is earned.

Benjamin Franklin, author, printer, scientist,
inventor, diplomat

Studying this chapter will help you to

➤ explain organizations and organization structure;

➤ organize work tasks into jobs and positions;

➤ organize jobs and positions into departments;

➤ explain delegation;

➤ explain factors that affect how work is organized;

➤ compare and contrast mechanistic and organic structures; and

➤ understand how the informal organization, contract workers, union workers, and medical jobs with physicians complicate organizing work.

HERE'S WHAT HAPPENED

Throughout Partners HealthCare's long history and extensive growth, managers had been organizing work into tasks, jobs, positions, departments, divisions, and other groupings to achieve the healthcare organization's (HCO's) mission and goals. After Partners' managers developed new strategic plans and goals for telehealth services, they had to reorganize the HCO's work to implement those plans. They assigned new specific tasks to specific jobs, including primary care physician, cardiologist, diabetes educator, telehealth nurse, pharmacist, equipment technician, project specialist, Center for Connected Health director, and others. Managers decided how much authority to delegate to lower-level positions in the hierarchy (organization chart). Many positions and work groups were specialized, and managers grouped them into departments and coordinated their work to accomplish shared goals. In doing all this, managers carefully considered internal and external factors that determined how work should be organized. Figuring out how to organize work is one way that managers added value to Partners HealthCare. As a result, managers helped the organization achieve goals, satisfy stakeholders, and improve population health in the Boston region.

In chapter 2, we learned terms and concepts for organizing work that are important parts of management theory. This chapter further applies those concepts and shows how they are used in the wide variety of HCOs.

After managers at Partners HealthCare developed plans for their organization (described in the opening vignette), they faced a complex question: How should they organize work and workers to accomplish those plans? It was not a multiple-choice question with just one correct answer. It was a complex puzzle for which different managers might choose different answers based on their unique interpretation of the situation. Remember contingency theory from chapter 2? The best way to organize is contingent (dependent) on factors such as organization size, environment, plans, and technology, which managers must try to perceive and interpret. There is no single best way to organize. Rather, there are many possible ways to organize—and each has strengths and weaknesses. Managers must consider the pros and cons of different organization forms and decide which would be best for the HCO now. Later, they should reconsider the HCO's organization form when its size, environment, plans, and other factors change.

Organizing is the second of the five main functions of management described in this book. Several of the management roles described by Henry Mintzberg in chapter 2 involve organizing: liaison, entrepreneur, disturbance handler, and resource allocator. Managers at all levels must organize the work and workers for which they are responsible. Even managers of small departments or sections of a department must understand how to formally organize work so that they can achieve their area's goals.

This chapter first defines organizations and then explains how hundreds of work tasks are organized into jobs and positions, which are organized into departments. Managers organize by using the principles of organization structure explained in this chapter. Organizing work in HCOs is too complex a subject to address in one chapter. This chapter explains how to organize jobs and departments. Chapter 5 describes structural designs for organizing departments into entire organizations. Chapter 6 discusses how to organize groups and teams needed to coordinate positions and departments. These chapters also explain complications that arise when organizing HCOs. Together, these three chapters provide a practical introduction to how managers organize HCOs. The organizing principles may be applied to an entire organization, to a division or department within an organization, and to a smaller section or work unit within a department.

ORGANIZATIONS

Organizations are "social entities that are goal-directed, designed as deliberately structured and coordinated activity systems, and are linked to the external environment" (Daft 2016, 642). What does this mean?

♦ An organization is a social entity—it has people.

♦ An organization is goal directed—it pursues a purpose.

♦ An organization is deliberately structured and coordinated—it is intentionally set up, organized, and arranged.

♦ An organization is an activity system—it is alive with people doing things that affect each other.

♦ An organization is linked to the external environment—it connects and interacts with its surroundings.

ORGANIZING WORK IN HEALTHCARE ORGANIZATIONS

An organization (as defined here) undertakes deliberately structured activity. Managers intentionally organize, or structure, the activities, tasks, and work into systems that become the **formal organization**. This creates the **organization structure** of jobs, reporting relationships, vertical hierarchy, spans of control, groupings of jobs into departments and an entire organization, and systems for coordination and communication (Daft 2016).

This structured activity can involve managers at various levels performing five types of organizing (Daft 2016) that are explained in chapters 4–6:

1. Work tasks must be grouped into job positions. Managers at all levels do this for their particular work units and areas of responsibility.

2. Jobs must be organized (grouped) into work units, such as teams and departments. Middle and top managers do this.

organizations
Social entities that are goal-directed, designed as deliberately structured and coordinated activity systems, and linked to the external environment.

formal organization
The official organization as approved by managers and stated in written documents.

organization structure
The reporting relationships, vertical hierarchy, spans of control, groupings of jobs into departments and an entire organization, and systems for coordination and communication.

3. Departments must be organized (grouped) into an entire organization. Top managers do this.

4. Work must be coordinated among and across job positions and departments. Managers throughout the organization do this.

5. The organization must be linked to other organizations and people in its environment. Managers throughout the organization do this.

Managers do not necessarily organize work in this sequence one step at a time. Nor do they always use all five types of organizing to achieve every goal or plan. Entrepreneurs who start an entirely new diagnostic testing business will have to do all five types of organizing. Years later, in the same organization, the managers might do only the first and second types of organizing when they want to add one new position in one existing department. Because these five types of organizing interact, managers may use several of them simultaneously until everything fits together.

Sometimes HCO managers might not first organize tasks into jobs and then jobs into a department. They might first add a department and then decide which jobs and positions are needed for it. Let's consider a hospital that wants to recruit physicians. First, suppose the hospital adds one new physician recruiter in its existing medical staff affairs office. That works out well, so another recruiter is added, and then a secretary, and then another recruiter. Eventually, managers organize those four positions into a new, separate department of physician recruitment. Alternatively, suppose that in the strategic planning process, managers decide the hospital must become more active in physician recruiting. They decide to create a new department of physician recruitment. Later, to implement this goal, managers decide which tasks, jobs, and positions are needed for the new department.

After organizing HCOs in these five ways, managers are not done organizing. They often will need to reorganize to better achieve the HCO's mission, vision, goals, strategies, and plans. Recall that HCOs are open systems—open to their environments. Frequent changes in the external environment force changes in how HCOs should be organized. For example, accreditors, health insurers, businesses (which pay for health insurance for their employees), and government agencies in the external environment have demanded that HCOs improve the patient experience (as discussed in chapter 1). This external pressure has led many HCOs to reorganize their tasks, jobs, departments, and work coordination. The Partners HealthCare scenario at the beginning of this chapter also provides an example.

ORGANIZING TASKS INTO JOBS AND POSITIONS

Managers must decide which work tasks and responsibilities should be assigned to which jobs and positions, along with the authority, reporting relationships, and qualifications for each job. These elements interact, so it is hard to determine one without the others. A good starting point is to consider which tasks to combine into a certain job and then figure out the other parts of the job.

In this chapter, **job** and **position** have been used somewhat interchangeably. These two terms have similar yet slightly different meanings. "A job consists of a group of activities and duties that entail natural units of work that are similar and related" (Fottler 2015, 143). Some jobs, such as president, are performed by just one person. Other jobs, such as nurse, might be performed by two, three, or many more people, depending on the volume of nursing work. For example, a department might have two, three, or more nurse positions, each filled by a separate person. "A position consists of certain duties and responsibilities that are performed by only one employee" (Fottler 2015, 144). Thus, five people may fill five distinct nurse positions and all perform the nurse job.

Organizing particular tasks into a job creates division of work and specialization. Think of a job you had and list the specific tasks you did. Also think of the tasks workers did when you went to a doctor's office for a checkup, an urgent care facility for a minor injury, or a hospice to visit a relative. Hundreds of tasks are done in HCOs, and managers usually (but not always) organize tasks into specific jobs so that work is not left to chance. Certain jobs are accountable for completing certain tasks. (After managers divide work into specialized jobs, they must coordinate all the specialized jobs toward common goals, as explained in chapter 5.)

Managers can use the *verb–noun* approach to organize tasks into a job. Here are examples: *arrange appointments* of all outpatients, *calculate* biweekly *payroll* of nonsalaried employees, and *ensure* patients' *protection* from radiation. This approach indicates what a worker is supposed to do. Another approach is to state the outcome for which a job is accountable. Here are examples: accountable for appointments of all outpatients, accountable for biweekly payroll of nonsalaried employees, and accountable for patients' protection from radiation. Managers should avoid task descriptions that are too brief or vague, such as *appointments, payroll,* and *protection.*

When assigning tasks to jobs, managers decide how wide or narrow to design a job. A job with many tasks is wider and less specialized than a job with fewer tasks. There is no "one best way" for a manager to determine how wide or narrow to make a job. The manager of a personal care home's maintenance department in Ithaca might follow the "practice makes perfect" guideline and have a narrow range of repeated tasks that a worker presumably becomes very good at (the scientific management approach discussed in chapter 2). This division of work would have separate, narrow jobs for carpentry, plumbing, electrical work, and painting in a personal care home. But narrow, repetitive jobs can become boring, and workers may eventually feel less motivated doing them day after day. Thus, the manager may decide to add tasks to broaden jobs (the human relations approach described in chapter 2). He might assign all maintenance tasks to all of the maintenance jobs and have less division of work and specialization.

job
A group of activities and duties that entail natural units of work that are similar and related; may be performed by more than one person.

position
A group of activities and duties that are performed by only one person.

Managers also must decide how precisely or loosely to identify job tasks and responsibilities. When their tasks are defined too precisely, employees may have difficulty adapting to changing situations. Thus, a trend has been to broadly define core job tasks in a general way with less specificity of assigned tasks. This approach allows flexibility amid changing organization needs and circumstances (McConnell 2018). It enables an employee to temporarily shift to an urgent problem or flex a bit to meet a customer's unusual request.

The questions of how specialized jobs should be and how many tasks to include in them affect all jobs throughout an HCO—including managerial jobs. Vice president (VP) titles in large hospitals reflect specialization and division of work: VP of financial affairs, VP of human resources, VP of patient experience, and others. A C-suite of hospital executive offices may include specialized executives, such as chief executive officer, chief operating officer, chief finance officer, chief nursing officer, chief information officer, chief medical officer, chief quality officer, and others. Alternatively, a small hospital might have only one VP without specialization. Where and when tasks are performed also affect division of work, specialization, and how tasks are organized. Tasks for a weekend nurse may be similar to but not all the same as tasks for a nurse who works weekdays. The tasks of a hospital physical therapist may slightly differ from tasks of a physical therapist in a sports medicine clinic. In addition to assigning specific tasks to each specific job, managers identify other elements of each job needed to organize work and create organization structure (McConnell 2018). Did managers at the organizations where you worked do the following?

◆ Managers decide how much authority to delegate to each job—for example, to spend money, to enter notes in medical records, to sign contracts, or to schedule patients. Each job must have sufficient authority to take actions, use resources, make decisions, and perform tasks that have been assigned to the job. Delegation of authority is explained later in this chapter.

◆ Managers establish reporting relationships for each job (as explained later in this chapter). Reporting relationships identify

— the position (e.g., supervisor, manager, lead, boss) to which a given position directly reports; and

— the positions (e.g., subordinates, direct reports), if any, that directly report to a given position.

◆ Managers identify other positions and jobs with which a position must coordinate (other than the immediate supervisor). For example, patient care jobs usually must coordinate their work with other patient care jobs. An accountant in the finance department might be required to coordinate with an employee benefits manager in the human resources department.

◆ Managers determine the qualifications needed to perform a job, such as education, experience, competencies, licensure, attitudes, behaviors, and other characteristics (further explained in chapter 7).

ORGANIZING JOBS AND POSITIONS INTO DEPARTMENTS

Another step in organizing work (to accomplish goals) is **departmentalization**, the organization of jobs and positions into departments or other groups. A manager must decide on what basis to departmentalize. A department (or bureau, division, section, office) can be organized by grouping jobs that share one or more factors (Dunn 2016). For example, managers might group together jobs that

departmentalization
Organization of jobs and work into departments, bureaus, divisions, sections, offices, and other formal groups.

◆ perform the same activities and tasks (e.g., payroll tasks),

◆ use the same equipment and technology (e.g., telehealth equipment),

◆ serve the same type of customers (e.g., female patients),

◆ create the same product or service (e.g., emergency care),

◆ work in the same place (e.g., the downtown site), or

◆ work at the same time (e.g., night shift).

For example, managers at Sarah Bush Lincoln Health System in Mattoon, Illinois, formed a care coordination department. It includes care coordinators, physician practice navigators, and health coaches who perform care coordination activities and tasks to improve population health (Hegwer 2016b).

As a department manager, you will apply management theory principles you learned in chapter 2 to design your department's report-

✓ CHECK IT OUT ONLINE

The US Department of Labor publishes the *Occupational Outlook Handbook*, which contains information about hundreds of jobs, including many in healthcare. This resource is available online at www.bls.gov/ooh/. The online handbook describes which tasks and work are designed into different healthcare jobs. You can search the handbook to learn more about the healthcare jobs mentioned in your classes and those you encounter throughout your career. Check it out online and see what you discover.

ing relationships (vertical hierarchy), span of control, line and staff positions, unity of command, and (de)centralization. We will study the application of management theory principles by using an example of positions in the sales department of a health insurance company. The sales manager, Kayla, must decide the *reporting relationships* of workers in her department. She decides that all four sales representatives will report directly to

organization chart
Visual portrayal of
vertical hierarchy,
departments, span
of control, reporting
relationships, and flow
of authority.

her, as shown in the **organization chart** in exhibit 4.1. This creates *vertical hierarchy* for the department.

When establishing reporting relationships and vertical hierarchy, the department manager also determines the *span of control* (how many workers report directly to a manager). If all four sales reps and one secretary report to Kayla, her span of control is five, which is reasonable. Suppose that, over time, the department grows and hires nine more sales reps who also report to Kayla. Her span of 14 could be too many for her to effectively manage. She would not have enough time to manage all the workers, her decisions would be delayed, and the sales reps would feel their boss is unavailable and uninterested in them. As department manager, Kayla should consider adding another level of management—a supervisor level—between the sales reps and herself. This adds a level to the vertical hierarchy, as shown in exhibit 4.2. All sales reps now report to either the East Region supervisor or the West Region supervisor. Kayla's span of control is now only three (two regional supervisors and one secretary). Kayla will have to delegate sufficient authority and responsibility to the supervisors so that they can make decisions without having to consult her too often. Delegation of that authority to the supervisors will enable closer supervision of the sales reps, which might be needed to achieve the planned sales goals.

Like many aspects of management, the "best" approach is contingent on several factors (Walston 2017). Recall from chapter 2 that research has found that different departments

Exhibit 4.1
Department
Organization Chart
with Two Levels
in the Vertical
Hierarchy

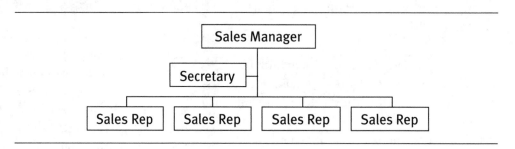

Exhibit 4.2
Department
Organization Chart
with Three Levels
in the Vertical
Hierarchy

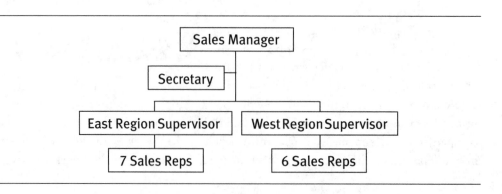

face different contingencies and thus should be organized with different degrees of centralization, specialization, division of work, chain of command, and so forth. The variety and standardization of work, the amount and frequency of change in work, workers' education levels and abilities, workers' physical locations, and external pressures all affect span of control. So too do the manager's abilities, management style, and methods of monitoring subordinates (Dunn 2016). If all the workers do similar work that is simple, repetitive, and easily explained in procedural rules, a manager might capably supervise ten or more workers. However, if workers do many different tasks that are complex, hard to explain, unpredictable, and nonroutine, then more supervision is needed and a manager should have a smaller span of control. If the department's environment changes often and unpredictably, a smaller span of control will allow more frequent supervision to help workers adjust. Workers who are more educated, better trained, and more professional require less supervision and thus permit the manager a wider span of control. Smaller spans of control require more supervisory personnel and thus more expense, which is an important factor to consider.

Organizing jobs into a department also involves deciding which jobs are *line* positions and which are *staff* positions. In exhibits 4.1 and 4.2, the sales reps are line positions in the vertical chain of command because they contribute directly to accomplishing the department's sales goals. The secretary is in a staff position outside the vertical chain of command. That position supports the line positions and indirectly helps to achieve the department's sales goals. Staff positions may provide assistance to relieve the workload of line positions, or staff may provide a specialized ability that line positions do not have (Dunn 2016). People in staff jobs offer advice and support to people in line jobs who make decisions. Staff jobs generally do not have much authority for making decisions. However, they may have power based on expertise, such as a Medicare reimbursement specialist, as discussed in chapter 10.

Unity of command is considered when organizing jobs in a department. According to this principle, a worker reports to—and takes directions from—a single boss. This approach makes sense, and workers like it. However, sometimes it is not realistic, even in a sales office—and especially in HCOs, as we will see later. In exhibit 4.1, four sales reps each report only to the sales manager and follow unity of command. The secretary reports directly to the sales manager yet most likely also assists and takes direction from the four sales reps. Direct contact between the sales reps and secretary enables them to work together rather than by communication through the sales manager. This makes better use of the sales manager's time and reduces miscommunications, delays, and other problems. However, it places more demands on the secretary and may require more meetings to resolve conflict if all four sales reps tell the secretary their work should be done first.

The manager must also decide how much to *centralize and decentralize authority* for making decisions. Recall that with decentralization, a manager **delegates authority** to a subordinate (lower-level) position to make decisions. Decentralization empowers the lower position by granting it authority to make decisions, take actions, and use resources needed to perform

delegate authority
Give authority to a subordinate position to make decisions and take actions.

the job. How much decentralization depends on the tasks and responsibilities assigned to a job, the people (manager and subordinate) involved, the type of work, and other factors. Certainly, the manager must delegate enough authority to enable subordinates to perform tasks and fulfill responsibilities assigned to their jobs. Kayla, as sales manager, can keep all authority centralized for some decisions and tasks (e.g., choosing the Salesperson of the Year award winner) so that only she does them. Yet she can simultaneously decentralize authority to sales reps for other decisions and tasks (e.g., scheduling sales calls, preparing contract proposals). The manager must delegate enough authority to lower-level positions, share enough information with those employees, and trust them so they can do the jobs they are responsible for (as assigned by the manager). Then the manager should get out of the way, avoid micromanaging, and hold them accountable for the delegated work. Appropriate delegation often enables lower-level employees to be more productive, motivated, and satisfied (Walston 2017).

When delegating authority, Kayla must consider possible problems. For example, she should realize that each sales rep probably will not do the work exactly the same way as she and other sales reps would do it. Decentralization increases variation and decreases standardization at lower levels of the organization. Is that acceptable to her? Kayla must think carefully about which authority to delegate to which subordinates. She might want to assign more tasks and delegate more authority to one sales rep (Josh) for his professional growth so he can cover for Kayla when she is away. However, other sales reps might then feel left out and think Kayla is unfair. Later chapters on leadership will offer more advice about delegating.

In summary, when delegating authority, the following things must happen (Dunn 2016; Walston 2017):

1. A manager must ensure that the employee knows what job the manager expects to be done.

2. The manager must grant the employee authority for the tasks, decisions, resources, and actions needed to do the job.

3. The employee must then accept responsibility and authority to do the job and be held accountable for it.

4. The manager must trust the employee to do the job and keep the manager informed with periodic reports.

After authority is delegated to lower positions, the manager position still has authority too. Delegating authority is like sharing knowledge—it increases the number of positions and people that have it, rather than taking it from one and giving it to another (Dunn 2016). Further, the manager is still responsible for the work delegated to lower-level employees. If those employees do not fulfill their assignments, the manager is ultimately responsible and must do the work herself.

Notice how Partners HealthCare used these organizing principles in the Here's What Happened at the beginning of this chapter. Managers brought together specialized jobs (e.g., diabetes educator, telehealth nurse, equipment technician) and created a Center for Connected Health with responsibility for developing patient-centered telehealth services. A director was given authority for the center, and authority for patient care decisions was delegated to lower-level patient care staff.

FACTORS THAT INFLUENCE ORGANIZING WORK

An HCO's environment (external factors) and the organization itself (internal factors) affect how managers organize work. Prior strategic planning, discussed in chapter 3, analyzed both types of factors. Take a few minutes to jot down examples of how the external environment and the organization itself might affect how work is organized. Then read the following example.

New technology invented in the external environment creates new ways of performing existing tasks—and sometimes entirely new tasks—that must be organized into jobs. The invention of digital communication led to the redesign of jobs to use electronic health records rather than traditional paper records. Digital "writing" slowed down physicians in hospital emergency departments, so many of those departments hired digital scribes. A scribe goes into the emergency room with the physician (and the patient) and writes all the digital medical records in real time while the physician treats the patient. After caring for the patient, the physician reviews, edits, and signs the digital record. Thus, because of a technological innovation in the external environment, a new digital scribe job was created and the tasks of the emergency room physician job changed. Artificial intelligence, chatbots, and virtual assistants developed in the external environment are further changing tasks and work in HCOs (Schawbel 2017).

mechanistic
Emphasizing specialized, rigid tasks; centralized decisions; strict hierarchy, control, and rules; and vertical communication and interaction.

organic
Emphasizing shared flexible tasks; teamwork; decentralized decisions; loose hierarchy, control, and rules; and horizontal communication and interaction.

EXTERNAL FACTORS

Recall from chapter 2 that contingency theory arose from studies that found one type of organization structure works best if the external environment is mostly stable and predictable, whereas a different organization structure works best if the external environment changes quickly and unpredictably. A **mechanistic** structure fits best with a stable, predictable environment, while an **organic** structure fits best with an unstable, changing environment. Characteristics of mechanistic and organic organizations are shown in exhibit 4.3.

These two organization structures are idealized types, and organizations are not entirely one or the other. They blend the two types and could be mostly one type or the other. Many managers feel their environments have become more unstable and unpredictable, so they have reorganized their HCOs to become more organic. The organic model seems more alive and natural than the mechanistic form. On the other hand, elements of

	Stable, Predictable Environment	Unstable, Unpredictable Environment
EXHIBIT 4.3 Environment and Structure	*Mechanistic structure is best.*	*Organic structure is best.*
	Separate, specialized, rigid tasks	Shared, flexible tasks adjusted by teamwork
	Centralized decisions	Decentralized decisions
	Strict vertical hierarchy, tight control, narrow span of control, many rules	Loose, flatter hierarchy; loose control; wide span of control; few rules
	Vertical communication and interaction	Diffuse horizontal communication and interaction

Sources: Data from Daft (2016) and Walston (2017).

mechanistic structure are being used to organize some patient care work, as noted in the Check It Out Online sidebar.

 CHECK IT OUT ONLINE

Healthcare workers often follow care protocols that list standardized work processes for specific health problems. These protocols are based on scientific evidence and best practices to help organize work by healthcare workers. Search online for "standard care protocols" or "hospital care protocols" to find examples of standardized work processes in healthcare. Check it out online and see what you discover.

You might want to quickly review in chapter 1 the sectors of the external environment and the healthcare trends and future developments. Thinking about these will help you understand the many external factors that affect how work and jobs are organized and why work and jobs are being reorganized. In recent years, stakeholders outside of HCOs have demanded—and reimbursement has changed to reward—better value, clinical quality, customer satisfaction, patient experience, patient safety, and transitions throughout the continuum of care. These external forces have been driving changes in how HCOs organize their work, jobs, and structure. Some of these changes are described in the Using Chapter 4 in the Real World sidebar and following bullet points (Bosko and Gulotta 2016; Hegwer 2016a; McConnell 2018; Radick 2016; Walston 2017):

◆ Reorganization to be more patient centered (rather than provider centered) for the patient's convenience

◆ Workflow analysis and redesign to streamline and facilitate prompt, seamless patient care among different jobs, departments, and facilities

◆ New tasks organized into new jobs such as chronic disease educators, population health coaches, care coordinators, medical practice facilitators, and patient experience officers

◆ Scripted tasks and behaviors (sometimes embedded in electronic health records) for staff to follow when interacting with patients and families

◆ Shifting more work to primary care and other ambulatory services in the continuum of care

◆ Data analytics, clinical information technology, and artificial intelligence to improve clinical care work processes and provide decision support for clinical care

 USING CHAPTER 4 IN THE REAL WORLD

Collecting payment from a medical group's patients may be difficult, awkward, and stressful for everyone involved. Front desk staff can better perform this task if the job has been designed well. The American Medical Association (AMA) offers scripts for this purpose. The scripts give staff standard approaches to collecting payment that allow for a courteous, respectful patient experience. Here is one script (AMA 2015):

Script 3: For collecting payment from patient upon check-out
After the appointment, the medical staff walks the patient to the front desk, says goodbye to the patient and quickly exits the area. The patient is now ready for check-out. Reviewing the patient's insurance eligibility verification response, say: *"According to your insurance benefit coverage details, your fee today is $310."*

Look directly at the patient and say, *"How would you like to pay for that—by check, cash or credit card?"*

Then wait and allow the patient to answer. . . . Look at the patient directly and allow them to answer. Do not speak until the patient has responded to your question. If a patient says they cannot pay the entire amount at the time of service, follow up by asking, *"How much are you able to pay today?"*

Thank the patient for whatever amount he or she can pay, and follow up by saying, *"And when do you anticipate paying the balance of today's visit?"*

Be sure the patient commits to a date for that payment and, again, wait for the patient to respond. . . . Make sure you address the *entire balance*, not just one payment, and then put the new payment arrangement in writing. This creates an agreement that the patient is more apt to abide by, as opposed to an oral agreement.

INTERNAL FACTORS

An HCO's size, its goals, and worker motivation are internal factors to consider when organizing tasks into jobs. In a small HCO, there may not be much division of work into specializations. Because larger HCOs have more work, more workers are hired, which allows for more specialization and, in turn, requires more coordination. In a small HCO, there is not enough medical imaging work for a full-time computed tomography (CT) tech, a full-time magnetic resonance imaging (MRI) tech, and so forth. So the HCO may have unspecialized imaging technicians who have broader responsibilities and perform CT, MRI, and radiology. Extensive growth in the medical imaging workload and number of employees could lead to specialization, division of work, and need for coordination. Conversely, if a large HCO downsizes during an economic recession, the fewer remaining workers may be expected to do whatever needs to be done with less specialization.

An HCO's goals also influence how work is organized. If the HCO has a goal to improve the quality of medical imaging, managers may create narrower medical imaging jobs that specialize in just one modality (e.g., CT or MRI) and staff those jobs with workers who are experts in that modality. Assuming that practice makes perfect, this specialization would improve quality. Also, specialization generally reduces errors and the need to redo work, which could help achieve an efficiency goal. In contrast, if the goal is to be responsive to customers' unique preferences to improve their patient experience, managers may organize jobs flexibly to allow workers to interact with customers and adjust to their needs. Doing so calls for more decentralization of authority to frontline service workers so they can make decisions quickly for customers. It also calls for fewer rigid rules.

When designing jobs, managers must also think about worker motivation. If jobs are too repetitive and only follow a simple step-by-step process, workers may become unmotivated. Jobs in which workers perform tasks alone may demotivate people who need social interaction. Jobs with rigidly organized narrow tasks and no opportunity for creativity demotivate people who need growth or self-expression. We will learn more about motivation in later chapters on staffing, leading, and motivating. For now, realize that job design affects—and therefore should consider—motivation.

Jobs can be organized in multiple ways. Some approaches focus on getting the work done, producing the products and services, and achieving the goals. Other approaches focus on keeping workers satisfied, enabling employees to grow, and fulfilling human needs. Each approach has advantages and disadvantages, and a manager must try to balance all considerations when organizing work. After deciding on an approach and implementing it, the manager should periodically evaluate the results and reorganize if necessary.

A FEW COMPLICATIONS

Managers can use the methods and principles explained in this chapter to organize work in HCOs. When doing so, they should consider four possible complications—the informal organization, contract workers, unionized workers, and medical jobs with physicians.

TRY IT, APPLY IT

Suppose you are the manager of a college health and wellness center. (You may think creatively about its mission and services.) Brainstorm and list at least 15 tasks that your center performs. Use the verb–noun approach to list the tasks. Then organize the tasks into jobs. Which jobs will perform which tasks? Compare your ideas with those of other students.

INFORMAL ORGANIZATION

This chapter has focused on the formal organization—the organization shown in the official bylaws, charts, job descriptions, policies, and other documents. However, managers must realize that after they formally organize work and workers, the workers will not always follow the formal organization. They often create and follow their own unofficial, **informal organization**, which coexists with the official, formal organization. Employees use their own unwritten and informal rules, work procedures, behaviors, expectations, and communication networks (e.g., the grapevine) to create their informal organization. Managers should understand that the informal organization can support—or disrupt—the formal organization. The informal organization is powerful and influential and often reflects how work is really done and how employees really feel about the organization (McConnell 2018).

Informal groups and unofficial arrangements arise from shared interests and social relationships among people who work together (Dunn 2016). Groups may form among the third-shift personnel in a skilled nursing facility, the information technology staff in a health insurance firm, or the therapists in a rehabilitation center. Coworkers with common interests or friendships outside the HCO may also create informal groups at work. Members of these groups talk, gossip, share opinions, support each other, and report what they have heard (true and untrue) elsewhere in the organization. They interact both at work and outside of work via social media, informal gatherings, recreational activities, and other opportunities. Group members help each other gain satisfaction and fulfill certain needs, such as the need for friendship, belonging, security, acceptance, status, comfort, emotional support, affiliation, reinforcement of one's beliefs, sympathy, camaraderie, and collective power.

Informal groups have their own rules, culture, and behavioral norms that specify what members of the group are supposed to do. These expectations may conflict with an HCO's official goals, job descriptions, and work plans. The groups strongly influence members who want to remain in the group and gain its benefits. The informal leader lacks formal authority yet influences others by using informal reward power and coercive power

informal organization
Workers' own unofficial and unwritten work rules, procedures, expectations, agreements, and communication networks (e.g., the grapevine), which coexist and may conflict with the official ones of the formal organization.

in the group. If a group member does not support the group's rules, then the leader and other group members may discipline that member using ridicule, avoidance, rejection, or other punishments.

Just as the formal organization has smaller parts, such as departments, so too does the informal organization. The basic unit is the small group—a few workers who share contact, interaction, feelings, and friendship. Depending on the size of the organization, there may be dozens of small groups in the informal organization. Small groups may form in each formal department of an organization and also around specific interests, such as "the parking problem." An employee may belong to more than one small group in the informal organization that coexists with the formal organization.

The informal organization, its groups, and its leaders can greatly influence employees to support—or oppose—the tasks, jobs, departments, and decisions of the formal organization (Dunn 2016). For example, the informal organization may support or oppose a change in the work schedule and job tasks at an outpatient therapy clinic. Managers in the formal organization may struggle to implement changes if the informal organization does not support the changes. Formal organization leaders should recognize this fact and work with informal leaders to gain this support. They must figure out who the informal group's leaders are and understand the group's norms, viewpoints, and expectations. Then they must develop collaborative working relationships with the informal group and its leaders. The formal leader must turn the informal leader into an ally rather than a rival. Later chapters provide more information about informal organizations.

CONTRACT WORKERS

Sometimes, not all the workers in an HCO are actual employees of the organization. For example, when a hospital is unable to fill vacant nurse positions, it might contract with a staffing agency for nurses. The agency hires its own nurses and contracts with businesses that need temporary nursing staff. The hospital pays the agency a fee, and the agency provides temporary workers (sometimes called *travel workers*). Temp agencies provide contract workers for dozens of job specialties, sometimes for a day and sometimes for much longer.

The contract between the agency and the HCO formally identifies the work responsibilities, required clearances to work, supervision, authority, and other aspects of the relationships among the worker, agency, and HCO. Even so, questions and conflicts can and do arise. The HCO might feel the agency worker lacks the skills or behaviors needed for the job, or the worker might feel the HCO demands more work than the contract allows. A contract therapist will feel more loyalty to the Therapists 'R' Us agency than to the HCO she is assigned to.

Another type of contract worker is someone, usually with specialized expertise, who negotiates his own contract with an HCO rather than working for a staffing agency or being hired as an employee. Biomedical engineers, medical physicists, and speech therapists are examples. These contract arrangements can be useful in some situations, but they complicate the department's and HCO's formal organization. When a hospital in Spartanburg developed a new radiation treatment center for cancer, it contracted with a full-time medical physicist. Along with job responsibilities, the written contract described how that position fit into the organization. The contract stated which manager the position reported to, identified what authority the position held, and explained how the position was required to coordinate with management, employees, and the medical staff.

In today's "gig economy," the contract worker concept has many variations, and employers are increasing their use of gig workers (Schawbel 2017). HCOs use freelance, per diem, temporary, part-time, and on-call arrangements and jobs. All of these approaches require managers to properly organize the relationships between the workers and HCOs.

Unionized Workers

Some workers in HCOs may vote to be represented by a labor union regarding their jobs, work, rules, schedules, compensation, and other terms of employment. For example, some clinical workers, maintenance workers, clerical workers, and others are represented by unions. Although it is not part of the official organization, the union controls unionized workers and their relationship with the employer. Unions obtain authority through employee elections and negotiated contracts (backed by labor laws) to control aspects of who works when, where, and how. After employees vote to be represented by a labor union, HCO managers alone cannot organize the work, tasks, and jobs. Instead, managers must use collective bargaining and negotiate with the union to jointly decide the terms and conditions of work for the represented workers (Malvey and Raffenaud 2015). Union rules control how HCO managers and employees communicate and interact with each other and how union representatives and HCO managers resolve workplace disputes. Unions complicate how work is organized into jobs and departments because managers must make such decisions jointly with the union. Labor unions are discussed in more detail in chapter 8.

Medical Jobs with Physicians

In hospitals, medical practices, outpatient surgery centers, health insurance companies, and some other HCOs, certain tasks, jobs, and positions must be performed by a physician. Some of these jobs involve medical work, such as surgeon, radiologist, anesthesiologist, and hospitalist. Others are administrative yet also involve medical work, such as vice president of medical affairs, medical director of quality care, and cardiology medical director. These jobs require a physician with appropriate medical expertise, a license to practice medicine, and other qualifications that only a physician would have. For these jobs, the HCO may hire and pay a physician, may contract with and pay a physician (see the "Contract Workers" section earlier in this chapter), or may grant the physician privileges to work in the HCO without being paid by the HCO. (In the last case, the physician is paid by patients and their insurance plans.) Positions that require a physician can make HCOs very different from other organizations. These positions make organization structure and management more complex because they do not fit neatly with the traditional chain of command, organization chart, and use of management authority.

Let's consider hospitals, because they have many kinds of medical jobs with physicians. A hospital generally does not hire a physician through the human resources department—the way it hires most employees. A physician applies to the hospital for medical staff privileges in a specialty such as neurology, orthopedics, or cardiology. She specifies the kinds of medical work and procedures for which she is requesting privileges. She submits her credentials (e.g., medical school degree, years of residency training, license, recommendation letters) and provides evidence of competency to perform her specified medical work. The medical staff office collects all this information and forwards it to the medical staff credentials committee for review. The credentials committee then makes a recommendation to the board of directors for consideration. The board decides whether to grant the physician the requested privileges to practice the requested kinds of medical work in that hospital.

Hospitals also have hospital-based physician (HBP) positions, such as pathologist, emergency physician, and hospitalist. Although there are variations, physicians in these positions work in and directly for the hospital rather than in their own private medical practice in the community. Physicians in these jobs might be employed by or contract with (and be paid by) the hospital to provide their services. Or, they might provide services in hospitals but bill patients and insurers for those services. In general, HBPs have authority and responsibility for their medical work but not for administrative work unless it is specifically required in their contract or assigned to them by managers.

In a variation of this scenario, a hospital or hospital system hires physicians as employees to work in medical offices (rather than in the hospital itself). Hospitals and their systems often own and operate primary care and medical specialty practices. The physicians are hired as employees and practice ambulatory medicine. They are office-based physicians, working for a hospital (system). If a patient needs to be admitted to the hospital, the patient is cared for by a HBP hospitalist who practices inpatient medical care. Like HBPs, the office-based physicians have authority and responsibility for medical work but not for administrative work unless it is specifically assigned to them by managers.

Where does medicine end and administration begin? Good question. **The boundary between medicine and administration is fuzzy.** Unity of command can be routinely violated if HBPs and administrative managers both direct the same laboratory technicians or the same emergency nurses. Managers and physicians share responsibility for the quality of patient care, but problems arise when physicians feel that anything affecting medical care is a medical matter and within their sole authority. If a radiologist claims authority to fire a technologist who made a mistake, the manager can say that is an administrative matter. On the other hand, managers must be careful about how involved they get in medical matters. If a physician asks a nonphysician manager, "And where did *you* go to medical school?" the physician likely believes the manager has become too involved in something that requires medical expertise. Yet, the administrative manager can—and must—require physicians to comply with hospital medical staff bylaws, rules, and standards. Usually, boundaries and responsibilities are understood and respected so that work proceeds smoothly. When managers take the lead with respectful, candid, and open dialogue, physicians can become integral parts of the management hierarchy with agreement on authority, coordination, organizing, and other matters. For this structure to work, the manager must cultivate a professional relationship with the physician leader based on trust, honesty, and ability.

Some physicians who work in a hospital are not hired, contracted, or paid by the hospital. The hospital grants privileges to these independent physicians to provide care to patients in the hospital; these physicians then bill the patients (and insurance plans) for payment. For example, a neurosurgeon is granted surgical privileges to perform neurosurgery on his patients in the hospital and collect payment for his services from those patients and their insurance plans. That physician most likely has a medical office practice in the community where he sees patients. He might also have privileges to perform neurosurgery on patients at other hospitals. The percentage of physicians in independent practice has been declining, while the percentage in interdependent practice (with a hospital) has been growing.

Do administrative managers have authority over the surgeon? Well, not entirely. In the hospital organization chart, the surgeon does not report to the operating room (OR) manager as the scrub nurses do. In many hospitals, the physicians are in a medical hierarchy different from the usual administrative hierarchy (organization chart). This medical hierarchy (explained more in chapter 5) usually reports to the chief of the medical staff or perhaps to the CEO and ultimately is accountable to the board of directors in the chain of command. Physicians do have more autonomy than other workers in deciding *how* they will perform their work. The manager can specify how the OR custodian should clean the room after a surgical case, but the manager cannot specify how the surgeon should perform the surgery. Hospital managers may, however, dictate which equipment and supplies are used in the OR to ensure consistency and efficient purchasing practices. In addition, the hospital neither employs nor pays the independent surgeon, which reduces the manager's power and influence over that physician. Yet, the manager does have authority to ensure the surgeon complies with hospital bylaws, policies, and standards. When the hospital grants a physician privileges to practice in the hospital, the privileges require this compliance, and the physician agrees.

In HCOs, medicine and management are gradually merging, resulting in less separation of medical and administrative matters. New payment methods—such as payment based on value, clinical quality, and customer satisfaction—are causing medicine and management to become more interdependent. Hospital managers must develop effective working relationships with physicians who are becoming more involved in leading, managing, and integrating clinical care across the continuum. Further, regardless of how integrated or separate medicine and management are, the physician has medical expertise on medical matters. A manager cannot direct a physician the way she directs nonphysician workers. Remember that physicians are physicians, which means they have autonomy, influence, and expectations based on medical expertise.

ONE MORE TIME

Organizations, including HCOs, are "social entities that are goal-directed, designed as deliberately structured and coordinated activity systems, and are linked to the external environment" (Daft 2016, 642). Managers deliberately structure HCOs by organizing tasks into jobs, organizing jobs into departments, and organizing departments into an entire organization. To accomplish this, managers use management theory, concepts, and principles including specialization, division of work, authority, reporting relationships, vertical hierarchy, chain of command, span of control, line and staff positions, unity of command, departmentalization, delegation, and decentralization. These elements are used to organize work and jobs.

There is no single best way to organize—it is contingent on external factors in the environment and internal factors in the HCO. Mechanistic structure works best in a stable environment, while organic structure is best for unstable environments. Organizations blend both approaches to fit with their environments and other contingency factors. When organizing HCOs, managers must consider the informal organization, contract workers, unionized workers, and medical jobs with physicians—which all complicate organizing HCOs.

(T) FOR YOUR TOOLBOX

- Organization structure and charts
- Specialization and division of work
- Vertical hierarchy (chain of command)
- Reporting relationships
- Span of control

- Line and staff positions
- Unity of command
- Departmentalization
- Delegation of authority and decentralization
- Mechanistic and organic structure

FOR DISCUSSION

1. Organizing work into distinct jobs requires managers to make decisions about tasks, responsibilities, authority, specialization, spans of control, reporting relationships, qualifications, and other matters. Which of these decisions do you think would be easiest to make? Why? Which would be hardest? Why?

2. Discuss how specific internal factors and specific external factors affect how work should be organized.

3. Compare and contrast mechanistic and organic structures. Why might an HCO be partly organic and partly mechanistic?

4. Discuss how the informal organization affects managing an HCO. How can HCO managers try to work with rather than against the informal organization?

5. How do medical jobs and work done by physicians affect how managers manage HCOs?

CASE STUDY QUESTIONS

These questions refer to the Integrative Case Studies at the back of this book.

1. Disparities in Care at Southern Regional Health System case: Explain how an informal organization may exist at SRHS. Then explain how the informal organization might affect Mr. Hank's efforts to reduce disparities in patient care at SRHS.

2. Hospice Goes Hollywood case: Describe how some complications in management and organization (explained in this chapter) may affect what happens in this case.

3. "I Can't Do It All!" case: Using this chapter, explain how you think Mr. Brice should organize work at Healthdyne. Describe how he should write tasks in vice presidents' job descriptions, delegate authority to vice presidents, and decentralize decision making.

4. The Rocky Road to Patient Satisfaction at Leonard-Griggs case: Explain how an informal organization may exist in this case. Then explain how the informal organization might affect Ms. Ratcliff's plans.

5. The Rocky Road to Patient Satisfaction at Leonard-Griggs case: Which tasks are evident in the intern's job? Which tasks are being added to the jobs of office personnel? Using terms, concepts, and methods from this chapter, explain how you would improve the way work is assigned and authority delegated in this case.

RIVERBEND ORTHOPEDICS MINI CASE STUDY

Riverbend Orthopedics is a busy group practice with expanded services for orthopedic care. It has seven physicians and a podiatrist, plus about 70 other employees. At its big, new clinic building, Riverbend provides extensive orthopedic care. Several technicians provide diagnostic medical imaging, from basic X-rays to magnetic resonance images. The physicians perform surgery in their own outpatient surgery center with Riverbend's own operating nurses and technicians. Therapy is provided by three physical therapists and one part-time contracted occupational therapist. In addition to staff providing actual patient care, the clinic has staff for financial management, medical records, human resources, information systems/technology, building maintenance, and other administrative matters. Occasional marketing work is done by an advertising company. Legal work is outsourced to a law firm. Riverbend is managed by a new president, Ms. Garcia. She and Riverbend have set a goal of achieving "Excellent" ratings for patient experience from at least 90 percent of Riverbend's patients this year.

One of Riverbend's physicians, Dr. Barr, argues that because he is a physician, he must be granted autonomy to practice medicine the way he prefers to practice (i.e., for the physician's convenience).

MINI CASE STUDY QUESTIONS

1. Explain how Ms. Garcia could apply tools, methods, concepts, and principles of organizing from this chapter to help achieve the goal. You may make reasonable assumptions and inferences.

2. Using what you learned in this chapter, describe how you think Ms. Garcia should work with Dr. Barr and other physicians to achieve Riverbend's goal. You may make reasonable assumptions and inferences.

REFERENCES

American Medical Association (AMA). 2015. "Scripts to Help Your Practice Collect Patient Payment at the Time of Service." Accessed May 9, 2018. www.stepsforward.org/Static/images/modules/20/downloadable/poc-scripts.pdf.

Bosko, T., and B. Gulotta. 2016. "Improving Care Across the Continuum." *Journal of Healthcare Management* 61 (2): 90–93.

Daft, R. L. 2016. *Organization Theory and Design*, 12th ed. Mason, OH: South-Western Cengage.

Dunn, R. T. 2016. *Dunn and Haimann's Healthcare Management*, 10th ed. Chicago: Health Administration Press.

Fottler, M. D. 2015. "Job Analysis and Job Design." In *Human Resources in Healthcare*, 4th ed., edited by B. J. Fried and M. D. Fottler, 143–80. Chicago: Health Administration Press.

Hegwer, L. R. 2016a. "5 Ways to Support Clinical Integration." *Healthcare Executive* 31 (1): 18–25.

———. 2016b. "6 Business Imperatives for Population Health Management." *Healthcare Executive* 31 (4): 11–28.

Malvey, D., and A. Raffenaud. 2015. "Managing with Organized Labor." In *Human Resources in Healthcare*, 4th ed., edited by B. J. Fried and M. D. Fottler, 389–426. Chicago: Health Administration Press.

McConnell, C. R. 2018. *Umiker's Management Skills for the New Health Care Supervisor*, 7th ed. Burlington, MA: Jones & Bartlett Learning.

Radick, L. E. 2016. "Improving the Patient Experience." *Healthcare Executive* 31 (6): 32–38.

Schawbel, D. 2017. "Workplace Trends You'll See in 2018." Published November 1. www.forbes.com/sites/danschawbel/2017/11/01/10-workplace-trends-youll-see-in-2018/.

Walston, S. L. 2017. *Organizational Behavior and Leadership in Healthcare: Leadership Perspectives and Management Applications*. Chicago: Health Administration Press.

CHAPTER 5

ORGANIZING: ORGANIZATIONS

Form follows function.

Louis Sullivan, architect

LEARNING OBJECTIVES

Studying this chapter will help you to

➤ organize positions and departments into complete organizations;

➤ describe, compare, and contrast five different organization structures;

➤ examine the governing body atop the organization;

➤ coordinate work internally throughout an organization;

➤ coordinate the organization with external organizations; and

➤ explain medical staff organization in hospitals.

HERE'S WHAT HAPPENED

Partners HealthCare is a large, complex organization governed by a board of directors. The corporate-level senior management includes the president/CEO, executive vice president (EVP) of administration and finance, VP of graduate medical education, VP of population health management, VP of human resources, VP of communications, chief clinical officer, chief strategy officer, chief information officer, chief quality and safety officer, senior medical director, and others. Below them are middle managers and lower-level managers responsible for an array of departments. Each department has employees; larger departments also have levels of management. Partners owns and operates academic medical centers, hospitals, physician practices, managed care plans, community health centers, rehabilitation facilities, clinics, hospices, research institutes, and other healthcare organizations (HCOs). Each has an organization structure of managers, departments, and positions. Dozens of committees, teams, and groups—such as transitions teams and a strategy implementation group—help coordinate the many parts into a whole. In addition to this internal organization structure, Partners organizes itself to connect and coordinate with its external environment. Partners forms interorganizational relationships to link with colleges and universities, insurance companies, suppliers, city government, grant funders, and others in its environment. Managers decide how to organize to fulfill their HCOs' mission and goals.

As we continue to study the real-world example of Partners HealthCare, we learn that it created organization structures to achieve its goals and mission. Many managers organize work tasks into positions and departments. Higher-level managers organize departments into an entire organization. They must then coordinate the departments throughout the organization. Managers apply the principles of hierarchy, span of control, delegation of authority, centralization, line and staff positions, and departmentalization to create the whole organization. Managers also decide how to organize work and positions to connect with the external environment. Newer and lower-level managers must understand this structure to know how their own work unit or department fits into the bigger picture and interacts with other parts of the organization. No department exists independently!

This chapter first provides background information about forming entire organizations and the relevant factors managers should consider. Five forms of organization structure for HCOs are presented, along with their advantages and disadvantages. The chapter then explains methods for coordinating departments within an HCO and for coordinating an HCO with external organizations. Finally, the chapter describes complications that might arise in an HCO and affect how the organization is designed. One complication is the organized medical staff—a unique organization structure found in hospitals.

ORGANIZATION STRUCTURES

Much of an organization's structure is reflected in its organization chart. This chapter explains (and illustrates with organization charts) five different forms of organization structure that are used by HCOs:

1. Functional structure

2. Divisional structure

3. Matrix structure

4. Horizontal structure

5. Network structure

Each of these general models has pros and cons. Many HCOs mix elements of these structural forms to create their own hybrid form.

Which structural form is best? It depends, as you might have guessed. This chapter's opening quote suggests that an organization's form depends on its function or purpose. Just as the form of a building depends on the building's purpose, the form of an organization depends on the organization's purpose. That is why managers must first plan the mission, goals, and purpose of the organization. The structural form of a university organization is different from that of a health insurance organization partly because the organizations have different purposes. What else determines the appropriate structural form? Recall from chapter 4 that an organization may be organic, mechanistic, or a mixture of both types, depending on its external environment, mission, goals, size, work technology, and culture (Daft 2016).

When determining organization structure, managers must consider differentiation among departments and work units. Each department is specialized to perform work that differs from other departments' work. The emergency, housekeeping, and administration departments do different work, and each department interacts with different parts of the external environment, pursues different goals, and uses different resources and production methods. Thus, the departments are organized differently. Further, employees in each department have different knowledge, skills, attitudes, behaviors, values, and ways of thinking. **Differentiation**—the differences in departments' structures and how their workers think and feel—helps to achieve specialized types of work (Daft 2016). However, differentiated departments eventually must be integrated (coordinated) to work together toward the organization's overall purpose. Without integration, differentiated workers and departments will work only toward their own department goals and not toward overall organization goals. Integrating departments is explained further in this chapter's section on coordination.

differentiation
Differences in departments' structures and how their workers think and feel.

The five organization charts shown in this chapter show five different approaches to organizing departments into a formal organization. Boxes, circles, and other shapes represent positions, departments, and other organization components. Vertical lines between boxes in a chart show the vertical hierarchy (chain of command), reporting relationships, flow of authority, and communication up and down the hierarchy. Boxes also may be connected with horizontal lines to show horizontal relationships. Higher boxes in a chart represent positions with more authority and responsibility. Of course, just drawing boxes and lines does not make an organization. The charts simply represent managers' ideas about how they want the organization to be structured. To create the desired organization in real life, managers must implement their ideas. Managers create the structure by organizing, staffing, leading, controlling, and doing other work explained throughout this book. When managers create and maintain accurate charts, employees can use the charts to understand how their organization works and how they fit into it (Dunn 2016).

Planning and organizing are closely connected. Chapter 3 taught us that managers must first assess changes, opportunities, and threats in the environment and adapt the HCO to those changes. Adaptation often requires a change in organization structure, such as from a functional to a divisional form. Second, in the planning process, managers assess the HCO's strengths and weaknesses, which may reveal that the HCO is not working well because it is not organized well. Perhaps middle managers do not have enough authority to act quickly, or perhaps departments are isolated rather than coordinated. If so, then managers will have to redesign the organization. Third, as chapter 3 explained, managers establish goals and then develop plans to implement them. Implementation often includes redesigning the organization structure so that the HCO can achieve the goals. In chapter 3, we read that Partners HealthCare set a goal to reduce the number of readmitted patients. To achieve that goal, managers had to apply organizing principles to redesign tasks, positions, departments, and the organization structure. The Using Chapter 5 in the Real World sidebar gives another example of redesign to achieve goals.

functional structure
An organization structure that organizes departments and positions according to the functions workers perform and the workers' abilities.

FUNCTIONAL STRUCTURE

The **functional structure** organizes departments and positions according to the functions workers perform and the workers' abilities (Daft 2016). In exhibit 5.1, the finance functions are organized under a VP of finance, health services functions are organized under a VP of health services, and so on. The vertical hierarchy and chain of command is clear, allowing for much control. This approach consolidates each kind of expertise into one part of the organization. Specialization is strong, so knowledge and skill are strengthened for finance, for marketing, and for human resources. However, specialization limits

USING CHAPTER 5 IN THE REAL WORLD

At rural Western Maryland Health System (WMHS), chronic disease care had been provided through separate, disease-specific clinics—a diabetes clinic, a heart disease clinic, and so forth. This organization structure caused duplication of costly staff, such as nurse practitioners, dietitians, and pharmacists. Patients with multiple chronic diseases had to schedule multiple appointments and go to different clinics. Then external changes in insurance payments and incentives drove WMHS to reduce duplication while achieving quality standards. To do this, managers redesigned their organization structure. They formed a Center for Clinical Resources that organized care for all common chronic diseases in one place (physically and organizationally). This change simplified how patients accessed care for multiple chronic conditions. It increased sharing of staff and efficiency. The new organization structure enabled staff to coordinate their care for patients with several chronic diseases. Staff could now better help patients understand how to manage all their medications, perform all their self-care, and follow all their dietary requirements. These improvements reduced expensive emergency department visits, reduced hospital admissions, and reduced total costs by almost $15 million. Managers changed the organization structure to achieve cost and quality goals and thereby adapt to change in the external environment (Van Dyke 2016).

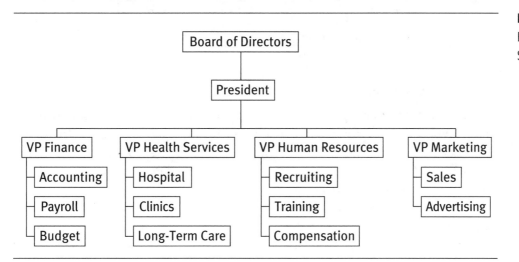

Exhibit 5.1
Functional Structure

employees' understanding of the whole organization and requires much coordination. Horizontal coordination methods (discussed later in this chapter) are needed to improve collaboration between workers under different functional VPs. For example, liaisons could be assigned to coordinate the finance and health services functions to help manage the costs of health services.

Many HCOs use the functional structure. It is common in smaller, newer organizations. This form is not effective for larger, diversified HCOs in rapidly changing environments because decision making is too centralized (at the top) and becomes too slow. The advantages and disadvantages of the functional form are as follows (Daft 2016; Dunn 2016):

Advantages

- Specialized positions grouped in departments

- Efficiency, economies of scale, and cost control

- Development of in-depth knowledge and abilities

- Most effective with only a few products and low complexity

Disadvantages

- Slow decision making and innovation

- Slow adaptation to changing environment

- Functional "silos" focus on their own functional work

- Inadequate horizontal department coordination

DIVISIONAL STRUCTURE

divisional structure
An organization structure that organizes departments and positions to focus on particular groups of customers or services.

The **divisional structure** organizes departments and positions to focus on groups of customers, products, or services rather than on (functional) types of workers (Daft 2016). For example, when an HCO in Towson grows and broadens its range of services, it may change from a functional to a divisional form. Compare and contrast these two forms in exhibit 5.2. What changes do you see?

Positions and departments are reorganized into a hospital division, a clinics division, and a long-term care division. Each division is designed to focus on one type of customer, such as customers who need hospital services. Each division is headed by a separate VP

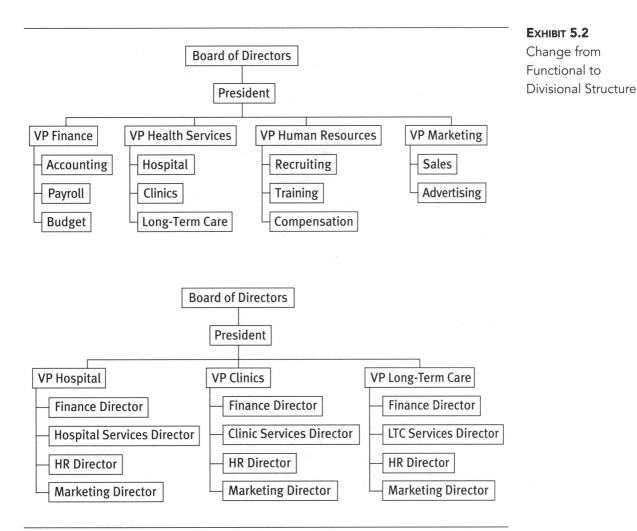

Exhibit 5.2
Change from
Functional to
Divisional Structure

who has appropriate stature and authority. What else do you see? Each division now has its own finance director (and staff), health services director (and staff), human resources director (and staff), and marketing director (and staff). The finance experts are no longer all grouped together as they were in the functional form. Each division now has its own finance knowledge, abilities, and expertise to quickly respond to its own financial affairs and those of its customers. Changes in the environment do not affect hospital, clinic, and long-term care services the same way. The divisional structure recognizes this and gives each division the staff, resources, and decentralized authority to monitor its environment and adjust itself as needed. Doing so may increase the total expense of staff and other resources.

The HCO must evaluate the increased cost compared to improved sales, revenue, patient experience, and market share. The advantages and disadvantages of the divisional form are the following (Daft 2016; Dunn 2016):

Advantages

◆ Ability to adapt to changing environment

◆ Better patient experience and customer satisfaction

◆ Decentralized, faster decisions

◆ Coordination of functions within each product/service division

◆ Good for larger organizations with several main products/services

Disadvantages

◆ Less efficiency and economies of scale

◆ Product/service "silos" that focus on their own product/service

◆ Less coordination and synergy among all products/services

◆ Less development of in-depth functional expertise

◆ Potential duplication of resources

MATRIX STRUCTURE

matrix structure
An organization structure that organizes work by combining functional and divisional structures; uses vertical and horizontal authority to manage workers.

The **matrix structure** combines the functional and divisional forms by superimposing horizontal coordination structure on top of vertical hierarchy structure (Dunn 2016). This structure can help an organization achieve efficiency (using vertical lines of authority) while also achieving quality and satisfaction for specific groups of customers, products, and services (using horizontal lines of authority). A matrix organization has advantages of both the functional and divisional forms. This approach is useful when an HCO must simultaneously

◆ efficiently share costly staff and resources among multiple products, services, and customers, and

◆ coordinate staff and resources to create quality products/services and improve customer satisfaction (Daft 2016; Walston 2017).

Examine carefully exhibit 5.3. What's going on in this organization? Functional management positions exist for functions such as human resources, marketing, and finance. The functional managers report up the functional vertical hierarchy to the president. These managers have authority over the lower-level employees who are permanently assigned to them, such as the marketing employees who work under the VP of marketing. These employees all have functional expertise, such as marketing expertise or nursing expertise. On the left side of the organization chart are several divisional managers, who commonly are called product/service line managers. Each of these managers is responsible for a specific product/service (e.g., cardiology, neurology) or group of customers. To meet goals set for a service line (e.g., surgery), the service line manager uses horizontal authority to manage the workers assigned to her service by the functional managers. Imagine Diana is the surgery service line manager at a hospital in San Diego. She must manage employees assigned to surgery by functional managers. That can be challenging.

The matrix structure offers no unity of command for the functional workers. For example, the VP of marketing assigns Sara (a marketing employee) to work on cardiology services. Sara works for—and is accountable to—the cardiology manager and the VP of marketing. Some employees may even report to more than one divisional manager. The VP of marketing might assign Sara to work part-time for the cardiology manager and part-time for the neurology manager. Sara then would have three bosses.

EXHIBIT 5.3
Matrix Structure

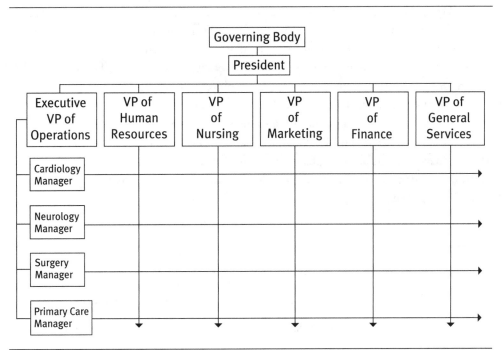

Source: Adapted from Daft (2016).

Often, HCOs that adopt product/service line management organize into a matrix form. For each clinical service, a service line manager has the authority to adapt that service to unique changes in technology, customer preferences, and other factors affecting that service. The service line manager horizontally coordinates the marketing, finance, service production, and other functions across the service line to achieve goals for that service line. The functional and divisional managers often share authority to lead the same workers, which requires effective interpersonal, conflict resolution, and communication skills.

Some large, complex healthcare systems operate multiple smaller HCOs at different sites that cover much or all of the continuum of care. These systems increasingly are adopting variations of the matrix form in which service line managers coordinate care across all facilities at all locations involved in a specific type of care (Buell 2016). For example, an orthopedic service line integrates all orthopedic care (e.g., diagnostic, surgical, rehabilitative, chronic) delivered to orthopedic patients in dispersed facilities, settings, and locations of the large healthcare system. Each service line may be led by a service line manager or by a dyad (physician and administrator). Allina Health, a large health system based in Minneapolis that has 13 hospitals, uses clinical service lines as its main organization structure to provide care at multiple sites throughout the continuum (Van Dyke 2016). Matrix structures are likely to be used by accountable care organizations to integrate various HCOs and services across the continuum of care (Walston 2017).

Managers use a variation of the matrix design for project management in HCOs (Dunn 2016). Senior managers assign a project manager to each project. The project managers replace the service line managers in the matrix chart. Each project manager forms a project team using permanent functional employees from finance, marketing, and other areas to provide skills needed for the project. Employees work their "regular" job while also serving on one or more project teams led by project managers. Outside stakeholders, such as an architect or supply vendor, might also be on project teams.

HCOs can and do create structural variations to fit their unique organization needs. Thus, managers might blend a mostly functional form with the matrix form for just a few medical service lines. The advantages and disadvantages of the matrix form are as follows (Daft 2016; Dunn 2016):

Advantages

◆ Development of both functional and product/service expertise

◆ Efficient, shared use of staff while improving customer satisfaction

◆ Ability to adapt to external changes affecting individual products/services

◆ Coordination and communication across the organization

Disadvantages

◆ No unity of command; more than one boss for each worker

◆ Potential for confusion, stress, and conflict among workers

◆ Well-developed skills required for communication and conflict resolution

◆ Time and expense required to train staff to work in a matrix

◆ Frequent conflict, requiring time and meetings to resolve

HORIZONTAL STRUCTURE

The **horizontal structure** organizes work into several horizontal core processes that are performed by self-managed, multidisciplinary teams of workers. "A process refers to an organized group of related tasks and activities that work together to transform inputs into outputs that create value for customers" (Daft 2016, 116). Examples of core processes are supply chain logistics, new product development, customer acquisition, and order fulfillment. Healthways, a company that improves health and well-being for employers, health plans, and health systems, is organized around five core processes: (1) understand the market, (2) build value solutions and products, (3) acquire and retain customers, (4) deliver solutions and add value, and (5) manage the business (Cummings and Worley 2015).

In the horizontal structure, core processes are performed by self-managed teams of empowered workers who have the necessary functional skills (Cummings and Worley 2015; Daft 2016). Teams have authority to make most decisions without vertical chain-of-command supervision. A process owner is accountable to senior management for the process team's overall performance, but this position does not use vertical chain-of-command supervision. Instead, the process owner focuses on facilitating the work process and coordinating workers. Team members are trained to perform multiple process activities so they can help throughout the process. This training also prepares workers to use data, resources, policies, and management methods to manage their process. Workers have the authority to use their judgment and make decisions to create value for customers. The process team's performance is measured according to how well it creates value and increases customer satisfaction.

This structure eliminates traditional department boundaries and vertical hierarchy that may hamper coordination, flexibility, and decision making. As shown in exhibit 5.4, teams, not positions and departments, are the basic component of organizing the horizontal form (Cummings and Worley 2015; Daft 2016). Each team thoroughly understands its customers and their expectations. The team designs its process to create value and ensure customer satisfaction. A team's workers have varied functional expertise yet continually interact, coordinate, and communicate with each other to perform the team's process. Thus,

horizontal structure
An organization structure that organizes work into core processes that are performed by self-managed, multidisciplinary teams of workers.

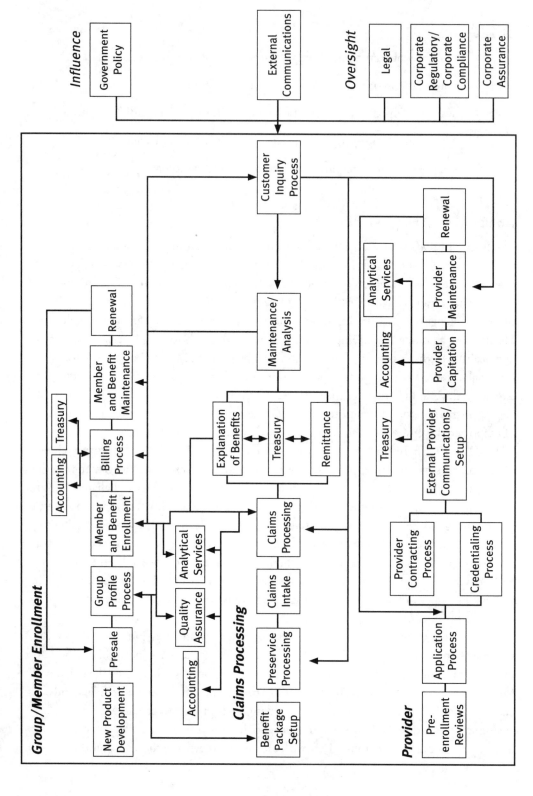

EXHIBIT 5.4
Horizontal Structure

workflow and coordination are faster, more agile, and better able to adapt to changes in the external environment, including customers' needs.

Organizations with highly interdependent activities and a strong customer focus should consider this form; so, too, should organizations in uncertain and changing external environments. This newer horizontal structure—also called *process, boundaryless,* and *team-based* structure—has become more common in recent years (Cummings and Worley 2015). The advantages and disadvantages of the horizontal form are as follows (Cummings and Worley 2015; Daft 2016; Dunn 2016):

Advantages

◆ Intense focus on creating value for customers

◆ Flexibility, efficiency, speed, responsiveness to customers

◆ Focus on the organization rather than own department

◆ Much teamwork and coordination

◆ Integration of varied tasks, activities, and expertise

◆ Fewer layers of management

◆ More responsibility and growth for employees

Disadvantages

◆ Risk of worse performance if organized around wrong core processes

◆ Extensive change of organization structure and management

◆ Resistance by managers and staff specialists

◆ Significant training requirements for new skills, culture, and knowledge

◆ Limited development of in-depth functional expertise

NETWORK STRUCTURE

Managers of organizations that use the **network structure** (also called *modular structure*) outsource tasks, jobs, functions, and departments to other organizations (Daft 2016). The organizations all connect via interpersonal relationships, trust, contracts, information systems, and telecommunications (Cummings and Worley 2015). The top manager is similar to a general contractor who subcontracts (outsources) most work to other organizations. The organization might do only what it specializes in and outsource everything

network structure
An organization structure that organizes work by outsourcing much of it to a network of other organizations connected by interpersonal relationships, contracts, and information systems.

else. For example, a urology group practice focuses on doing urology. The urologists could outsource financial management, information technology, legal services, human resources tasks, marketing, and administration to other organizations. As shown in exhibit 5.5, the network form does not have a vertical hierarchy.

The network structure is a matter of degree; most HCOs contract out at least some work. For a new ambulatory surgical center, this approach enables a fast start, flexibility, and quick growth through partner organizations such as a law firm, an accounting firm, and an advertising firm. Years later, when it is much bigger, the HCO probably will still outsource some work (e.g., legal work) rather than hire its own staff (e.g., an attorney). Even large HCOs contract out some work. For example, many contract with language interpretation companies to communicate with patients who do not know the local prevailing language.

The network structure is used by all sizes of organizations. In large ones, such as global pharmaceutical firms, the network becomes very complex, dynamic, and dispersed. Managers spend much of their time managing the network. They may add new partner organizations, change the amount of work sent to others, renegotiate agreements, strengthen

EXHIBIT 5.5
Network Structure

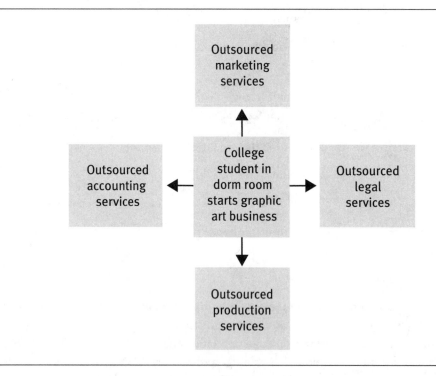

coordination among partners, monitor performance, and make other adjustments to the network. Many HCOs outsource work using a network approach that is so seamless that patients and others do not realize it exists. A manager should always remember that the network approach creates dependencies and risk. Success depends on organizations in the network. Lousy performance by any of them weakens the network. The advantages and disadvantages of the network form are listed here (Cummings and Worley 2015; Daft 2016; Dunn 2016).

Advantages

◆ Quick access to expertise, systems, facilities, and equipment with minimal investment

◆ Flexibility to grow, shrink, and adjust to rapidly changing external environments

◆ Useful for organization specialization and innovation

◆ Less time spent on managing a large, complex organization hierarchy

Disadvantages

◆ Dependence on other organizations for critical services

◆ Risk of failure if outsource partner performs poorly

◆ Time and expense to choose partners, negotiate contracts, and manage relationships

◆ Potentially weaker employee loyalty and commitment

HYBRID STRUCTURES

The five organization structures explained in this chapter are just a starting point. **Managers often create custom structures by combining elements of more than one organization structure.** They might start with functional and then add matrix structure for the ob-gyn service line and for the outpatient surgery service line. Or, top managers might create a divisional structure in which each division has its own finance staff and marketing staff, but then take a functional approach in centralizing human resources to ensure consistency of employment practices. The possibilities and variations are endless. If you've seen one HCO organization chart, you surely haven't seen them all!

✓ **CHECK IT OUT ONLINE**

Search for *healthcare organization charts* online and see the wide variety of charts for HCOs. They come in many sizes, structures, designs, and shapes—including circular and triangular! You'll find charts for specific types of HCOs such as health insurance companies, medical groups, home care businesses, consulting firms, hospitals, nursing homes, and others. Some are the actual organization charts of real HCOs. Check it out online and see what you discover.

GOVERNING BODY

Most HCOs (except for small ones) have a governing body at the top of the organization structure. It may be called the board of trustees, board of directors, board of governors, or something similar. The board acts on behalf of the organization's owners to do what is best for the owners. The owners may be investors, shareholders, citizens, a city, a church, or others. They elect or appoint a board to act on their behalf and to ensure the organization fulfills the owners' responsibilities. Board members are entrusted with the following responsibilities to govern the HCO for the owners (White and Griffith 2019):

1. The board ensures management capability by hiring and monitoring the performance of the president/CEO, establishing policies for hiring and developing other managers, and maintaining a succession plan.

2. The board establishes the HCO's mission, goals, vision, values, and strategy each year. It then approves necessary budgets and implementation plans, including major policies.

3. The board monitors the HCO's performance compared to preset plans, budgets, and targets and ensures implementation of plans to achieve goals. When target performance levels are not met, the board requires explanation and corrective action.

4. If an HCO has a medical staff, the board approves medical staff bylaws, appoints physicians, and monitors their performance.

5. The board reviews its own performance and that of individual members. It ensures that board governance is effective.

Most boards have some members from outside the HCO, such as a realtor or banker, and some from inside the HCO, such as the CEO (and chief of staff if there is a medical staff). The board chooses and appoints its own members. A board might seek people who can bring a certain perspective to the board, such as a physician or a patient. Boards also seek people who can contribute particular expertise, such as in strategic planning or fundraising. To fulfill its responsibilities, the board appoints members to committees, such as for finance, strategic planning, and quality.

COORDINATION WITHIN AND BEYOND A HEALTHCARE ORGANIZATION

Recall from chapter 2 that coordination is connecting individual tasks, activities, jobs, departments, and people to work together toward a common purpose. We learned how Partners HealthCare does this in the opening Here's What Happened. Coordination is essential because organizations have become more complex and work has become more specialized and divided up. As mentioned in chapter 1, healthcare stakeholders are demanding better clinical integration of patient care, as well as better patient experience for the nonclinical aspects of healthcare. All of that requires better coordination. Yet, changes in jobs and staffing—such as telecommuting, job sharing, flexible work schedules, and a growing number of workers in organizations—create challenges for coordination (Dunn 2016).

Coordination is needed because individual departments affect other departments. For example, the human resources department of an assisted living facility in Orlando must coordinate with all other departments to ensure the right kinds of workers are hired when needed. When departments must share resources (e.g., staff, equipment, office space, information), coordination is essential. Think back to the matrix organization structure, in which staff members are shared among parts of the organization. The departments must coordinate carefully to share workers.

Because HCOs are open systems, they must also coordinate their work with other organizations in the external environment. An HCO in Fayetteville must acquire labor, supplies, information, and perhaps government approvals from other organizations. And, it must have customers, clients, and others who use its products and services. The HCO must organize jobs and departments to connect and coordinate with parts of the environment such as schools, the state department of health, office supply companies, banks, health insurance companies, and others.

Coordination occurs in four directions. An organization needs vertical, horizontal, and diagonal internal coordination (i.e., within the organization). It also needs external coordination (i.e., with other organizations).

- ◆ Vertical coordination connects work up and down the vertical hierarchy in an organization.

- ◆ Horizontal coordination connects work sideways across an organization.

- ◆ Diagonal coordination simultaneously connects work vertically and horizontally in an organization.

- ◆ External coordination connects work with other organizations.

Coordination Structures and Processes

How can healthcare managers strengthen coordination for their HCOs? They can create structures and processes that enable employees to exchange information! Coordination depends on people sharing information, and specific organization structures and processes enable such sharing. The chapter's opening Here's What Happened and the Using Chapter 5 in the Real World sidebar gave examples of coordination processes, and examples for an academic medical center are in the following list. Managers must understand all these methods and decide which ones will work best for the kind of coordination required. Many HCOs have been redesigning their organizations to strengthen horizontal coordination by including interdisciplinary teams and project teams. The team approach fits well with millennials, who may like to work in teams.

◆ *Hierarchical referral.* This is the chain of command used by supervisors and subordinates to exchange information up and down a vertical hierarchy (Daft 2016). The chemotherapy cancer treatment supervisor tells a subordinate nurse which patients she will serve today. During the day, that nurse informs the supervisor of progress on the patient schedule and about an equipment problem in Room 4.

◆ *Mutual adjustment.* Workers who do not have a supervisor–subordinate relationship informally exchange information to coordinate their work (Mintzberg 1983). They adjust their work and themselves to each other. A maintenance worker and a nurse confer to decide when to replace a light bulb in the ceiling above a patient's bed.

◆ *Rules, plans, and protocols.* These coordinate workers for recurring situations or problems. They tell what should be done so workers do not have to ask the supervisor (and perhaps wait for a reply). Work is often coordinated by rules, plans, protocols, and procedures (Daft 2016), which may create standardized outputs and standardized processes. For example, a protocol tells the primary care team which specialists should be consulted for a new diabetic patient.

◆ *Information systems.* Electronic information systems are used to gather, analyze, arrange, and report information throughout an organization and to other organizations. Each person can decide which information to send to whom to coordinate vertically, horizontally, diagonally, or externally. Wikis, electronic whiteboards, collaborative document-editing tools, meeting management groupware, and project management software may be useful. At the end of each week, the director of medical education uses the management information system to report key performance indicators to selected physicians, department staff, and other stakeholders.

◆ *Liaison.* A liaison is an employee of one department whose job includes coordinating that department's work with another department (Daft 2016). This liaison may have a particular type of expertise to share with the other department that helps coordinate the departments. For example, a purchasing specialist from the supply chain department serves as a part-time liaison to the emergency department to coordinate purchasing and inventory of costly supplies.

◆ *Full-time integrator.* This job devotes all of its time to coordinating multiple departments or other organization units. The **integrator** does not directly supervise these departments, nor is the integrator an employee of any of the departments (Daft 2016). The product/service line managers shown in matrix organizations in this chapter are full-time integrators. So, too, are the project managers described in chapter 3 and earlier in this chapter. For example, a project manager integrates employees from six departments to jointly implement the expansion and relocation of the data analytics department. Note that although a job whose title includes the word *coordinator* might seem to be a full-time integrator job, in some cases the job does not really include much coordination work (Dunn 2016).

integrator
A person who works full-time coordinating the work of multiple departments toward a common purpose.

◆ *Task forces, teams, committees, councils, and other groups.* These groups bring together representatives of multiple departments (and other parts of an organization) to directly coordinate the departments' work (Daft 2016). Members exchange information, plan activities, and make joint decisions to coordinate their activities. Groups can be expanded to include people from outside the organization. Task forces are temporary; teams, committees, and councils tend to do longer-term work (Daft 2016). For example, the faculty diversity committee coordinates the work of academic departments and professional staff to increase diversity of the faculty.

◆ *Relational coordination.* When organizations use relational coordination, "people share information freely across departmental boundaries, and people interact on a continuous basis to share knowledge and solve problems" (Daft 2016, 100). A culture of openness, trust, teamwork, and flexibility, along with an extensive web of cooperative working relationships among employees, creates the coordination. Much time and effort are needed to gradually develop such coordination. For example, senior clinical managers established shared performance goals and shared performance rewards to develop more relational coordination among the clinical services.

◆ *Boundary spanners.* These employees coordinate their organization with organizations in the external environment. They do so by working across the boundary of their own organization. They might send information from their organization into the external environment and other organizations. Or, they might gather information from external organizations and bring it into their own organization (Daft 2016). Recall from chapter 1 that the environment may be divided conceptually into sectors for human resources, supplies, funds, customers, and so forth. Specific jobs can coordinate an organization with specific sectors of the environment. For example, a talent recruiter from the medical center met with staff at several local colleges (in the human resources sector) to discuss job opportunities for graduates.

◆ *Contracts and other agreements.* Organizations commit to contracts to coordinate their work with that of other organizations. Two people representing two organizations may reach a simple agreement with a brief meeting and handshake. Managers and attorneys negotiate complex contracts that require several meetings and many pages of terms and conditions. For example, the contract between the medical center and construction company coordinated ten months of work to build a genetics research laboratory.

Managers also formally connect their HCO with other organizations by using interorganizational structures such as alliances, mergers, joint ventures, accountable care organizations, hospital systems, supply chains, networks, and independent practice associations. An HCO uses these interorganizational structures to link with one or more other organizations in its environment to achieve its goals. These structures may connect two or more organizations . . . sometimes hundreds!

As we read in chapter 1, many HCOs are joining with others, and this trend will continue. For example, in this chapter we saw that Partners HealthCare is made up of numerous HCOs that together form an integrated health system. Blue Cross health insurance companies throughout the country are members of the national Blue Cross Blue Shield Association. Many independent physician practices in western New York State have joined the Greater Rochester Independent Practice Association (2017) to gain access to customizable care management services and tools. In these interorganizational arrangements, independent HCOs give some of their power and resources to the alliance, joint venture, or network. In return, they expect to gain benefits such as cheaper prices for equipment, access to innovations, or better reimbursement payments. HCOs use legal documents, bylaws, contracts, and other mechanisms to structure these new organizations and coordinate work among the member HCOs.

Recalling a trend reported in chapter 1, HCOs are implementing coordination methods to integrate clinical care throughout the continuum (Hegwer 2016). Care historically has been fragmented, but now managers are strengthening coordination because of payment changes that reward coordinated care. Managers and clinicians use standardized care plans that specify how care is to be coordinated with other members of the healthcare

TRY IT, APPLY IT

Your college or university is an organization with many units, such as departments, centers, offices, and so forth. Which parts have to coordinate with others? Which coordination methods are used? Think about how your college or university would use the coordination methods discussed in this chapter. Describe a situation in which hierarchical referral would be used to coordinate work. Then describe a situation in which mutual adjustment would be used. Try to do the same for rules, information systems, liaisons, full-time integrators, committees, relational coordination, boundary spanners, and contracts. Then discuss your ideas with other students.

team. Electronic medical records and other information technologies communicate information to staff to help them coordinate care. Liaisons and integrators—such as transition care specialists, practice facilitators, and service line managers—coordinate care across multiple departments, facilities, and locations. Interdisciplinary teams and other groups coordinate care among multiple departments and professions. Alliances and joint ventures connect HCOs with other organizations (both HCOs and non-HCOs) in their communities to coordinate care throughout the continuum. Managers use these methods to better coordinate transitions of care, in which a patient moves from one facility (e.g., primary care office) to another (e.g., hospital) and then another (e.g., rehabilitation center) and then home. Gaps in transition coordination were common in the past and resulted in higher costs and poorer health (Bosko and Gulotta 2016). Now managers use coordinating structures and processes described in this chapter to avoid gaps during transitions and thereby improve population health.

COMPLICATIONS

Managers can use the models and principles explained earlier in this chapter to organize HCOs. When doing so, they should consider two complications that occur in some HCOs.

CONTRACT DEPARTMENTS

Do you remember learning in chapter 4 about contract workers who fill positions in HCOs? In some cases, these contract workers are not limited to just a few temps from a nursing agency. An even more interesting—and potentially complicated—situation is when an HCO contracts with an outside company to operate an entire department, such as food service or housekeeping. This type of contracting is similar to the network outsourcing approach except that the external company puts its own employee in the HCO's department manager position (e.g., food service manager). In some arrangements, the outside company installs its own workers in other positions (e.g., dietitian, lead cook). People in these positions work inside the HCO with HCO workers but work for (and are paid by) the outside company. Here, too, the unity of command can be violated. The HCO's top managers must decide how much authority to delegate to the food service manager if the position is held by an outside person who is not on the HCO payroll. Coordination with other parts of the HCO may be awkward if other employees question the food service manager's loyalties. These arrangements work fine in many HCOs, but they can cause problems and confusion if not organized well. **Top managers must devote care and attention to formally stating how the contract workers (and department) fit in the organization structure.**

PHYSICIANS AND THE ORGANIZED MEDICAL STAFF IN A HOSPITAL

As we learned in chapter 4, medical positions and physicians can complicate how managers organize HCOs. In this chapter, we study another aspect of physicians in HCOs: the organized medical staff of a hospital. Although hospitals are not all alike, the following discussion offers a general explanation of the medical staff structure. However, keep in mind that because of external forces, hospitals are trying new approaches to integrate the medical staff with their management hierarchy. The separation of the clinical structure and administrative structure has been disappearing. There is much variety, and if you've seen one hospital organization chart . . . you've seen one hospital organization chart.

A hospital has a bureaucratic structure designed by managers using the organizing principles explained in this chapter. It also has a medical staff structure comprising physicians (and, if hospital bylaws allow, dentists and other clinical professionals). Together, these structures are sometimes referred to as a *dual structure*. The medical staff is organized into departments and divisions for medical specialties (e.g., oncology) and subspecialties (e.g., dermatologic oncology). The hospital board of directors delegates to the medical staff the authority and responsibility for medical care in the hospital. The board of directors also dictates that physicians and the medical staff must comply with hospital bylaws, policies, and standards. These are generally based on laws, regulations, accreditation requirements, national or state guidelines, professional norms, and other external criteria. Physicians design their medical staff structure and expect some degree of autonomy.

The organized medical staff is essential to fulfill the hospital's goals and mission. Yet, the medical staff structure may or may not be shown in detail on a hospital organization chart. The structure might be depicted by a medical staff box connected to a board of director's box or a CEO box at the top. In a large academic medical center, the medical staff often consists of the medical school faculty organized as a separate entity that contracts with the hospital—shown on the main organization chart as a box connected to the top of the administrative structure. Sometimes the two structures are separate and appear this way on the organization chart. In other hospitals, the two structures are partly or almost completely blended together into one structure. For example, physicians and the medical staff hierarchy and committees may be shown reporting to a VP of medical affairs, who reports to the hospital CEO. Another approach is to appoint both a physician (as a clinical comanager) and a nonphysician (as an administrative comanager) for each medical department or service line (e.g., neurology, cardiology, pediatrics). Many structural variations exist.

In recent years, the trend has been to combine the clinical and management structures more tightly for better interaction and accountability. This combination enables physicians and hospitals to improve patient care, strengthen finances, manage population health, and adapt to the external environment and demands of stakeholders. The medical staff and the management team appoint liaisons to each other's committees, councils, and departments to help coordinate their work. The chief of the medical staff and a few other physicians may serve on the board of directors. Administrative representatives attend meetings of the medical staff and its departments and committees. In the administrative structure, some departments or service lines have a nonphysician administrative manager and a physician as codirectors (in a dyad model). A hospital might assign codirectors to specific problems that involve both medicine and administration, such as patient safety or patient care quality. Disagreements are inevitable, so leaders of the medical staff and management team (sometimes with the board of directors) must be ready to resolve conflicts. These two structures—the traditional organization hierarchy and the medical staff hierarchy—coexist and together form the total hospital organization.

Within the medical staff are physicians with different relationships to the hospital, as mentioned in chapter 4. Some physicians are based in the hospital, such as radiologists, emergency physicians, and hospitalists. Others are based in the community in their physician office practices. They all must obtain hospital privileges to perform medical work in the hospital. Some physicians work in the hospital's administrative structure—such as a VP of medical affairs—and are employed and paid by the hospital.

Confused? If so, you are not alone. Even experienced hospital managers sometimes feel a bit confused, because there are

- different types of hospitals,

- different types of jobs and positions filled by physicians in hospitals,

- different types of relationships between hospitals and physicians, and

- both administrative and medical staff structures that are interrelated in varying ways.

To make things even more interesting, these relationships are continually evolving to adapt to the trends and developments in healthcare discussed in chapter 1.

This discussion of physicians and the medical staff in an HCO has revealed several general points. First, physicians may fit into a hospital organization structure in a variety of ways. Managers should not assume all physician–hospital relationships are alike. They must examine and understand each one individually.

Second, physicians have authority and responsibility for medical care, whereas managers have authority and responsibility for administrative matters. However, the boundary between medicine and administration is blurred, which creates conflicts between managers and physicians. Hospital patient care employees may be directed by both physicians and managers, so unity of command can be violated.

Third, hospitals have an administrative hierarchy (shown in the hospital organization chart) and a medical staff hierarchy (not always shown in the hospital organization chart). These hierarchies have been merging in recent years. Several organization structures are used to coordinate the medical staff and administration, including medical–management committees, physician–administrator dyads, appointment of managers to medical staff committees, and liaisons between the medical staff and administration. Medical staff representation on the hospital board of directors is an organization structure that provides direct input from the medical staff to the board for policies that affect the practice of medicine.

Also recall from chapter 4 that physicians have power and influence based on their medical expertise, which confers high status and affects their relationships with others. Managers, of course, have their own expertise—management—and the authority of their positions. Yet, they should be careful about when and how they assert their managerial authority while working with physicians, who expect autonomy based on professional expertise. Ongoing collegial discussion can resolve problems, though managers must sometimes assert authority—for example, to obtain physicians' compliance with accreditation standards and licensure requirements.

ONE MORE TIME

Managers must decide how to organize and coordinate work to accomplish goals and adapt to the external environment. Thus, organizing is closely tied to planning. Lower-level managers organize tasks into positions and departments; higher-level managers organize departments into an entire organization. They decide which departments to group with others for close interaction, and they arrange coordination of departments throughout the organization. Because it is an open system, the organization must be linked to other organizations and people in its environment. Managers use hierarchy, span of control, delegation of authority, centralization, line and staff positions, and departmentalization to create the whole organization.

Managers organize HCOs to generally follow one of five structures:

1. *Functional structure* organizes departments and positions according to the functions workers perform and the abilities they use.
2. *Divisional structure* organizes departments and positions to focus on particular groups of customers or services.
3. *Matrix structure* organizes work by combining functional and divisional forms; it uses vertical and horizontal authority to manage workers.
4. *Horizontal structure* organizes work into core processes that are performed by workers in self-managed teams.
5. *Network structure* organizes work by outsourcing much of it to a network of other organizations connected by interpersonal relationships, contracts, and information systems.

Each of these five structural forms has pros and cons. Managers often combine elements of more than one organization form to create a mixed hybrid structure. Thus, much variation exists as HCOs organize based on their unique combination of environment, mission, goals, size, work, technology, and culture.

HCO managers coordinate departments vertically, horizontally, diagonally, and with external organizations using various structures and processes. These include hierarchical referral; mutual adjustment; rules, plans, and protocols; information systems; liaison roles; full-time integrators; task forces, teams, committees, councils, and other groups; relational coordination; boundary spanners; and contracts and other agreements. Most HCOs have a governing body (or board) at the top of the organization structure to act on behalf of the owners and take ultimate responsibility for the organization. Contract departments in HCOs and the medical staff structure in hospitals complicate how these organizations are managed.

(T) FOR YOUR TOOLBOX

- Functional structure
- Divisional structure
- Matrix structure

- Horizontal structure
- Network structure
- Coordination structures and processes

FOR DISCUSSION

1. Discuss the pros and cons of the functional structure versus the divisional structure.

2. Explain the matrix structure. What are its pros and cons?

3. Discuss what you believe are the most important responsibilities of a governing board.

4. Describe at least four ways managers can coordinate work among departments within an HCO.

5. Some HCOs do not design their organization structure using just one of the five structures discussed in this chapter. Instead, they begin with one structure and then modify it—sometimes creating a unique organization structure. Why might that be a good idea?

6. In a hospital, how does the medical staff complicate the traditional management organization hierarchy? What challenges does the medical staff create for administrative managers?

CASE STUDY QUESTIONS

These questions refer to the Integrative Case Studies at the back of this book.

1. "I Can't Do It All!" case: Based on the information in this case, draw a functional organization chart for Healthdyne. Assume Healthdyne grows and Mr. Brice wants to reorganize Healthdyne with a West Region and an East Region. Draw a new organization chart for Healthdyne.

2. Managing the Patient Experience case: Explain how various coordination methods from this chapter could be used to coordinate patient experience work at Academic Medical Center.

3. The Rocky Road to Patient Satisfaction at Leonard-Griggs case: Based on the information in this case, draw an organization chart for Leonard-Griggs. Use one of the five organization structures presented in chapter 5, or a variation of one. Explain the rationale for your chart.

RIVERBEND ORTHOPEDICS MINI CASE STUDY

Riverbend Orthopedics is a busy group practice with expanded services for orthopedic care. It has seven physicians and a podiatrist, plus about 70 other employees. At its big, new clinic building, Riverbend provides extensive orthopedic care. Several technicians provide diagnostic medical imaging, from basic X-rays to magnetic resonance images. The physicians perform surgery in their own outpatient surgery center with Riverbend's own operating nurses and technicians. Therapy is provided by three physical therapists and one part-time contracted occupational therapist. In addition to staff providing actual patient care, the clinic has staff for financial management, medical records, human resources, information systems/technology, building maintenance, and other administrative matters. Occasional marketing work is done by an advertising company. Legal work is outsourced to a law firm. Riverbend is managed by a new president, Ms. Garcia. She and Riverbend have set a goal of achieving "Excellent" ratings for patient experience from at least 90 percent of Riverbend's patients this year.

During a conversation at lunch, Dr. Chen tells you he thinks more coordination is needed to reach the patient experience goal. He asks you about tools and methods to consider for improving coordination at Riverbend Orthopedics.

Mini Case Study Questions

1. Using information from the case and chapter, draw an organization chart for Riverbend Orthopedics. Explain your organization structure. You may make reasonable assumptions and inferences.

2. What would you tell Dr. Chen for improving coordination?

REFERENCES

Bosko, T., and B. Gulotta. 2016. "Improving Care Across the Continuum." *Journal of Healthcare Management* 61 (2): 90–93.

Buell, J. M. 2016. "Clinical Integration: The Future Is Here." *Healthcare Executive* 31 (1): 10–16.

Cummings, T. G., and C. G. Worley. 2015. *Organization Development and Change*, 10th ed. Stamford, CT: Cengage Learning.

Daft, R. L. 2016. *Organization Theory and Design,* 12th ed. Mason, OH: South-Western Cengage.

Dunn, R. T. 2016. *Dunn and Haimann's Healthcare Management*, 10th ed. Chicago: Health Administration Press.

Greater Rochester Independent Practice Association. 2017. "About Greater Rochester Independent Practice Association." Accessed November 26. www.gripa.org/About/Our-Story.

Hegwer, L. R. 2016. "5 Ways to Support Clinical Integration." *Healthcare Executive* 31 (1): 18–25.

Mintzberg, H. 1983. *Structure in Fives: Designing Effective Organizations.* Englewood Cliffs, NJ: Prentice-Hall.

Van Dyke, M. 2016. "Leading in an Era of Value: 3 Key Strategies for Success." *Healthcare Executive* 31 (6): 20–28.

Walston, S. L. 2017. *Organizational Behavior and Leadership in Healthcare: Leadership Perspectives and Management Applications*. Chicago: Health Administration Press.

White, K. R., and J. R. Griffith. 2019. *The Well-Managed Healthcare Organization*, 9th ed. Chicago: Health Administration Press.

CHAPTER 6

ORGANIZING: GROUPS AND TEAMS

Coming together is a beginning. Keeping together is progress. Working together is success.

Henry Ford, founder of the Ford Motor Company
and inventor of the factory assembly line

LEARNING OBJECTIVES

Studying this chapter will help you to

➤ describe characteristics of groups and teams,

➤ state the purposes of groups and teams,

➤ explain structural characteristics that affect the performance of groups and teams,

➤ explain process characteristics that affect the performance of groups and teams,

➤ recognize helpful and harmful roles played by members of groups and teams,

➤ understand how to make groups and teams effective, and

➤ comprehend how to make group meetings effective.

HERE'S WHAT HAPPENED

Partners HealthCare had established goals to improve population health and adapt to changing payment incentives. To accomplish these goals, managers organized teams, committees, and other groups of workers. For example, Partners had a strategy implementation group and transition teams. When organizing them, managers had to make important decisions about the group and teams to ensure their success. For example, for the strategy group, key decisions probably included the purpose of the group, whom to assign to the group, how much authority it should have, and to whom it would be accountable. Managers, or the group members themselves, had to decide who should chair (lead) the group, how often it should meet, with whom it would communicate, and how it would make its decisions. Managers had to orient new members to their committee roles. Potential conflict among group members (e.g., because of differences in professional viewpoints) could have deterred them from working together. Partners HealthCare's managers—and the strategy implementation group's members—had to use group structures and processes to enable the group to perform well. The group was then able to achieve its purpose and help Partners achieve its organization goals. The same was true for the transition teams.

This chapter, the third about organizing, helps us understand why and how healthcare organizations (HCOs) organize people into groups such as teams, committees, huddles, task forces, and councils. As we learned in chapters 4 and 5, organizing groups is a form of coordination that HCOs use to achieve goals. We saw that Partners HealthCare used these types of groups. It would be hard to imagine how even a small HCO—much less a large, complex one—could succeed without organized groups, teams, committees, and similar organization structures. Although they often are not shown on organization charts, these structures are essential to contemporary organizations—including HCOs. What are some teams, committees, and task forces you have heard of in HCOs?

Managers at all levels of an HCO must create and participate in groups and teams. Top managers must support groups and promote teamwork throughout accountable care organizations, medical practices, health insurance companies, pharmaceutical firms, assisted living centers, mental health clinics, community health alliances, and other HCOs. Managers at lower levels must do the same within their own departments and work sections. When you are a new manager, consider volunteering for teams and committees to become more widely known in your HCO. Working with employees outside your department or work unit will give you opportunities to grow professionally, learn more about your HCO, and develop rewarding work relationships with others. This chapter will improve your teamwork skills, which are important for healthcare management jobs.

You may have belonged to some clubs, teams, groups, and committees that were effective and fun and some that were not. Why do group experiences vary? Good groups and teams are not automatically good; they are good because managers created them properly. How can managers do that? In this chapter we learn how, beginning with basic ideas about groups and teams and their purposes. Next, we study how managers create group structures and processes that strongly affect a group's success or failure. We also examine roles group members perform that may help or harm the group. All these things matter for a group, whether it is a board of directors, a children's health task force, or an air ambulance team. In this chapter, you will acquire more tools to use when managing HCOs.

This chapter focuses on formal groups and teams—the ones that appear in organizations' official written documents and are created by top managers. We know from chapter 4 that there is also an informal organization, which includes informal groups that managers do not create. Although this chapter explains what managers can do to create and manage their organization's formal groups, most of these concepts and methods also apply to informal groups.

GROUPS AND TEAMS

A **group** is "two or more people who interact with each other and share a common purpose" (Johnson and Rossow 2019, 100). A **team** is a special kind of group whose members share a common goal and accountability for outcomes and coordinate tasks, skills, and resources interdependently (Griffin, Phillips, and Gully 2017, 254). Teams tend to be smaller than groups. HCOs often have interprofessional teams with members from multiple departments and professions. A **committee** is a formal group with an official purpose and official relationships with other parts of the organization (Dunn 2016, 357). These terms are not precisely defined and sometimes are used interchangeably when it is not important to distinguish among them (Griffin, Phillips, and Gully 2017). This book uses that approach.

Additional characteristics of groups include the following (Dunn 2016; Griffin, Phillips, and Gully 2017; Johnson and Rossow 2019):

- ◆ Some have line authority to make decisions; others only make recommendations.

- ◆ They vary in how much they are self-directed and able to manage themselves.

- ◆ Some exist within a single functional department of an organization, yet many have members from multiple functional departments (i.e., are cross-functional), multiple disciplines (i.e., are interdisciplinary), or multiple organizations (i.e., are interorganizational).

- ◆ They exist at all levels of hierarchy, from the board of directors on down.

- ◆ They may be permanent (standing) for ongoing work, or they may be temporary (ad hoc) for specific, one-time work.

group
Two or more people who interact with each other and share a common purpose.

team
A special kind of group whose members share a common goal and accountability for outcomes and coordinate tasks, skills, and resources interdependently.

committee
A formal group with an official purpose and official relationships with other parts of the organization.

♦   Some exist in a building with members interacting in person, while others (virtual groups) exist in cyberspace with members interacting electronically.

Why do HCOs have groups and teams? Groups can help HCOs do the following (Dunn 2016; Griffin, Phillips, and Gully 2017; Johnson and Rossow 2019):

♦   Combine and coordinate work that is fragmented because of division of work and specialized expertise

♦   Enable workers to grow, try new roles, and develop professionally

♦   Expand workers' knowledge of their HCO beyond their own departments

♦   Enable workers to share and exchange skills, knowledge, and organization learning

♦   Build commitment (through participation) to solutions, changes, and new plans

♦   Obtain input, representation, and support of stakeholders, interest groups, and constituents

♦   Improve problem solving and decision making by bringing in diverse and necessary input, points of view, experience, and expertise

♦   Strengthen working relationships and camaraderie among employees

Teams are likely to become more common in HCOs because they can help integrate clinical care and coordinate projects. Another reason is the number of workers entering the workforce who like to work in teams and may ask about it in job interviews (Schawbel 2016).

In addition to advantages, groups and teams also pose certain disadvantages (McConnell 2018). Starting a team and preparing it to work effectively can require many organization resources. Group meetings take time and might require workers to be in a conference room rather than caring for patients or doing other essential work. Some teams have too many meetings that last too long. Group decision making is slower than individual decision making. As a result, groups may become stagnant and bureaucratic and thereby impede needed change. A committee might even be known as "the graveyard" if proposals are sent there and never heard of again.

GROUPS AND TEAMS IN HEALTHCARE ORGANIZATIONS

HCOs have many types of groups, teams, committees, councils, and task forces. The following examples illustrate this variety: Population Health Coordination Council, Diversity in Healthcare Group, Board of Directors Planning Committee, Telehealth Installation

Team, Interdisciplinary Practice Committee, Data Analytics Task Force, Cross-Functional Readmissions Committee, Patient Experience Subcommittee, and Virtual Care Team.

Although groups and teams form in most types of organizations, they seem to be especially common in HCOs. Why? Healthcare is multidisciplinary, involving disciplines such as nursing, pharmacy, occupational therapy, social work, medicine, dietetics, and dozens of others. Many disciplines have specialties. For example, nurses specialize in pediatric nursing, emergency nursing, psychiatric nursing, and so forth. C-suite managers specialize in finance, marketing, diversity, operations, patient experience, ethics, and more. In addition, healthcare work is often performed on weekdays and weekends, sometimes in two or three shifts per day and in different locations. Teams overcome this division by coordinating and integrating their work (as discussed in chapters 2 and 5). **Managers create groups to coordinate work among many different professions, disciplines, departments, shifts, and locations.** For example, Christiana Care Health System in Delaware has an interdisciplinary team that includes a medical director, nurse care coordinators, pharmacists, social workers, and support staff to improve population health (Buell 2018).

As noted earlier—and worth repeating—groups and teams are not automatically good. They become good partly because of what managers do. Managers first create the *structures* of a group. Then managers and team members create the *processes* of that group. This chapter explains how. The structures and processes described in the following sections strongly affect a group's performance and effectiveness.

STRUCTURES OF GROUPS AND TEAMS

When you form a group, think carefully about these seven structural characteristics: purpose, size, membership, relation to organization structure, authority, leader, and culture. The characteristics are interrelated and affect group performance. Choose them wisely so your group can succeed. These seven characteristics are explained in the following sections (Albritton and Fried 2015; Dunn 2016; Fried, Topping, and Edmondson 2012; Griffin, Phillips, and Gully 2017).

PURPOSE

Each group must have a clear purpose, which is sometimes called its *charge* or *mandate*. This charge will guide the group in many ways, such as determining who should be in the group, how often it will meet, which resources it will need, and whether it is temporary or ongoing. When group members have a clear purpose, they can focus rather than drift aimlessly or shift from one direction to another. With a purpose as a target, a group can also measure progress more easily. A group's purpose is usually stated (at least in rough-draft form) when people first decide the group is needed. The written statement of purpose usually comes from the manager who formally creates the group and holds it accountable for achieving its purpose.

Managers should devote careful thought and effort to writing the group's statement of purpose. That effort will pay off later by giving clear guidance to the group and its members. The group should periodically update its purpose, if needed, to reflect changing situations.

SIZE

The size of a group strongly influences how well it performs. In this chapter's opening Here's What Happened, for example, managers at Partners HealthCare had to decide how big the strategy implementation group should be to achieve its goals. Pop quiz: What size is best? If you said, "It depends," you are correct! Bonus question: What does it depend on?

Managers should consider several factors when they determine the size of a group, team, or committee. They must weigh the advantages and disadvantages of a big group against those of a small group. The best size depends on the group's purpose. For example, the purpose might require certain departments, stakeholders, or others to be represented and able to participate. If the group's purpose is to coordinate the work of seven departments, then the group should include at least seven people, one to represent each department. The group must be big enough to include members with the needed expertise, such as data analytics or e-health. If the group's purpose is to advise and make recommendations to others who will then make a decision, a larger number of members will bring a wider range of views and information. To build support for a strategic plan, a large planning group allows more people to participate so that they will be more likely to support the final plan. When a great deal of work must be accomplished, a large group can allocate tasks among more members.

Although big groups offer advantages, they also have disadvantages. Because they have more members than small groups, big groups require more time and effort for all members to become comfortable working with each other. Even then, big groups are hard to manage because there is less cohesion and cooperation among members. Smaller splinter groups and informal groups often emerge within large groups. If this happens, it may signal a need to subdivide a large group into several smaller subgroups, each focused on a part of the full group's purpose. More time and effort are also needed for large groups to meet, discuss issues, gather input, resolve differences, and reach decisions. Costs rapidly increase in big groups because the salary meter continues to run during meetings and costs for food, supplies, and other resources increase. In large groups, communication and interaction become more formal and controlled and require more administrative support.

These disadvantages of large groups reveal the advantages of small groups. Exhibit 6.1 lists the advantages of big groups and small groups. According to Dunn (2016), four to nine members is a good size for a committee. Dye (2017) says there is no ideal size for a team, but a range of 6 to 11 members is generally appropriate. Jeff Bezos, founder and CEO of Amazon, believes a team should be small enough to feed with two pizzas (Choi 2016)!

Advantages of Big Groups	Advantages of Small Groups
More opportunity to obtain diverse views, ideas, expertise, and input	Easier and faster to reach agreement
More people committed to the group's purpose and work	Less time needed for members to get acquainted and be comfortable with each other
More stakeholders who feel they have a say and are represented	More group cohesiveness and cooperation; time for all members to speak
Tasks and work spread among more people	Less formality, fewer administrative tasks, easier to manage
Better for solving complex problems	Less costly

EXHIBIT 6.1
Group Sizes and Advantages

Sources: Dunn (2016); Fried, Topping, and Edmondson (2012); Griffin, Phillips, and Gully (2017).

MEMBERSHIP

The membership (composition) of a group strongly affects the group's performance. Partners HealthCare had to think carefully about the composition of its strategy implementation group and its transition teams. Managers might choose (or recommend) the members of a committee, team, or council. Alternatively, people in a department, division, or other part of an HCO might choose someone to represent them in a group. For example, the social services department might choose its employee, Olivia, to represent the department on the consumer engagement team. Those who choose or elect members to serve in groups should consider these questions:

◆ Who can provide the pertinent knowledge, skills, and attitudes this team needs?

◆ Who works well with people in groups (or could after training and coaching)?

◆ Who has sufficient time for the team while still doing her regular job?

◆ Who could add diversity to a committee?

◆ Who might grow professionally from group membership?

◆ Who can represent certain stakeholders, constituents, and groups on this committee?

◆ Who is needed for this team to comply with applicable requirements, laws, and standards?

◆ Who can perform helpful task and maintenance roles and avoid harmful personal roles?

Exhibit 6.2 shows three types of roles that group and team members may perform (in much the same way people perform roles in a movie or school play). When group members perform *task roles*, they *help* their group achieve its tasks and purpose. When they perform *maintenance roles*, they *help* group members maintain good feelings about the group and about working with group members. In contrast, when group members perform *personal roles*, they try to fulfill personal needs in ways that may *harm* the group. Which of these roles have you seen group members perform? Task and maintenance roles increase members' satisfaction with the group and increase group effectiveness; personal roles do not. When managers pick people to serve in groups, they should consider not only people's technical skills but also the roles people could contribute to the group. (As a new manager who wants to succeed, be sure you perform task and maintenance roles but not personal roles.)

Managers should also consider the diversity of team membership. Diverse members can bring diverse ideas, viewpoints, attitudes, and values that can lead to innovative solutions to complex problems. When membership is diverse, members may become more aware of biases and limited information that block thinking (Johnson and Rossow 2019). Diversity can help open people's perspectives to enable better problem solving and decision making.

Although group membership diversity has advantages, it also has disadvantages. Diverse members will have varied attitudes, beliefs, and preferences regarding authority, hierarchy, communication, decision making, and other aspects of group interaction and behavior (Griffin, Phillips, and Gully 2017). This, along with diversity of team members' ages, education levels, statuses, and cultures, may impede (at least initially) group trust, communication, participation, cohesiveness, and decision making. Thus, a manager who appoints a committee of diverse members should provide sufficient time, training, and activities to strengthen members' trust in one another and to encourage interaction and communication. (A later section of this chapter, and chapters 7, 8, and 15, all offer ideas for how to do this.) A related factor is group membership duration. Membership should be long enough to allow group members the time and interaction needed to develop trust and cohesiveness (Johnson and Rossow 2019). Then the group can realize the benefits of diverse membership.

RELATION TO ORGANIZATION STRUCTURE

Another structural feature of a group is the way it relates to the HCO's overall organization structure and hierarchy. This relationship affects how the team performs and how effective it can be. A committee that ties into the formal organization at a high level is perceived as more important and powerful than a committee that is accountable to a lower level of the

Exhibit 6.2
Roles of Group
Members

Task roles help the group achieve its tasks and purpose.

Role/Function	Actions and Behaviors
Leader	Leads the group by performing multiple task and maintenance roles
Initiator	Suggests new tasks, directions, problems, solutions, procedures
Information seeker	Requests relevant facts, opinions, data
Information giver	Provides relevant facts, opinions, data
Clarifier	Clarifies and explains terms, ideas, issues, opinions, data
Elaborator	Explains in depth, giving examples, details, interpretations, implications
Devil's advocate	Argues for alternative choices, raises contrary opinions, forces debate
Evaluator	Judges ideas, information, progress, results
Synthesizer	Combines and summarizes ideas
Agreement tester	States possible agreement, asks if members agree
Energizer	Stimulates members, urges progress
Orienter	Keeps discussion on track, redirects the group to stay on task
Recorder	Takes notes, prepares records

Maintenance roles help group members maintain good feelings about the group and about working with group members.

Role/Function	Actions and Behaviors
Encourager	Praises others, affirms others' contributions, recognizes others
Harmonizer	Smooths over conflict, reconciles disagreements, reduces stress, eases tension
Compromiser	Offers or accepts compromises, admits own mistakes, changes opinion to maintain cohesion
Facilitator	Invites participation of members, suggests procedures for discussions, keeps communication open for all
Observer	Monitors and comments on feelings of the group and how it functions
Follower	Accepts ideas, goes along with the group

Personal roles do not help the group; rather, they help members fulfill personal needs.

Role/Function	Actions and Behaviors
Aggressor	Attacks others, attacks the group, harshly disagrees
Blocker	Opposes the group's ideas, impedes progress, is overly negative
Dominator	Tries to dominate and control the group, asserts authority
Help seeker	Seeks help with personal problems, seeks sympathy and support
Recognition seeker	Calls attention to self, seeks praise and recognition
Special interest seeker	Speaks up for a different group's interests

Sources: Adapted from Daft (2016); Dunn (2016); Dye (2017); Fried, Rundall, and Topping (2000); Myers and Anderson (2008).

TRY IT, APPLY IT

When you read through the group roles in exhibit 6.2, did it bring to mind people you know? Do you know someone who is a natural initiator, clarifier, energizer, harmonizer, or observer? Perhaps you also know a blocker or dominator. To strengthen your understanding of roles in groups, try to think of someone you know who could perform each of the task and maintenance roles. Those are people to have in a group or on a team!

HCO. The high-level association will provide more political clout and resources, which could help the group succeed. After all, a group cannot perform well if it does not have sufficient resources and support from higher-level managers. Team members' main jobs also create links to different departments, divisions, and work units in the HCO's structure.

When a manager creates a committee, task force, or team, the manager must decide to whom it will be accountable. For Partners HealthCare, the top managers had to decide to whom the strategy implementation group would be accountable (perhaps the chief strategy officer) and to whom it would report its work (perhaps the senior management team).

AUTHORITY

When creating a task force, team, committee, or other group in an HCO, managers must decide what (if any) authority the group will have. Will a patient safety team have authority to *establish* a policy requiring nurses to repeat verbal orders from a physician (to ensure the orders were heard correctly)? Or will the committee only have authority to *recommend* that policy? Perhaps the committee will only have authority to *advise* nurses to repeat verbal orders. How about an HCO's employee picnic task force—how much authority will it have to spend funds? At a healthcare consulting firm, the summer picnic task force wanted unlimited authority, but the managing partner authorized it to spend only up to $2,000; a higher amount would need further approval. Authority might vary over time or because of other factors. For example, a new task force might initially have little authority but be given more authority after it becomes more proficient.

LEADER

The leader position—and the person who serves in that position—is yet another structural feature of a group. This position may be called the committee chair, group lead, task force director, team captain, or some other title.

Suppose the president of a medical group practice in Columbus creates an employee advisory council to inform managers about employees' concerns. Will the president appoint the council chair, or will the council members elect their own leader? For standing committees that continue for years, how long should someone serve as chair? What duties and authority will the leader have? The more clearly these details are stated at the beginning, the better the group can perform. Depending on a group's size and purpose, it might have more than one leader. For example, large formal committees and councils might have a chair, a vice chair, and a secretary. The responsibilities of each leader position should be clearly defined and shared with all group members.

Another consideration is who will serve in the formal leader position(s). Imagine a medical school's ethics council in Miami that has a chair position with designated responsibilities. Who should be the chair? Earlier, we learned about task roles, maintenance roles, and personal roles in groups. How well a group leader performs task and maintenance roles will strongly affect the group's success. Ideally, a group's formal leader position will be filled by someone with the right knowledge, skills, abilities, and role behaviors.

Besides the formal leader, a group may have an unofficial, informal leader (as we learned in chapter 4). A committee member with high energy who likes to socialize may become an informal leader. So, too, might a team member who has relevant expertise. Suppose a patient care council has 20 members, including 4 nurses. The nurses might sit together at council meetings, text each other between meetings, and let the most experienced nurse be their informal leader.

CULTURE

The final structural feature of a group, team, or committee is its culture—the values, attitudes, and norms (behaviors) that are considered proper and guide the group's members. A group might value risk-taking and thinking outside the box, or it might not. A committee should establish its expected behaviors, such as "no side conversations during meetings" and "make new members feel welcome." Culture may include sensitive issues such as trust, conflict, civility, and respect. A culture that supports collegial disagreement will enable people to safely express different points of view. The culture should fit the purpose of the group and should not strongly conflict with the HCO's overall culture. For example, if a strategic planning team is to brainstorm new ideas, its culture must not be rigid and stifling. Group members must believe it is OK to ask "stupid" questions and suggest "crazy" ideas. A group's culture will also affect how members feel about being part of the group and whether they continue to actively participate. If a committee's culture allows physicians to behave in an arrogant manner toward other members, then nonphysicians will not fully participate in the committee.

Managers and group members must decide what the culture of the group should be and then take steps to establish it. The group culture is likely to be based on the group's history, traditions, purpose, and situation, as well as on members' personalities (Griffin, Phillips, and Gully 2017). If a group establishes and embraces its culture, then those values and norms will strongly influence the group's effectiveness. More information about this is provided later in this chapter and in chapter 11 on culture in HCOs.

PROCESSES OF GROUPS AND TEAMS

Besides structure, groups and teams in HCOs must have processes to do their work. Structure only creates a committee; processes make the committee come to life with activity. Listen closely to a team and you will hear the hum of activity; with some teams, you might also hear shouting, cheering, arguing, and other sounds! When you are on a team or committee, think about five processes: developing, leading, communicating and interacting, decision making, and learning. Group leaders and members together create these processes, which all affect group performance. In addition, these processes may affect structure, such as by shaping the group's culture. The following sections explain the five group processes (Albritton and Fried 2015; Dunn 2016; Griffin, Phillips, and Gully 2017; McConnell 2018; Walston 2017).

DEVELOPING

As Henry Ford's quote at the beginning of this chapter implies, groups of workers go through stages. Before actually working together, they first come together and then progress toward staying together. Bruce Tuckman incorporated those ideas in a team development model that is still commonly used today (Tuckman 1965; Tuckman and Jensen 1977). The model provides a broad understanding of groups and suggests that groups go through five stages of development: forming, storming, norming, performing, and adjourning. Although it does not portray every group, the model does provide a useful guide for understanding how to manage and participate in groups. The five stages of the team development model involve the following (Dunn 2016; Griffin, Phillips, and Gully 2017; Johnson and Rossow 2019; McConnell 2018):

1. Forming Stage

   ◆ Members get acquainted, act polite, and try to figure out what is OK and not OK.

   ◆ Members learn the group's purpose, roles, and behaviors.

   ◆ Members reduce barriers with icebreakers (e.g., self-introductions, interviewing and then introducing other members, scavenger hunt, team-building exercises).

◆ The leader should set a positive tone and stimulate new thinking and motivation.

2. Storming Stage

   ◆ Members more openly express opinions and argue about the group's goals, methods, rules, and tasks; conflicts arise.

   ◆ Some members strive for control, creating conflict.

   ◆ The leader should demonstrate cooperation and teamwork and emphasize team purpose.

3. Norming Stage

   ◆ Members figure out how to work together and agree on rules; expected norms (behaviors); a code of conduct; and methods for decision making and cooperating and communicating with each other.

   ◆ Cooperation increases, conflict decreases, members socialize, and the group feels more cohesive.

   ◆ The leader should emphasize the group's goals and purpose.

4. Performing Stage

   ◆ Members have figured out how to work together and now focus on achieving the team's purpose and goals.

   ◆ Members plan how to accomplish goals, divide up work, and assign tasks.

   ◆ Members perform their tasks, evaluate progress, and make adjustments as needed.

   ◆ The leader should guide progress toward goals and motivate members.

5. Adjourning Stage

   ◆ After the group finishes its goals and purpose, members celebrate what they achieved.

   ◆ If members worked well together, they may mourn the end of their team, feel sadness about not meeting again, and express farewells.

   ◆ The leader should help members reach closure.

Think about teams or groups you have participated in. Are some aspects of this model familiar based on what those groups did? Managers use this model to understand group behavior, realizing that some groups may not go through all five stages or develop in a linear way. For example, some housekeeping workers at a personal care home who already know each other could be appointed to a department task force to create a new work schedule. Because they know each other, they will not have to go through the forming stage. Members may quickly progress to the performing stage. Alternatively, if an ongoing community advisory board expands its purpose and increases its size from 7 to 15 members, it should back up and redo the earlier forming stage.

Many local, regional, national, and global HCOs, such as healthcare systems, nursing home chains, hospital management companies, and pharmaceutical firms, use virtual teams. Managers who lead or serve on virtual teams in cyberspace should be especially sensitive to how members progress through these stages of development. Some group members—particularly those who have not been in a virtual group before—may struggle with getting to know and becoming comfortable with each other if their technology does not allow them to see body language and facial expressions. Members may argue more about rules for communicating and norms for interacting. A section later in this chapter tells how to create effective virtual teams.

Some groups are very diverse with respect to members' demographics, experiences, cultures, and other characteristics. A new culturally diverse team might experience stereotyping, distrust, conflict, and communication problems. Here, too, extra time, effort, training, and support will likely be needed as the team moves through the stages of development (Griffin, Phillips, and Gully 2017). Managers should provide plenty of time and opportunity—formally and informally, planned and unplanned—for members to become acquainted professionally and personally (Dye 2017). Managers, groups, and teams often do not realize how much time and effort are needed in the forming stage to begin the team building that should continue through later stages.

LEADING

Leading greatly affects group performance. We learned earlier that small groups may have a single leader, such as team captain, committee chair, or task force director. Larger groups may have multiple leaders, including a chair, vice chair, and secretary. These *structural positions* are different from the *process behaviors and actions* that leaders actually use for leading. The leader should engage in task and maintenance roles, activities, and behaviors (listed in exhibit 6.2) to lead the group to achieve its purpose and lead members to maintain good feelings about the group. The leader should explain the group's purpose and goals, divide up the work, arrange assignments, resolve conflicts, and motivate everyone to help the group succeed. In addition to performing many task and maintenance roles, the leader should interact effectively with each member. This may involve more indirect leadership (e.g., facilitating discussions and resolving conflicts) and less direct leadership (e.g., giving orders).

Sometimes the leader may let one or more team members lead (Albritton and Fried 2015). For example, the formal leader may let a member with specific expertise (e.g., social media savvy) lead the group when it must handle a specific matter (e.g., a social media problem). This approach strengthens the group by actively involving more members, using their expertise, and enabling them to develop leadership skills for the future. When leading a group, the formal leader must also identify informal leaders and work effectively with them. Chapters 9, 10, and 11 are about leading and offer useful advice about leading groups and teams.

COMMUNICATING AND INTERACTING

Because group members must communicate and interact with people both inside and outside their group, communication processes are important to the group's success. Ideally, all team members will easily communicate with each other in meetings, one-to-one conversations, and other interactions. However, we know that does not always happen because of biases, communication preferences, personal relationships, differences in age or status, and other factors. If members are not comfortable interacting with each other, then communication can become limited, as shown in exhibit 6.3. In other groups, some members may communicate with one or two other members but not the whole group; this also restricts communication.

Leaders must help their group communicate and interact well so that group members—and the group itself—can be effective. Too little interaction or communication

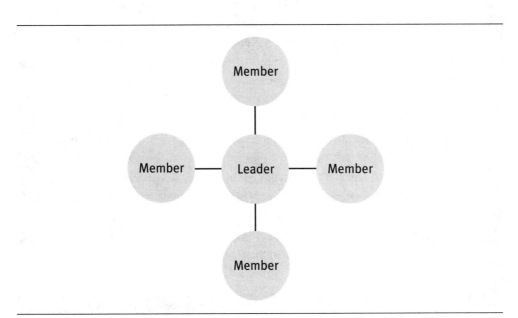

EXHIBIT 6.3
Limited Communication Among Group Members

among members will reduce trust, cohesiveness, and effectiveness. However, too much interaction or communication could overload group members and cause them to back away from the group.

Effective processes are also needed for the group to communicate and interact with people outside the group. For example, think of a group of hospital staff members who are planning how the hospital should adjust to value-based reimbursement. That group must communicate with other people, departments, and groups inside the hospital. In addition, the group will have to communicate and interact with people outside the hospital. Why? To obtain resources, information, and expertise from outsiders and to coordinate its work with other parts of the hospital and with other organizations.

Communication processes must be created by teams and their members. These processes can by enhanced by methods and technologies such as meetings, social media, huddles, conference calls, documents, e-mail, intranets, and blogs. The chair of a community health council in Richmond could use multiple processes to help members communicate

 USING CHAPTER 6 IN THE REAL WORLD

At Bellin Health Systems, based in Green Bay, Wisconsin, medical office patient care teams huddle for 5 to 10 minutes each day prior to seeing the first patient. The huddle includes providers and care team coordinators, as well as a patient access representative, nurse, and behavioral health consultant if available. A care team coordinator leads the huddle by quickly discussing plans for the day, scheduled patients and their needs, potential staffing issues, continuity of care, opportunities for extra patients, and availability of medical records from other facilities. These daily huddles help the team communicate and interact to improve team performance and enhance the patient experience (Bellin Health Systems 2014).

Cone Health and its accountable care organization, based in Greensboro, North Carolina, use multiple committees and teams to improve coordination of clinical care. An operating committee of physicians and managers oversees daily operations. Five subcommittees guide credentialing, contracting and finance, medical management, quality, and health information exchange. Teams focus on helping providers avoid readmissions, surgical-site infections, and other problems. The senior vice president for quality and patient safety at Cone Health believes that clinical integration is about connecting the people who can improve care throughout the continuum. Teams and committees help do that (Hegwer 2016).

and encourage them to interact. The task and maintenance roles (shown in exhibit 6.2) also can strengthen communication and interaction processes in groups. When members perform those roles (and avoid the harmful personal roles), they improve their group's communication and interaction. For example, throughout many HCOs, small teams briefly huddle each morning to enhance patient experience, safety, care, and service. In these quick (usually stand-up) huddles, employees discuss the schedule, safety concerns, patient convenience, and related topics. Problems are identified, addressed, and monitored in subsequent huddles. Successes may be quickly announced and celebrated. The Using Chapter 6 in the Real World sidebar gives examples of teams and committees improving communication, interaction, and coordination at two HCOs. Chapter 15 includes more information about effective communication.

DECISION MAKING

How are decisions made in groups you participate in? Do members vote? Does the leader try to build consensus for an idea that everyone generally agrees with? Or perhaps the leader obtains input from members and then makes the decision alone. Decision making in groups can range from autocratic decisions made by the group leader to democratic decisions made by all members. This subject is more fully addressed in chapter 13 on decision making. For now, remember that groups can use various processes to make decisions. A single committee may use different decision processes for different decisions because of different leadership, time urgency, members, and other factors. Each approach has pros and cons. Decision by consensus agreement strengthens group support of the decision. However, more time and discussion are needed to reach a consensus decision than to make a decision by majority vote (or by an autocratic leader). A consensus decision might not be possible for a radical, innovative decision that could be made by a committee chair deciding alone after consultative input from the group. Members must use decision-making processes that best fit the group given its goals, time, resources, and members' ability to make decisions. Group members can become better at making decisions through training, coaching, and experience.

Group members and leaders should watch for two possible problems when making decisions. The first occurs when responsibility for a group decision is spread among group members so that no single individual is accountable. This situation is reflected in the saying "When it is everybody's decision, it is nobody's decision." Knowing they will not be held individually responsible, members might take group decision making less seriously than individual decision making. Thus, group leaders must create and reinforce individual as well as group accountability for decisions, such as by calling on each person to individually state a choice.

Second, groups should strive to avoid **groupthink**. This is a process in which group members quickly agree without considering diverse ideas and thoughtful analysis; it is

groupthink
A process in which group members quickly agree without considering diverse ideas and thoughtful analysis, usually to maintain group harmony.

usually done to maintain group harmony. Groupthink can cause group members to avoid the different ideas, critical thinking, and discussion needed for effective problem solving and decisions (Dunn 2016). It occurs when leaders and group norms (developed in the norming stage) so strongly support group harmony that they block critical thinking and debate. Members think, "We must all get along," so they do not disagree with each other. Yet, some tactful disagreement is good for organizations to prevent quick, superficial, and ineffective decisions. Groups potentially can make better decisions than individuals because groups bring a wider range of information, experiences, perspectives, and insights to the decision. Groupthink can block these potential benefits, so group leaders should create team norms that support critical thinking and diverse ideas. They should encourage productive disagreement early in the decision-making process.

LEARNING

A final important group process is group learning (Fried, Topping, and Edmondson 2012). The team must learn as a team. That is not the same as individual learning by individual members. The group must reflect on its structure and processes to learn how it is doing as a group. Based on what it learns about itself, the group then can improve its structures and processes.

For example, suppose a safety-net primary care clinic in Chicago appoints a new fundraising committee to obtain $50,000 in donations. The group comprises 13 members, some of whom do not know the others. The group will have to develop itself, lead itself, communicate within and beyond itself, and make decisions. How well does the group perform all these duties? Kiera feels there is not enough communication between the leader and herself. Travis thinks the group's members have been blindly guessing how much local businesses will donate rather than carefully analyzing data. Colleen and Taylor feel the group is struggling and might not reach its goal. Group learning is needed. The group should openly discuss its processes and how it is doing. The leader, through discussion or confidential surveys, can ask group members for feedback about the group's processes and outcomes and seek suggestions for improvement. (The following Check It Out Online box describes a group self-assessment survey to help guide group learning.) To overcome weak processes, the group can engage in team-building exercises and training in group processes (e.g., communicating, decision making). The group can reaffirm its norms or, if necessary, return to the norming stage to develop new norms. It might have to change its structures, such as by reducing its size or strengthening leadership authority. People do not automatically work well as a group. They must learn how to work together as a group. **The group learning process enables a group to evaluate itself, learn about itself, and then adjust its structures and processes to improve group performance.**

EFFECTIVE GROUPS AND TEAMS

To create effective groups and teams, managers and groups can establish the structures and perform the processes discussed earlier in this chapter. When necessary, managers and group members can adjust team size, membership, culture, communication, and other structures and processes. These structures and processes that influence a group's effectiveness are mostly internal to the group.

Factors external to a group in an HCO also influence that group's effectiveness. These factors outside a group often are still inside the group's HCO. For example, suppose an HCO in Milwaukee provides outpatient lab tests, medical imaging, and cardiology tests. Within this business, an equipment committee decides which equipment to buy each year. The equipment committee will be influenced by factors outside the committee yet inside other parts of the HCO. The business's managers, financial situation, political relationships, workload, and competing priorities are in the HCO yet outside the committee and will affect the committee's performance. The group must monitor and understand these factors. Further, many factors outside the HCO in its external environment will also influence the group's effectiveness. Recall factors and trends in the environment described in chapter 1, such as customers' preferences, laws, competitors, and new scientific discoveries. Prior discussion of the communication and interaction process said groups interact with their environments to gather information and resources. That process should also include understanding and adjusting to forces and factors in the external environment that affect the group.

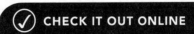

CHECK IT OUT ONLINE

If you are part of a team or group, consider taking an online assessment of your group. The MindTools website offers a Team Effectiveness Assessment with 15 questions (www.mindtools.com/pages/article/newTMM_84.htm). After answering the questions, you can click the Calculate My Total button to learn the results. Then check the brief guide that explains how to interpret your results to better understand how your team functions and performs. Team members can use this assessment to guide team learning and improvement. Check it out online and see what you discover.

Some HCOs employ consultants to improve effectiveness of groups and teams. For example, to support the developing and learning processes, managers may use consultants for training, coaching, and mentoring to ensure team members have the skills needed to work in groups. Many employees have excellent knowledge and technical skills for their jobs but lack skills for group decision making, communicating, and interpersonal relations. By providing time, funds, and other resources for this, managers demonstrate commitment to the group's success. Going further, Cummings and Worley (2015) explain that organization development (OD) consultants help businesses create effective groups such as self-managed work teams. In these teams, each member can perform most or all tasks performed by the team so each person can help anywhere. The team is designed to manage itself to complete a product or service or a major component of a larger production process;

it is the horizontal structure discussed in chapter 5. To shift to this type of organization design and team requires very extensive, ongoing change and redesign of work over months or even years. OD consultants use their expertise to create self-managed work teams by focusing on individual group members, on the group, and on how the group connects with other parts of its organization.

Effective Virtual Teams

Creating an effective virtual team is especially challenging because members usually are separated in time and space with less opportunity for communication and interaction. Depending on the technology, they might not be able to see or hear each other. Thus, the processes described earlier in this chapter are harder to perform. Group members may feel only weakly connected to the team. In addition to what has already been stated for effective teams in general, virtual teams should consider the following (Griffin, Phillips, and Gully 2017):

- ◆ Use appropriate technology for each kind of team task, such as assigning work, writing documents, maintaining files, and conducting meetings. Wikis, electronic whiteboards, collaborative document-editing tools, meeting management groupware, and project management software may be useful.

- ◆ Establish appropriate degrees of security, access, anonymity, and synchrony.

- ◆ Spend extra time and effort to create mutual understanding, trust, respect, and collaboration among members.

- ◆ Emphasize unifying team goals, purpose, values, and expectations.

- ◆ Involve experienced virtual team members in coaching members with less experience.

- ◆ When choosing team members, select people with the skills and attitudes that will enable them to succeed on a virtual team.

- ◆ Early in the life of the team, establish appropriate processes, procedures, rules, and even rituals to ensure proper virtual behavior by members.

Guidelines for Effective Meetings

What would groups (and HCOs) do without meetings? Because groups meet often (sometimes too often), managers should do their best to ensure that meetings are worthwhile. Employees gripe about meetings that are pointless, unproductive, and a waste of time. Managers who know how to make meetings worthwhile are rewarded with better results and happier employees. Managers should consider doing the following, using e-tools to simplify these activities when possible (Dunn 2016; Dye 2017; McConnell 2018):

◆ Before calling a meeting, ensure that a meeting is really needed.

◆ Plan the meeting and its agenda: what, why, who, where, when, and how.

◆ Send participants the agenda and necessary materials a few days early so they can prepare.

◆ Orient new group members before their first meeting.

◆ Arrange for someone to accurately record the minutes (and distribute them later).

◆ Respect people's time—begin on time, stay on time, and end on time.

◆ Set the tone and state ground rules and etiquette (e.g., listen, maintain confidentiality, avoid blaming, don't interrupt, don't have side conversations, be sure to participate, support each other, make decisions by consensus).

◆ State the purpose of the meeting.

◆ Lead the meeting, follow the agenda, and use time wisely to ensure all agenda items are covered.

◆ Respect everyone by leading a balanced discussion, seeking input from everyone, and performing appropriate task and maintenance roles.

◆ Don't use meeting time for matters that are better discussed by smaller subcommittees or in one-on-one conversations.

◆ Use time-outs, mediation, and separate conflict-resolution meetings if necessary.

◆ End on a positive note, summarize the meeting, review assignments, and thank participants.

◆ Follow through on decisions, assignments, and arrangements for the next meeting.

ONE MORE TIME

A group is two or more people who interact with each other and share a common purpose. A team is a special kind of group whose members share a common goal and accountability for outcomes, and coordinate tasks, skills, and resources interdependently. Managers use teams, committees, huddles, task forces, councils, and other groups to coordinate work, enable workers to grow, build commitment to changes and plans, obtain the input and support of stakeholders, and improve problem solving and decision making. At all levels of an HCO, managers must create, participate in, and support groups.

The success of teams, committees, and other groups requires appropriate group structures and processes. When forming a group, think carefully about seven structural characteristics (purpose, size, membership, relation to organization structure, authority, leader, culture) and five processes (developing, leading, communicating and interacting, decision making, and learning). Group development includes five stages—forming, storming, norming, performing, and adjourning. When group members perform task roles, they help their group achieve its tasks and purpose. When they perform maintenance roles, they help group members maintain good feelings about the group and about working with each other. Managers should nurture these roles in groups and discourage members from performing harmful personal roles to fulfill their own personal needs. Group members should periodically evaluate their group to identify and resolve possible problems. Virtual teams may need additional considerations, such as cyber ground rules and support for members new to virtual groups and meetings. Groups often have meetings, and leaders and members should follow tips for effective meetings to increase each meeting's value and outcomes.

(T) FOR YOUR TOOLBOX

- Group structures (purpose, size, membership, relation to organization structure, authority, leader, culture)
- Group processes (developing, leading, communicating and interacting, decision making, learning)
- Roles of group members (task, maintenance, personal)
- Team development model (forming, storming, norming, performing, and adjourning)
- Guidelines for effective meetings

For Discussion

1. Why are teams, committees, and other groups needed in HCOs?

2. Discuss structural factors that affect the performance of groups and teams.

3. Discuss process factors that affect the performance of groups and teams.

4. Name a group you belonged to that was fun and effective. Which structure characteristics and process characteristics do you think made the group fun and effective?

5. Looking at exhibit 6.2, consider all the task and maintenance roles used in groups. Which of those roles would come easily to you? Which roles would you like to develop in the future?

6. Which of the guidelines for effective meetings discussed in this chapter would come easily to you? Which would you like to further develop for your career?

Case Study Questions

These questions refer to the Integrative Case Studies at the back of this book.

1. Disparities in Care at Southern Regional Health System case: Suppose Mr. Hank wants to appoint a healthcare disparities committee to advise him on how to reduce healthcare disparities. Decide and describe, in as much detail as possible, what you think each of the seven structural characteristics should be for this committee. For example, write the committee's statement of purpose. Determine its size. Make up job titles to list members of the committee. Decide what authority the committee should have. Decide and describe the other structures.

2. Managing the Patient Experience case: Decide and describe, in as much detail as possible, what you think each of the seven structural characteristics should be for Mr. Jackson's multidisciplinary working group. For example, write the group's statement of purpose. Determine its size. Make up job titles to list members of the working group. Decide what authority the group should have. Decide and describe the other structures.

3. Rocky Road to Patient Satisfaction at Leonard-Griggs case: Suppose the executive director decides to create a team to plan and implement the survey. How could Ms. Ratcliff use the team development model with this new team? Describe problems that might arise during the team development process.

RIVERBEND ORTHOPEDICS MINI CASE STUDY

Riverbend Orthopedics is a busy group practice with expanded services for orthopedic care. It has seven physicians and a podiatrist, plus about 70 other employees. At its big, new clinic building, Riverbend provides extensive orthopedic care. Several technicians provide diagnostic medical imaging, from basic X-rays to magnetic resonance images. The physicians perform surgery in their own outpatient surgery center with Riverbend's own operating nurses and technicians. Therapy is provided by three physical therapists and one part-time contracted occupational therapist. In addition to staff providing actual patient care, the clinic has staff for financial management, medical records, human resources, information systems/technology, building maintenance, and other administrative matters. Occasional marketing work is done by an advertising company. Legal work is outsourced to a law firm. Riverbend is managed by a new president, Ms. Garcia. She and Riverbend have set a goal of achieving "Excellent" ratings for patient experience from at least 90 percent of Riverbend's patients this year.

Ms. Garcia has been cautious about forming groups, teams, and committees because she previously worked in an HCO that wasted much time with meetings that were not worthwhile. Yet she realizes that some groups are useful.

MINI CASE STUDY QUESTIONS

1. Using information from this chapter and other sources, describe groups, teams, and committees that Ms. Garcia might want to create at Riverbend Orthopedics. What would be the specific purpose of each group?

2. Explain to Ms. Garcia what could be done to ensure group meetings are worthwhile.

REFERENCES

Albritton, J., and B. J. Fried. 2015. "Human Resources Management: Practices for Quality and Patient Safety." In *Human Resources in Healthcare*, 4th ed., edited by B. J. Fried and M. D. Fottler, 503–35. Chicago: Health Administration Press.

Bellin Health Systems. 2014. "Bellin Health Huddles." Published September 1. www.steps forward.org/Static/images/modules/21/downloadable/Huddles.pdf.

Buell, J. M. 2018. "The Health Continuum: Leveraging IT to Optimize Care." *Healthcare Executive* 33 (1): 10–18.

Choi, J. 2016. "The Science Behind Why Small Teams Work More Productively: Jeff Bezos' 2 Pizza Rule." Buffer. Updated March 22. https://blog.bufferapp.com/small-teams-why-startups-often-win-against-google-and-facebook-the-science-behind-why-smaller-teams-get-more-done.

Cummings, T. G., and C. G. Worley. 2015. *Organization Development and Change*, 10th ed. Stamford, CT: Cengage Learning.

Daft, R. L. 2016. *Organization Theory and Design*, 12th ed. Mason, OH: South-Western Cengage.

Dunn, R. 2016. *Dunn and Haimann's Healthcare Management*, 10th ed. Chicago: Health Administration Press.

Dye, C. F. 2017. *Leadership in Healthcare,* 3rd ed. Chicago: Health Administration Press.

Fried, B. J., T. G. Rundall, and S. Topping. 2000. "Groups and Teams in Health Services Organizations." In *Health Care Management: Organization Design and Behavior*, 4th ed., edited by S. M. Shortell and A. D. Kaluzny, 154–90. Clifton Park, NY: Thomson Delmar Learning.

Fried, B. J., S. Topping, and A. C. Edmondson. 2012. "Teams and Team Effectiveness in Health Services Organizations." In *Shortell and Kaluzny's Health Care Management: Organization Design and Behavior,* 6th ed., edited by L. R. Burns, E. H. Bradley, and B. J. Weiner, 121–62. Clifton Park, NY: Delmar Cengage Learning.

Griffin, R. W., J. M. Phillips, and S. M. Gully. 2017. *Organizational Behavior: Managing People and Organizations*, 12th ed. Boston: Cengage Learning.

Hegwer, L. R. 2016. "5 Ways to Support Clinical Integration." *Healthcare Executive* 31 (1): 18–25.

Johnson, J. A., and C. C. Rossow (eds.). 2019. *Health Organizations: Theory, Behavior, and Development*, 2nd ed. Burlington, MA: Jones & Bartlett Learning.

McConnell, C. R. 2018. *Umiker's Management Skills for the New Health Care Supervisor*, 7th ed. Burlington, MA: Jones & Bartlett Learning.

Myers, S. A., and C. M. Anderson. 2008. *The Fundamentals of Small Group Communication.* Thousand Oaks, CA: Sage Publications.

Schawbel, D. 2016. "10 Workplace Trends You'll See in 2017." Published November 1. www. forbes.com/sites/danschawbel/2016/11/01/workplace-trends-2017/.

Tuckman, B. W. 1965. "Developmental Sequence in Small Groups." *Psychological Bulletin* 63 (6): 384–99.

Tuckman, B. W., and M. A. C. Jensen. 1977. "Stages of Small Group Development Revisited." *Group and Organizational Studies* 2: 419–27.

Walston, S. L. 2017. *Organizational Behavior and Leadership in Healthcare: Leadership Perspectives and Management Applications.* Chicago: Health Administration Press.

CHAPTER 7

STAFFING: OBTAINING EMPLOYEES

Our employees are our greatest asset.

Business slogan

HERE'S WHAT HAPPENED

Partners HealthCare revised its mission and developed ambitious goals to improve the quality and cost-effectiveness of patient care. More specifically, managers intended to use technology to improve four priority health conditions: diabetes, heart attack, stroke, and colorectal cancer. To achieve their goals, managers had to staff the organization. They planned which jobs were required (e.g., telemonitoring nurse) and how many positions were needed for each. They organized and designed jobs by identifying the tasks, responsibilities, authority, and qualifications required for each job. For example, the telemonitoring nurse job was responsible for monitoring remote patients' vital signs via telehealth technology, responding when the telehealth system signaled that vitals were abnormal, and guiding patients through biweekly heart education. Managers had to recruit applicants for the positions and evaluate the applicants using selection criteria. Careful selection of telemonitoring nurses was needed because some nurses prefer working with patients by standing at the bedside rather than by sitting at a monitor. After managers decided whom to hire for each position, they prepared job offers with compensation, starting dates, and other essential information. By performing the staffing function, managers progressed toward their goals for patient care.

staffing
Obtaining and retaining people to fill jobs and do work.

A s we see in the opening Here's What Happened, healthcare organization (HCO) managers must obtain people to do the work to achieve the HCO's mission and goals. This is part of the staffing function—the third of the five fundamental management functions we learned in chapter 2. We can think of **staffing** as the process of obtaining and retaining people to fill jobs and do the work. Previous chapters on planning (the first management function) and organizing (the second management function) referred to workers, employees, jobs, positions, and staff. Building on that discussion, this chapter and chapter 8 teach us how managers staff their organizations. Staffing requires managers to perform several of the management roles we studied in chapter 2: monitor, entrepreneur, disturbance handler, resource allocator, and negotiator.

As we learned in chapter 4, healthcare is often a service, and services are performed by people (rather than manufactured by machines). Most HCOs are labor intensive and depend on many people to perform the services. These people may be called staff, workers, employees, associates, personnel, human resources, workforce, or talent. Even though we might be impressed by the amazing medical equipment used in many HCOs, we must remember that people (human resources) are needed to operate the equipment (physical resources). Further, some medical work and much nonmedical work (e.g., management itself) does not involve fancy gadgets and equipment. **Healthcare is a service provided by people, so managers must excel at staffing.**

Many organizations, including HCOs, proclaim, "Employees are our greatest asset." How can managers *obtain* their "greatest asset"? How can managers then *retain* their "greatest asset" to avoid the time, expense, effort, and lost revenue of replacing workers (and avoid receiving negative comments on employer review websites such as Glassdoor)? Chapters 7 and 8 answer these questions. First, we identify seven staffing processes that HCOs use. Then we examine three special concerns for staffing HCOs. After considering this background, we study in more depth the seven staffing processes. The first three are explained in this chapter and focus on *obtaining* workers. The other four staffing processes are explored in the next chapter and focus on *retaining* workers. When you become a manager, you will soon become involved in staffing. Chapters 7 and 8 will help you prepare for that work.

The staffing of some HCOs includes physician jobs. As we learned in chapters 4 and 5, physician jobs may be quite different from other types of jobs. People who perform physician jobs might—or might not—be employed by the HCO where they work. If they are employed, they are usually obtained and retained differently than other employees are and in ways that are beyond the scope of this book. Thus, chapters 7 and 8 will focus on nonphysician staffing.

STAFFING PROCESSES

The management staffing function can be divided into seven processes that managers should perform. These processes are shown in exhibit 7.1 and entail the following (Fottler 2015b; French 2007; Fried and Gates 2015; McConnell 2018; Noe et al. 2016):

1. **Planning for staff**—forecasting the staff (workforce) the organization will require in the future and planning how to effectively obtain and retain that future staff

2. **Designing jobs and work**—determining the work tasks to be done by a job, along with the job's qualifications, supervision, working conditions, rules, and schedules

3. **Hiring staff**—recruiting and selecting people for jobs, which may include reassigning existing workers by promotion or transfer

4. **Developing staff**—helping employees acquire new knowledge, skills, attitudes, behaviors, and competencies for current and future jobs

5. **Appraising performance**—evaluating workers' job performance and discussing those evaluations with them

planning for staff
Forecasting the staff (workforce) the organization will require in the future and planning how to effectively obtain and retain that future staff.

designing jobs and work
Determining work tasks to be done by a job, along with the job's qualifications, supervision, working conditions, rules, and schedules.

hiring staff
Recruiting and selecting people for jobs, which may include reassigning existing workers by promotion or transfer.

developing staff
Helping employees acquire new knowledge, skills, attitudes, behaviors, and competencies for current and future jobs.

appraising performance
Evaluating workers' job performance and discussing those evaluations with them.

EXHIBIT 7.1
Seven Staffing
Processes

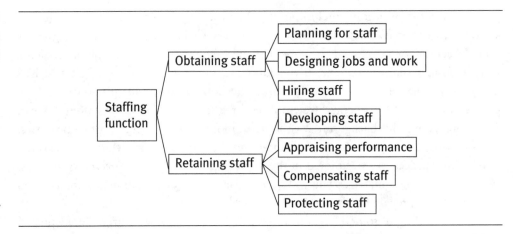

compensating staff
Determining and
giving wages, salaries,
incentives, and
benefits to workers.

protecting staff
Ensuring that workers
have proper and safe
work conditions, their
rights are protected,
and their opinions
are considered by
managers.

diversity
The range of human
differences that include
the primary (internal)
dimension such as
age, gender, race,
ethnicity, physical and
mental ability, and
sexual orientation
and the secondary
(external) dimension
such as thought styles,
religion, nationality,
socioeconomic status,
belief systems, military
experience, and
education.

6. **Compensating staff**—determining and giving wages, salaries, incentives, and benefits to workers

7. **Protecting staff**—ensuring that workers have proper and safe work conditions, their rights are protected, and their opinions are considered by managers

Which of these processes have you noticed in a summer job or part-time job during school?

As mentioned, this chapter studies the first three staffing processes, which get people in the door to start working. Chapter 8 explains the other four processes, which keep people working rather than walking out the door. **These seven staffing processes interact with and affect each other.** For example, designing a public health inspector's job may lead to developing current inspectors to perform new competencies, which then may lead to higher compensation for the inspectors. Also, all these processes can contribute to both obtaining and retaining staff. For example, hiring obtains staff, and if it is done well, the staff stay and are retained. Compensation must start high enough to hire people, and it must later increase to keep people.

Managers should ensure that all seven staffing processes are done well to help their HCOs survive and thrive. In doing so, they should keep in mind three special concerns: staff diversity and inclusion; centralized, decentralized, and outsourced staffing; and laws and regulations. These are explained in the following sections.

WORKFORCE DIVERSITY AND INCLUSION

Chapter 1 reported US demographic trends that indicate HCOs' labor supply and patient population will continue to become more diverse in multiple ways. "**Diversity** refers to the range of human differences that include the primary or internal dimension such as age, gender, race, ethnicity, physical and mental ability and sexual orientation; and the secondary or external dimension such as thought styles, religion, nationality, socio-economic status, belief systems, military experience and education" (Trustees of Boston College 2016). The primary, internal dimension may be referred to as *human diversity* and the secondary, external dimension as *cultural diversity* (Evans 2015). Together, these dimensions create differences among staff in many aspects of work, including status, communication, authority, teamwork, professional behaviors, and use of time.

A diverse workforce, including a diverse management team, can improve organization performance, population health, patient experience, community relationships, and other expectations of HCOs' stakeholders (who are also becoming more diverse). For example, many HCOs have been unable to hire enough nurses, pharmacists, and primary care physicians to fill job vacancies. However, HCOs that are open to a diverse workforce—and are perceived favorably by diverse workers—have a larger supply of labor from which to hire. Having positions filled (rather than vacant) enables better clinical performance, customer satisfaction, and patient experience. Also, patients may prefer providers and caregivers of their own ethnicity who understand how that ethnic group experiences disease and feels about medical care. These and other cultural factors affect patients, patient care, clinical outcomes, and community population health. A diverse workforce can help an HCO successfully compete in diverse communities, reduce disparities in patient care, and thereby achieve financial benefits (Evans 2015). A diverse workforce brings a wider range of ideas and innovations for managers and decision makers to consider. However, if diversity is not valued in an organization, it may create conflict, avoidance of coworkers, less teamwork, biased or constrained decisions, illegal actions, and other negative outcomes. Thus, managers must lead and manage their HCOs to value diversity and use it to strengthen the organization.

Hiring a diverse workforce is not enough; HCOs also must ensure inclusion of its workforce and staff. "**Inclusion** involves the active, intentional, and ongoing engagement of our diversity, where each person is valued, respected and supported for his or her distinctive skills, experiences and perspectives, to create a working and learning environment where everyone has an opportunity to experience personal fulfillment and participate fully" (Trustees of Boston College 2016). Many HCOs can do more to eliminate disparities, improve diversity, and be more inclusive. How can they do this? By applying management tools, methods, processes, and ideas from this book. For example, during strategic planning (chapter 3), an HCO can include diversity and inclusion in its mission, vision, values, and goals. When organizing its jobs, departments, and structure (chapters 4–6), the HCO can assign diversity and inclusion responsibilities to specific jobs and departments and then provide sufficient resources for them. When staffing the organization, an HCO can recruit a chief diversity officer, hire a diverse workforce, provide training to develop cultural competence for working with diverse populations, and appraise and reward employees based on how well they support diversity and practice inclusion. Later chapters in this book will provide more ideas to help you and your HCO reduce disparities,

inclusion
The active, intentional, and ongoing engagement of diversity, where each person is valued, respected, and supported for his or her distinctive skills, experiences, and perspectives, to create a working and learning environment where everyone has an opportunity to experience personal fulfillment and participate fully.

CHECK IT OUT ONLINE

The American Hospital Association, Institute for Diversity in Health Management, and National Center for Healthcare Leadership recently developed an assessment tool that HCO managers can use to ensure their organizations reflect the communities they serve (Institute for Diversity and Health Equity 2018):

A Diversity, Equity and Cultural Competency Assessment Tool for Leaders helps health care organizations assess their progress to create high-quality, inclusive, equitable and safe care environments aimed at eliminating health and health care disparities to improve the health and well-being of our neighbors and communities. *A Diversity, Equity and Cultural Competency Assessment Tool for Leaders* includes four sections:

- **Assessment Checklist:** A tool that hospital and health care leaders can use as a starting point in evaluating the equity, diversity, inclusion and cultural competency of their organization and identifying what activities and practices are in place or need to be implemented.
- **Action Steps:** A suggested "to do" list for how to use this tool to raise awareness within your organization.
- **Case Studies:** Examples of hospitals and health systems that are implementing leading practices. You will find a description of their activities, as well as information for the key contact within each organization so you can learn more.
- **Bibliography:** Resources to help you and others in your organization learn more about diversity and cultural competency.

The assessment tool is available at the Institute for Diversity and Health Equity website (www.diversityconnection.org/diversityconnection/membership/Resource%20Center%20Docs/Assessment%20Tool%20v4(20-page%20bklt).pdf). Check it out online and see what you discover.

increase diversity, and be more inclusive. By doing so, you will better serve your populations, employees, and stakeholders.

The Check It Out Online sidebar describes a useful resource for HCOs striving to become more diverse, inclusive, and culturally competent. The Using Chapter 7 in the Real World sidebar provides examples of how two HCOs have improved their workforce diversity.

In the United States, aging of the workforce, delayed retirements, and changing demographics have led to increased workforce diversity based on age and generation. An HCO may have workers born in five generations: traditionalists, baby boomers, Generation Xers, millennials (Generation Y), and the newly emerging Generation Z (Wagner 2017). The nonphysician workforce at Baptist Health Lexington in Kentucky consists of 29 percent baby boomers, 47 percent Generation Xers, 22 percent millennials, and 2 percent from the other two categories (Wagner 2017). Having five generations of workers is unusual and expands age diversity in the workforce. The workforce can also be diverse in terms of employment status, such as full-time, part-time, contract, per diem, freelance, and other kinds of "gig worker" status.

The generations have important differences (and similarities) in their attitudes and expectations about work. Managers staffing an HCO must understand, respect, and adapt to these differences. One size will not fit all generations with regard to an HCO's compensation plan, work schedules, company loyalty, performance reviews, career opportunities, and other staffing-related elements. Managers should first understand the differences (and similarities) among the generations of employees and then develop staffing processes for a wide variety of workers (Fottler 2015b).

USING CHAPTER 7 IN THE REAL WORLD

University Hospitals Health System (UH) is based in Cleveland and serves northeastern Ohio. To increase the diversity of its workforce, UH has partnered with community organizations that help train local people of diverse backgrounds for both healthcare and nonhealthcare jobs. By supporting these local partners, UH helps develop a diverse, local labor pool from which it can hire diverse workers. UH's governing board members are from diverse backgrounds, and the board monitors diversity and inclusion data (Hegwer 2016).

Henry Ford Health System in the Detroit metropolitan area actively develops its diversity, believing that doing so gives it a competitive advantage. System leaders provide diversity training, host book clubs, and use immersion strategies to engage and educate the HCO's workers. Each business unit has a diversity committee to handle diversity issues locally. Seven distinct resource groups support African-American leaders, LGBT (lesbian, gay, bisexual, and transgender) staff, women, millennials, Arab Americans, caregivers, and Latinos. Annual events and ceremonies celebrate diversity heroes and champions. Diverse teams provide a variety of perspectives that enable innovation. These and other diversity initiatives strengthen the organization (Hegwer 2016).

Centralized, Decentralized, and Outsourced Staffing

Top managers must decide if staffing will be done internally by the HCO's employees or outsourced to external consultants and companies. When the work is done internally, top managers must decide which portion of that work will be done by centralized human resources (HR) specialists and which will be done by decentralized line managers throughout the organization. In HCOs large enough to have HR specialists, these employees perform some staffing-related tasks and provide advice, tools, systems, and procedures to line managers that enable them to perform staffing work for their areas of responsibility. Some organizations decentralize much of the staffing work to department managers and do not have a traditional HR department (Fottler 2015b).

Let's consider a small HCO, such as a new home care business in Riverside. Initially, it might have only an owner-manager, a few nurses, and a clerical assistant. The owner-manager will likely do the staffing work, perhaps with help from an external consultant. When the business grows, the owner-manager might hire specialized HR employees to assist with staffing. When the HCO becomes even larger with more employees and staffing requirements, it might create an HR department with internal specialists for hiring, development, compensation, and other staffing processes. The home care business might use external consultants for some staffing work, such as comprehensive job analysis, recruitment of hard-to-find employees, and design of compensation plans. By this time, the HCO will have a management team with lower-level managers who make staffing decisions in their areas of responsibility, such as nursing, physical therapy, occupational therapy, and durable equipment. Eventually, the home care HCO might be acquired by a large health system or corporation with an advanced HR department or service center to support staffing of smaller acquired HCOs. Alternatively, some businesses have downsized their HR departments and shifted more staffing work to operating departments and outside staffing companies (Fottler 2015b). In each HCO, top managers have to decide which staffing work will be done at the centralized corporate level, which will be decentralized to lower levels throughout the entire organization, and which will be outsourced.

Line managers in a vertical hierarchy are usually responsible for staffing in their department or work unit (e.g., hospice). To do this, they are often supported by the HR department and specialists. A centralized HR department creates staffing programs, policies, and procedures for all managers to use with their employees throughout an HCO. For example, HR specialists may prepare an onboarding program for all new employees, create a social media approach to recruiting new staff, and design a performance evaluation rubric for appraising employees.

An HR department supports other departments with information systems, mobile apps, and other technology for staffing. The HR staff can manage databases for many aspects of staffing and thousands of applicants, employees, and former employees. This database management can help line managers identify approved positions, track applicants, measure diversity and inclusion, manage employees' benefits and compensation, identify which employees are due for performance appraisals, and track employee safety problems. Having centralized HR staff gives lower-level operating managers throughout an HCO the tools, methods, and systems they need for staffing their departments and work units. The centralized programs, policies, and procedures improve consistency and fairness throughout an HCO. However, line managers are ultimately responsible for staffing in their departments and work units.

Supervisors and managers can all benefit from working with HR staff and experts. Although managers should work closely with the expert HR staff, some do not. Why would managers turn down free, expert help? In HCOs, conflict sometimes arises between managers of departments (e.g., informatics, outpatient infusion, supply chain, community health education) and HR staff. Some managers might think the HR staff is bureaucratic and hinders the staffing process with too many forms and procedures. However, such forms and procedures can help HCOs avoid lawsuits, negative publicity on social media and job review sites, and difficulty recruiting workers in the future. Those forms and procedures also might prevent a manager from making a serious mistake that could reflect badly on the manager's performance.

LAWS AND REGULATIONS

Staffing is greatly influenced (actually, controlled) by laws, court decisions, and regulations at the national, state, and local levels of government. Laws and regulations affect how managers recruit staff, interview applicants, compensate employees, promote or discharge employees, and perform most aspects of staffing. For example, if you have had a job, you probably know that laws require workplace safety and forbid discrimination in hiring. In addition to these types of laws, state governments regulate and require licensure for many healthcare jobs. Exhibit 7.2 identifies important laws that affect staffing in HCOs (Dunn 2016).

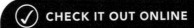

CHECK IT OUT ONLINE

The US Department of Labor has a practical online resource for employment laws (www.dol.gov/elaws/). It explains many laws and regulations affecting small businesses and workers. The guide is especially useful to people who need hands-on information on topics such as wages, benefits, safety, health, and nondiscrimination. This valuable resource can help you learn more about staffing laws now and during your career. Check it out online and see what you discover.

Labor law is complex, and it changes. Local, state, and federal governments may pass new laws and regulations, weaken or strengthen enforcement of existing laws, or revoke laws. Court decisions also cause changes in labor laws and regulations.

Managers and supervisors should educate themselves about legal aspects of staffing via training and online resources (see the Check It Out Online sidebar). HCO managers often consult HR specialists and labor attorneys; some large HCOs hire their own labor attorneys. **In addition to acting legally, fairly, and consistently, managers and supervisors should also carefully document all staffing processes, decisions, and actions.** Job applicants and employees might file lawsuits if they feel they were unfairly denied a job, promotion, pay raise, or even a preferred work schedule. The saying "If it isn't documented, it didn't happen" means managers must document their staffing actions in case a legal challenge arises.

PLANNING FOR STAFF

Now we begin studying in depth the seven staffing processes identified earlier in this chapter. The first is planning for staff. In chapter 3, we learned that during strategic planning, HCOs create a mission and goals along with implementation plans to achieve them. "A

EXHIBIT 7.2
Staffing Legislation

Legislation	Concern or Content	Administrative or Enforcement Agency
Fair Labor Standards Act of 1938	Minimum wage, overtime pay, and record keeping	US Department of Labor
Fair Employment Act of 1941	Prohibits discrimination[‡]	Committee on Fair Employment Practices
Equal Pay Act of 1963	Compensation relative to the sex of a worker	Equal Employment Opportunity Commission
Title VII of the Civil Rights Act of 1964[†]	Sex, color, race, religion, and national origin	Equal Employment Opportunity Commission
Age Discrimination in Employment Act of 1967 (amended 1978)	Age (protection for those 40 to 70 years old)	Equal Employment Opportunity Commission
Occupational Safety and Health Act of 1970	Workplace safety	Occupational Safety and Health Administration
Rehabilitation Act of 1973	People with disabilities	US Department of Labor
Employee Retirement Income Security Act of 1974	Pension and healthcare plan rules	US Department of Labor
Immigration Reform and Control Act of 1986	Employment eligibility verification	US Department of Labor
Employee Polygraph Protection Act of 1988	Prohibits use of polygraphs by most private employers	Secretary of Labor
Americans with Disabilities Act of 1990	People with disabilities	Equal Employment Opportunity Commission
Family and Medical Leave Act of 1993	Permits unpaid leave for certain reasons	Employment Standards Administration
Health Insurance Portability and Accountability Act of 1996	Health insurance coverage	US Department of Labor
Nursing Relief for Disadvantaged Areas Act of 1999	Permits temporary employment of alien/foreign RNs	US Department of Labor

Source: Dunn (2016, 401).

[†]As amended by the Equal Employment Opportunity Act of 1972, the Pregnancy Discrimination Act of 1978, and in 1991 when a cap on punitive damages was applied.

[‡]Applied to national defense industry.

critical need exists to elevate the discussion about workforce planning and development to ensure it becomes a standing, rather than crisis-driven, component of comprehensive strategic planning for hospitals and health systems" (McNally 2018). We will examine two broad activities managers use to plan for staffing:

1. Forecasting the organization's future required staff (workforce)

2. Planning how to obtain and retain the forecasted required staff (workforce)

To forecast the HCO's required staff (workforce), managers must forecast several factors based on input from supervisors, managers, and others:

◆ Expected turnover, retirements, resignations, and other departures, as well as promotions, transfers, and other transitions—all based on historical data, future plans, and good judgment

◆ Numbers and types of positions and workers—and their required qualifications and competencies—needed to achieve the organization's mission and goals for the coming years

To plan how to obtain and retain the required staff (workforce), managers must analyze internal and external factors, perhaps using a SWOT (strengths, weaknesses, opportunities, and threats) analysis that has been customized for staffing:

◆ The HCO's internal factors, strengths, and weaknesses pertaining to staff, such as funds to pay competitive wages, support for a diverse workforce, and working conditions that are attractive to Generation Z employees

◆ The HCO's external forces, threats, and opportunities pertaining to staff, such as changes in labor laws and regulations; changing availability of workers from four or five generations; customers' demands for empathetic staff; plans of nearby vocational schools; diversity of the local labor supply; and developments in artificial intelligence, robots, chatbots, and virtual assistants

Given these factors, managers can anticipate staffing needs and plan accordingly. How many retirees must be replaced next year, and in which positions? How many mental health counselors will be needed to staff the new primary care clinics? Given the nursing shortage in our area, should we contract with a nursing agency and freelance workers? Which changes in hiring could improve the diversity of our workforce? Which compensation and benefits would help retain millennials and Generation Z workers?

Which changes in staffing processes are needed to improve employees' engagement in their work and jobs?

As a result of the staff planning process, an HCO might determine it needs to hire three nurse practitioners, two data analysts, and one compliance officer, and eliminate two supply clerks. The HCO will probably change some staffing programs, policies, systems, methods, and tools so that it can obtain and retain the required workers. To accomplish this, the organization might plan the following types of changes to the other six staffing processes during the coming year:

◆ *Job designing.* Centralize the final approval of new job descriptions by the vice president of human resources.

◆ *Hiring.* Decentralize hiring decisions to department managers, and revise the policy for hiring military veterans.

◆ *Developing.* Develop workers' competencies for interacting with disabled clients.

◆ *Appraising.* Revise performance appraisal methods to require each employee to do a self-evaluation.

◆ *Compensating.* Revise the policy for using paid days off to better meet the needs of employees with young children.

◆ *Protecting.* Create a workforce diversity celebration to recognize and celebrate the diversity of the staff.

Staffing involves much work, especially in large businesses and HCOs. Performance management systems and other technology are available to help manage the hiring, developing, appraising, and other staffing activities for hundreds, thousands, or many more employees.

DESIGNING JOBS AND WORK

Recall from chapter 4 that the terms *job* and *position* are similar but not the same. "A *job* consists of a group of activities and duties that entail natural units of work that are similar and related" (Fottler 2015a, 143). Some jobs, such as president, are performed by just one person. Other jobs, such as nurse, are performed by more than one person if the amount of work is too much for one person. There are multiple nurse positions, and each is filled by a person who performs the nurse job. "A *position* consists of certain duties and responsibilities that are performed by only one employee" (Fottler 2015a, 144). Thus, five people may fill five nurse positions that all perform one nurse job.

Job Analysis

In chapter 4, we studied how work and jobs are designed as part of organizing work in an HCO. This task is also linked to staffing. Job and work design involves determining which tasks and activities must be done and how they should be organized into jobs, positions, teams, and work units. Workers in the healthcare industry perform hundreds of distinct jobs. For example, in the Here's What Happened at the beginning of this chapter, Partners HealthCare designed the telemonitoring nurse job to include monitoring patients' vital signs along with other tasks. Job analysis dissects jobs to identify the specific tasks, activities, and behaviors of each job and their relative frequencies.

Historically, job analysis assumed jobs were stable and constant. The analysis simply defined the tasks and activities of a job. Today, however, managers view jobs as more flexible and even adaptable to fit particular people and situations (Fottler 2015a; Noe et al. 2016). Many HCOs now use competency-based job analysis. A competency is a set of related knowledge, skills, and attitudes (e.g., interpersonal) associated with job performance (Fottler 2015a). Jobs also are being redesigned for team-based work and performance. HCOs have adopted these newer, flexible approaches to job analysis because internal and external factors (e.g., the trends described in chapter 1) cause continual change in HCOs. Because flexibility is needed, many job descriptions include the statement "Other duties as assigned."

Managers and HR staff analyze jobs using several methods, including observation, written surveys, and interviews. This information is used to create **job descriptions** (also called *position descriptions*). Although HCOs use different formats and content, all job descriptions state the job title and (in varying detail) the work to be done. Many job descriptions describe minimum qualifications, such as traits, education, skills, competencies, and licensures for the job. More detailed job descriptions may include authority, reporting relationships, equipment and materials used, working conditions, usual work schedule, mental and physical demands, interactions with others, and salary range (Dunn 2016; Fottler 2015a).

Line managers, including lower-level beginning supervisors, work closely with HR staff and top managers to do job analyses. Accuracy matters because job analyses guide other staffing processes used to obtain and retain staff. Managers use job analyses and job descriptions to

- plan how many of which types of jobs are needed,

- write announcements of specific job openings,

- decide which applicants could best perform various jobs,

- evaluate each employee's job performance,

- determine how to train and develop employees,

job description
A statement that indicates the job title and work to be done; often includes minimum qualifications and describes the job's authority, reporting relationships, equipment and materials used, working conditions, work schedule, mental and physical demands, interactions with others, and salary range. Also called *position description*.

◆   decide the pay for each job and worker,

◆   recognize potential dangers of some jobs, and

◆   perform the staffing processes in general.

Incorrect or sloppy job analysis can lead to bad hiring choices, employee lawsuits, poor organization performance, and an HCO's failure to achieve its goals. Think of the trends discussed in chapter 1 and recall that, for instance, HCOs are striving to improve population health, patients' engagement in their care, workforce diversity, patient safety, and mobile health. Adapting to such trends requires accurate job analyses.

WORK RULES AND SCHEDULES

Besides job descriptions (written from job analyses), designing jobs and work involves creating work rules, schedules, and standards of behavior. Managers are responsible for this, and sometimes workers participate in the process. Although people may feel that rules are confining, most employees desire the structure, predictability, and civility in their workplace that rules can provide. When creating rules, managers must balance the needs of the HCO with the needs of employees. For example, rules may limit socializing at work to ensure patient care is not delayed while employees discuss sports scores or weekend parties. Rules continually evolve to address issues, such as what employees may view online during work or tweet on Twitter after work. If two employees do not like each other, can one bully the other on Instagram? Managers may have to create work rules for such situations.

As a manager, you will have to create work schedules as part of job design. Scheduling can be challenging for any organization, especially for HCOs that operate 24/7. Is it Jose's turn to work weekends? Did Zainab work nights last month? Can Brittany work on New Year's Day? Managers must balance the needs of the HCO and patients with employees' schedules. Scheduling often permits some flexibility to let employees arrive (and depart) at different times. Some staff members may work five 8-hour days per week, whereas others may work four 10-hour days. HCOs may allow telecommuting and working from home or other remote sites. However, some organizations have reduced this option in favor of actual (not just virtual) human interaction among workers, which millennials and Generation Z may prefer (Schawbel 2017). Scheduling must consider full-time and part-time jobs and how they fit into a schedule. Contingent, temporary, gig, per diem, contract, and on-call workers may be assigned part of the schedule. Complications arise and must be addressed when an employee is on vacation or out sick. Managers should work closely with the HR department to ensure their department schedules adhere to labor laws and are consistent with the HCO's overall staffing policies.

Managers should remember that workers of different generations have varied preferences and expectations about their work schedule, work–life balance, family obligations, and control of their lives. The work schedule is a big factor in how employees feel about their job and employer.

Hiring Staff

After designing jobs and work, managers must obtain people to perform those jobs. For this task, HCO managers usually hire people as employees on the HCO's payroll. These employees may be full-time, part-time, on-call, per diem, permanent, temporary, seasonal, or some other status. Alternatively, some HCO managers contract with a healthcare staffing company (e.g., HealthCare Support), a temporary ("temp") staffing agency (e.g., Kelly Services), or some other outside business (e.g., Aramark) that assigns its own employees to the HCO, as we saw in chapter 5. In this chapter, we will focus on how an HCO's managers hire employees on the HCO's payroll, which is the most common approach to staffing HCOs. Even when putting people onto its payroll, the HCO might outsource some work to a recruiting company, a staffing search firm, or external consultant. Managers must continually decide how much staffing work to do internally and how much to outsource to specialists.

Hiring staff involves recruiting and selecting people for jobs, which may include reassigning existing workers by promotion or transfer. Some HCOs refer to this as *talent acquisition*. Perhaps you have been a job applicant and participated in this process. It includes

◆ recruiting applicants,

◆ selecting from among applicants,

◆ making a job offer, and

◆ sometimes reassigning a worker (e.g., promotion, transfer).

To begin recruitment, managers and HR staff should ensure that a current, accurate job description is available to guide recruitment and later selection. Then, upper management must authorize filling a vacant position (this authority may be delegated to HR staff). Vacant positions are not always filled right away, and a decision must be made about each vacancy. For example, if a decline in workload is expected, vacant positions may be frozen and not immediately filled. Later, when workload is forecasted to permanently increase, managers would probably approve hiring to fill those vacant positions.

Recruiting

HR staff (or contracted recruitment firms) perform most of the recruiting process. Larger HCOs with larger HR staffs may have one or more specialized recruiters. Smaller HCOs may handle recruiting or perhaps outsource this work to a recruiting company. Can you suggest ways to recruit people? How did you find out about jobs you have applied for? *Internal recruitment* seeks applicants from inside the HCO for promotion or transfer (Fried and Gates 2015). This approach uses the HCO's printed and electronic job boards and newsletters, networking among staff, and managers' conversations with current employees about open jobs.

Managers also use *external recruitment*, which seeks applicants from outside the HCO. This involves going to job fairs and professional conferences, networking beyond the HCO, and posting job openings on the HCO's website and job search websites. Additional methods for external recruitment include talking with representatives of schools and colleges, contacting former employees, using search firms and employment agencies, and placing ads in newspapers, professional newsletters, and trade magazines. Social media (e.g., Facebook, LinkedIn) and job websites (e.g., CareerBuilder, Glassdoor, Monster, TweetMy-Jobs, JobsInHealthcare, Health eCareers) are also useful and enable an HCO to "e-cruit" externally and easily reach many potential applicants. This approach creates a connection that goes beyond one-way methods. Many applicants respond well to recruiting via social media and mobile devices when these media and devices are optimized and designed for easy use. Such recruiting efforts may include virtual-reality previews of the job and organization that also are used at job fairs and professional conferences.

Managers will have to decide how extensively to recruit—internally, externally, or both? Locally, regionally, nationally, or globally? They must use appropriate recruitment processes and methods to obtain a strong applicant pool and achieve the HCO's diversity requirements and goals. According to Schawbel (2016), some businesses are trying to improve the recruiting and hiring experience because applicants who have had a bad experience share their stories on Glassdoor and other employer review websites.

What are the pros and cons of internal and external recruiting? Take a minute to jot down some ideas, and then read exhibit 7.3.

Managers and HR recruiters must prepare job announcements carefully when recruiting—especially for external applicants. The announcement should include a clear, realistic, and thorough description of the job and HCO so job seekers can properly decide whether or not to apply. Fried and Gates (2015) suggest giving potential applicants the following information:

◆ Required qualifications, such as education, experience, and preferences (that are legal)

◆ Job information, such as job title, department and company name, work to be done, work location and schedule, and compensation

◆ How to apply, such as whom to contact, what information to provide, and the deadline for applications

EXHIBIT **7.3**
Advantages and
Disadvantages
of Internal and
External Recruiting

Internal Recruiting

Advantages	Disadvantages
Applicant already familiar with HCO and thus more likely to fit in	Employee may apply for promotion and then be upset if not promoted
Applicant already known by the HCO	Employee may become boss of former coworkers, which can create problems
Employees see opportunities to grow, which strengthens employee morale and retention	Fewer new ideas, methods, innovations brought into the HCO from outside; inbreeding
Inexpensive	Small pool of potential applicants
Helps retain good employees	Creates a new vacancy
Fast	Employee may require extra coaching and mentoring to be fully prepared

External Recruiting

Advantages	Disadvantages
New ideas, methods, innovations brought into the HCO	Can be expensive for some methods
Large pool of potential applicants	HCO may be viewed as not supporting current employees, lowering morale
Applicant comes without awkward political relationships or problems with coworkers	Time and effort required to onboard and acculturate new employee
Can find applicants with all required competencies	Applicant not known by HCO, so more time and effort needed to select and hire
Creates awareness of the HCO	

Sources: Adapted from Fried and Gates (2015) and Noe et al. (2016).

This information may be provided in different ways, including online, in print, via multimedia, in person, in meetings, and in phone calls. Many companies offer this information in preapplication job previews for potential applicants before they apply. Doing so can save everyone time in the hiring process.

TRY IT, APPLY IT

Suppose you work at a small, suburban hospital near a big city such as Orlando, Detroit, or Las Vegas. The hospital's director of marketing will retire in six months, and a replacement must be hired. How could you recruit diverse applicants for this job? Use what you have learned in this chapter to outline a recruitment plan.

Here are several other ideas to keep in mind when recruiting:

◆   Offer incentives to applicants and to current employees who refer applicants.

◆   Focus the recruiting process on applicants and design the application process from their perspective; respect them by making it easy to apply for the job and by not contacting them at their current place of employment.

◆   While recruiting, subtly sell the HCO as a place to work by honestly identifying things an applicant might appreciate.

Managers should evaluate how effective their recruiting effort is. For example, they can measure the quantities and qualities of applicants overall (including specific types of diversity), for each job opening, and for internal and external recruiting. Recruitment time and cost per job opening also should be tracked.

SELECTING

Managers select the applicant to whom they will offer a job. A hiring decision has important short- and long-term consequences for the HCO, so managers should invest time and effort to make a wise selection. An unwise selection may lead to voluntary or forced turnover followed by repeating the costly, time-consuming hiring process. Other consequences may include tension and stress among coworkers, lost revenue, and delayed service for patients. The rest of this section describes a general approach to selection; many variations exist and depend on the organization's size.

The manager of the department with the job vacancy, plus the immediate supervisor for the vacant job, confer with HR staff. They must all agree on selection methods that comply with laws and the HCO's policies and that are appropriate for the particular staffing situation. Methods vary depending on the organization and the job. More time and assessment are needed to fill higher-level jobs. Some situations are more urgent than others. The immediate supervisor for the job must be involved in the selection, and commonly a team also participates (Fottler 2015b). This team might include future coworkers of the person to be hired, from both inside and outside the department. HR staff is responsible for ensuring compliance with laws, organization policies, and the job description (White and Griffith 2019).

Selection criteria help determine which applicant to hire. At first, a supervisor might say the person who can best perform the job should be hired. Someone else might suggest hiring a person who can perform the job well *and* is likely to stay with the organization for many years. Which criteria in the job description absolutely must be met (e.g., licensure)? Which criteria are important yet could be modified (e.g., two rather than three years of prior experience)?

The criteria almost always include fit. What is *fit*? Traditionally, organizations hired based on *applicant–job fit*, emphasizing how well someone could perform the job. Now managers also take into account *applicant–organization fit,* which considers an applicant's values, behaviors, attitudes, and overall work style (Fried and Gates 2015). For example, to what extent is an applicant competitive or cooperative? How well a new employee will fit into the organization and with other workers is more important now than it was in the past. Some companies hire applicants for fit and develop their skills afterward. However, research does not strongly show that better fit is related to better job performance (Fried and Gates 2015). Managers must also be careful that hiring for fit does not deter hiring for diversity or violate labor laws.

The rest of this section explains a general approach to selection that may be used with both internal applicants (for promotion or transfer) and external applicants (for new hires). This approach includes HR staff. If they are not available, then the manager and support staff would do the HR work. Of course, each company develops its own approach depending on the job to be filled.

After the HCO receives applications in response to its recruiting, HR screens them using preset criteria to select applications for further consideration. Pop quiz: What did we learn in the second staffing process that would provide useful standards for screening applications? Did you say *job descriptions*? These indicate basic qualifications, skills, and competencies applicants should have. Job descriptions can be used to eliminate unqualified applicants and identify qualified applicants for further consideration. HR staff or electronic scanners read each application (or resume) and compare it against criteria in the job description. Applicants who do not meet an essential requirement (e.g., having a nursing license) can be eliminated.

The hiring company and the applicant continue assessing each other. Many companies enable applicants to use electronic assessments, realistic job previews, and "tryouts" for the job (Fried and Gates 2015). These may be done online or in multimedia meetings with current employees. Applicants can learn more about the job and organization and what it would be like to actually work in that job and organization. The company presents the good and the bad about the job. Current employees may say what they like and dislike. Then applicants can better decide if they are still interested. They can answer their own questions: Would I fit well with that job in that HCO? Do I want to work there? Meanwhile, the hiring company further evaluates applicants by asking them legal job-related questions to more fully understand their skills, attitudes, behaviors, and fit with the job and the organization. After this interactive question-and-answer part of the job preview, the organization should have a better understanding of each applicant. Will this applicant fit well with our job and our HCO?

The hiring manager (or team) selects applicants who possess the required qualifications and seem to fit with the organization. In some cases, managers may choose someone who does not currently have all the required skills yet seems to fit the HCO well and could be trained to do the job tasks. This is the "hire for fit, train for skills" approach. In some cases, managers might give preference to internal candidates, which could strengthen overall employee retention in the HCO.

The HR staff may next arrange tests of applicants. One-third of organizations in the United States test for personality traits such as flexibility (Noe et al. 2016). A hiring manager might also test applicants to measure and learn about their knowledge, aptitude, skills, mental ability, and physical ability. Other tests may be used for drug screens, job-related medical problems, past criminal records, and fluency in English (Fried and Gates 2015). Managers should use tests that are valid, reliable, and not culturally biased.

Managers then interview candidates—perhaps three to five—selected from among the top candidates who also passed any necessary tests. The first interview may be done by telephone, teleconference, or videoconference, especially if the applicant lives far away. If that interview goes well, an on-site, face-to-face interview, which is more expensive and time-consuming, is arranged. Guidance from the HR staff is essential to help all interviewers understand how to conduct a fair, effective interview. For example, they must know which questions they may (and may not) ask during interviews. **Laws generally forbid questions about applicants' race, religion, age, country of origin, gender, marital status, family, health, disabilities, and personal lives.** The few exceptions (e.g., asking whether the applicant is legally old enough to work or legally eligible to work based on citizenship or work visa) must be narrowly and carefully worded (Fried and Gates 2015; McConnell 2018).

Interviews help the selection team understand applicants well enough to select someone. HCOs often hire based on applicants' traits (e.g., flexibility, initiative) rather than only technical skills (e.g., taking blood samples, writing code). Interviews, more than applications and resumes, enable managers to judge an applicant's fit. However, interviews are neither highly reliable nor highly valid (Fried and Gates 2015). Interviewers do not always ask all applicants the same questions in the same manner, which may lead to different responses. Interviewers also interpret applicants' answers and emotions differently. Some applicants look online to find and then rehearse recommended answers to common interview questions.

Managers in many HCOs use behavioral interviewing (also called *competency-based interviewing*) to predict how an applicant might fit in the organization and perform in a certain situation or role. This approach can help managers judge who has the required competencies. For example, during an interview, an HCO manager in Hattiesburg might say, "Conor, describe a situation in which you had to work on a team with people you did not know" or "Debbie, please tell me about a time when you helped a confused client." The manager judges the applicant based on the applicant's reported behavior in the job-related situations.

Effective interviews take much time and effort. The following tips can improve interviews and help managers make good choices (Dunn 2016; Fried and Gates 2015; McConnell 2018; Noe et al. 2016):

◆ Decide who (e.g., the manager, immediate supervisor, coworkers in the department) will participate in the interview and if they will meet with the applicant together or separately.

◆ Prepare by reviewing a current job description, the applicant's file, and other information.

◆ Contact applicants via their personal phone number or e-mail address; do not contact them at their current job.

◆ Give applicants sufficient advance notice to arrange time off from their current job and to prepare.

◆ Arrange a suitable time (without interruptions) and a comfortable place for everyone involved.

◆ Ensure the work site will leave a good impression on the applicant.

◆ Begin with brief chitchat to help the applicant relax.

◆ Ask questions that require more than a few words to answer.

◆ Ask questions that require answers that reflect how well the applicant *could* do the job (is capable), *would* do the job (is willing), and would fit in the job and organization.

◆ Ask situational questions for which the applicant must explain how she would handle a job-related situation.

◆ Avoid questions that are inappropriate, illegal, biased, or culturally insensitive.

◆ Allow time for the applicant to think before speaking, and wait for the applicant to answer.

◆ Listen closely for content and feeling; pay attention to the applicant's body language, voice, emotions, and responses.

◆ Be respectful, friendly, genuine, and professional toward the applicant.

◆ Gather information about the applicant's abilities, personality traits, and expectations.

◆ If an applicant gives only vague, safe, or socially acceptable answers, ask probing follow-up questions.

◆ Softly sell the job and the HCO, but do not overdo it or misrepresent anything.

◆ Be sure the applicant understands the job, expectations, schedule, pay and benefits, and what working at the HCO will be like.

◆ Ask for and fully answer the applicant's questions.

◆ Avoid taking many notes during the interview, but do write detailed notes soon afterward.

As a manager, you might interview applicants whose native language and culture differ from yours. You might participate in selection decisions that consider culturally diverse applicants. Such situations require careful communication, sensitivity, and emotional intelligence. The preceding guidelines can help ensure a fair, useful interview. Chapter 15, on professionalism, gives more advice on how to handle potential language and cultural barriers when interviewing and selecting people for jobs.

Promptly after each interview, the manager should gather feedback from everyone who interacted with (or even observed) the interviewee. Include HR staff, everyone who interviewed the applicant, and even a receptionist who observed how the applicant behaved while waiting outside the manager's office. These people should not let biases influence them. They should make thoughtful judgments based on evidence and avoid premature assumptions and safe political choices.

In most cases, the final selection decision is made by the immediate supervisor of the new employee (Dunn 2016; McConnell 2018). That person's decision should be based on extensive input from other selection team members, future coworkers, the direct supervisor's own boss, HR staff, and others who participated in the selection. Depending on the HCO's hiring process, a committee might make the final decision. Sometimes the choice is difficult; all candidates may have strengths and weaknesses and perhaps no candidate

---

→ TRY IT, APPLY IT

The recruitment plan you prepared for the Try It, Apply It earlier in this chapter was a huge success. Many applicants applied for the director of marketing job. Three diverse applicants have been chosen for in-depth interviews. Use what you learned in this chapter to plan how you will conduct the three interviews. Write an interview plan outlining (1) who will be involved, (2) where and when interviews will be held, (3) what will be done before and during interviews, and (4) seven questions to ask (and three questions not to ask). How would you make the interview convenient and appealing for the applicants?

---

stands out as the best. Some people might look qualified in an application but not perform well in a live interview. Managers should openly involve others in the selection process to obtain different perspectives.

If necessary, another interview can be arranged to further evaluate an applicant. Although a second interview requires more time, it can lead to better hiring decisions. Managers must strive to avoid poor decisions by being thorough. A bad choice will haunt the manager and hurt the HCO. Chapter 13 offers good advice on making decisions. As we will see, some managers use intuition in making decisions—including hiring decisions—and may rethink a preliminary decision if it does not feel right the next day.

At some point during the selection process, HR staff will perform reference checks to confirm information the application provided (e.g., college degree) and try to obtain new information (e.g., work ethic). The timing of reference checks varies depending on the situation. Confirmation of a college degree may be done early in the process by contacting the applicant's college. Talking to an applicant's current boss by phone may be done after obtaining the applicant's permission. If the applicant does not want her boss to know she is looking for a new job, this reference check might be done after the job offer has been made subject to satisfactory reference checks.

While it seems prudent to check references (and most managers do), this step is not a strong predictor of how well someone will perform in a new job (Fried and Gates 2015; Noe et al. 2016). Why is that? When asked to provide a list of references, applicants list people who will speak favorably. Also, references often are vague and rarely identify an applicant's weaknesses or past problems. In many businesses, HR policies do not allow much information to be shared about former employees (other than dates of employment and job title) for fear of being sued (McConnell 2018).

Because official references often are too vague or minimal to be useful, some hiring managers search online and look at social media to learn about applicants. Managers might do this during the initial screening process to verify applicants' prior employment and to gather information that may help them decide which applicants to interview. Later, a manager might informally contact someone on LinkedIn whom the applicant and manager both know. That approach may yield more information than an official reference. Members of a search committee might look for applicants on Facebook. Conceivably, a manager might not hire someone because of information obtained from social media. This raises ethical and legal issues related to privacy, justice, validity, and the employer's obligation to avoid hiring incompetent or dangerous workers. Arguably, only HR staff (not hiring managers) should conduct reference checks and obtain only references that the applicant has given written permission for (McConnell 2018).

Once the supervisor, manager, or team decides which applicant to hire, HR staff extends a firm job offer to the individual with a starting date and salary. The offer may be made subject to reference checks and background checks (e.g., for drug abuse or criminal conviction) if those were not already done. After the candidate accepts the job offer and clears all background verifications, the HR staff should ensure the HCO has documented the specific reasons each other applicant was not hired. This documentation is essential because, months or years later, the HCO might have to legally justify its hiring decision. However, if applicants call and ask why they were not hired, the HR staff should simply say that a more appropriate candidate was chosen, without going into detail (McConnell 2018). Giving reasons for rejection may be neither helpful nor needed, and it could lead to problems (Dunn 2016, 452). HR staff may just say the applicant's qualifications did not sufficiently match the job requirements.

ONE MORE TIME

The management function of staffing involves obtaining and retaining employees to do the work required to achieve the HCO's goals and mission. Staffing may be understood by studying seven interrelated processes. This chapter explained the first three processes (chapter 8 will explain the other four). While performing all staffing processes, managers should be attentive to three special concerns: staff diversity and inclusion; centralized, decentralized, and outsourced staffing; and laws and regulations.

First, managers plan for staff—forecasting the staff (workforce) the organization will require in the future and planning how to effectively obtain and retain that future staff. This work involves planning new approaches to the other staffing processes, such as new job design and job descriptions, new methods for hiring workers, new development of staff, new compensation methods, new ways to evaluate workers' performance, and new approaches for protecting employees.

Second, managers design jobs and work—determining the work tasks to be done by a job, along with qualifications, supervision, working conditions, rules, and schedules. HCOs have been shifting to more flexible job design to adapt to frequent changes in healthcare and external environments.

Third, managers hire staff—recruiting and selecting workers for jobs, which may include reassigning existing workers by promotion or transfer. Managers can recruit internally, externally, or both, using informative job announcements. When hiring for a job, managers use the current job description to evaluate applicants' qualifications and fit with the job and organization. Tests are also used to judge applicants. Several applicants are chosen for interviews with the job's immediate supervisor, a higher manager, future coworkers, and others. Based on candid input from interviewers, a final selection is made, usually by the person who will supervise the new employee. A job offer is then made by HR staff, subject to reference checks.

HR specialists, departments, or consultants often assist managers with the staffing function. The HR experts are usually responsible for creating programs, policies, procedures, methods, and tools that managers and supervisors throughout the HCO use to staff their individual departments. This approach creates consistency and fairness throughout the organization. It also helps managers comply with the many laws, court decisions, and regulations that affect how managers staff their HCOs.

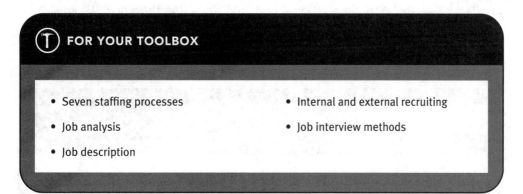

ⓣ FOR YOUR TOOLBOX

- Seven staffing processes
- Job analysis
- Job description
- Internal and external recruiting
- Job interview methods

FOR DISCUSSION

1. Briefly describe the seven processes that managers use to staff an HCO. Discuss how each process is necessary for an HCO to succeed.

2. Which information is typically included in a job description? How are job descriptions used with other staffing processes?

3. Discuss the advantages and disadvantages of internal recruiting for different jobs in HCOs. Then do the same for external recruiting.

4. Give examples of questions that are appropriate and not appropriate for a manager to ask an applicant during a job interview. Why are some questions inappropriate?

5. Reflect on the list of tips for effective job interviews (near the end of the chapter). Which of these tips do you feel are most important? Why?

CASE STUDY QUESTIONS

These questions refer to the Integrative Case Studies at the back of this book.

1. "I Can't Do It All!" case: Mr. Brice realizes he must make "serious changes" so that his vice presidents will make decisions. Explain how he could use staffing processes to increase and improve decision making by his vice presidents.

2. Increasing the Focus on Patient Safety at First Medical Center case: How could job design, job analysis, and job descriptions support the focus on patient safety at First Medical Center?

3. Managing the Patient Experience case: Consider the pros and cons of internal and external recruitment. How might Mr. Jackson's prior jobs and work experience affect his success as chief experience officer at Academic Medical Center?

4. Rocky Road to Patient Satisfaction at Leonard-Griggs case: How could Ms. Ratcliff and the manager of human resources use job design, job analysis, and job descriptions to implement the patient satisfaction surveys at the physician practices?

 RIVERBEND ORTHOPEDICS MINI CASE STUDY

Riverbend Orthopedics is a busy group practice with expanded services for orthopedic care. It has seven physicians and a podiatrist, plus about 70 other employees. At its big, new clinic building, Riverbend provides extensive orthopedic care. Several technicians provide diagnostic medical imaging, from basic X-rays to magnetic resonance images. The physicians perform surgery in their own outpatient surgery center with Riverbend's own operating nurses and technicians. Therapy is provided by three physical therapists and one part-time contracted occupational therapist. In addition to staff providing actual patient care, the clinic has staff for financial management, medical records, human resources, information systems/technology, building maintenance, and other

(continued)

RIVERBEND ORTHOPEDICS MINI CASE STUDY *(continued)*

administrative matters. Occasional marketing work is done by an advertising company. Legal work is outsourced to a law firm. Riverbend is managed by a new president, Ms. Garcia. She and Riverbend have set a goal of achieving "Excellent" ratings for patient experience from at least 90 percent of Riverbend's patients this year.

Riverbend currently has one HR manager with expertise in all aspects of HR and one compensation specialist. Ms. Garcia wants to obtain more HR support for staffing, but she is unsure whether to hire more HR specialists (full-time or part-time) or contract with an HR consulting firm for expertise when needed. Also, Ms. Garcia and Dr. Chen want to strengthen workforce diversity and inclusion at Riverbend.

MINI CASE STUDY QUESTIONS

1. Which factors and information should Ms. Garcia consider when deciding how to increase HR support for staffing Riverbend Orthopedics?

2. Suggest how Ms. Garcia and Dr. Chen could strengthen workforce diversity and inclusion at Riverbend Orthopedics. You may make reasonable assumptions and inferences.

REFERENCES

Dunn, R. T. 2016. *Dunn and Haimann's Healthcare Management*, 10th ed. Chicago: Health Administration Press.

Evans, R. M. 2015. "Workforce Diversity." In *Human Resources in Healthcare*, 4th ed., edited by B. J. Fried and M. D. Fottler, 123–42. Chicago: Health Administration Press.

Fottler, M. D. 2015a. "Job Analysis and Job Design." In *Human Resources in Healthcare*, 4th ed., edited by B. J. Fried and M. D. Fottler, 143–80. Chicago: Health Administration Press.

———. 2015b. "Strategic Human Resources Management." In *Human Resources in Healthcare*, 4th ed., edited by B. J. Fried and M. D. Fottler, 1–34. Chicago: Health Administration Press.

French, W. L. 2007. *Human Resources Management*, 6th ed. Boston: Houghton Mifflin Company.

Fried, B. J., and M. Gates. 2015. "Recruitment, Selection, and Retention." In *Human Resources in Healthcare*, 4th ed., edited by B. J. Fried and M. D. Fottler, 181–234. Chicago: Health Administration Press.

Hegwer, L. R. 2016. "Building High-Performing, Highly Diverse Teams and Organizations." *Healthcare Executive* 31 (6): 10–19.

Institute for Diversity and Health Equity. 2018. "Institute Resource Center: 'A Diversity, Equity and Cultural Competency Assessment Tool for Leaders.'" Accessed August 20. www.diversityconnection.org/diversityconnection/membership/Institute-Resource-Center.jsp.

McConnell, C. R. 2018. *Umiker's Management Skills for the New Health Care Supervisor*, 7th ed. Burlington, MA: Jones & Bartlett Learning.

McNally, K. 2018. "The Imperative for Strategic Workforce Planning and Development: Challenges and Opportunities." Published February 28. www.aha.org/news/insights-and-analysis/2018-02-28-imperative-strategic-workforce-planning-and-development.

Noe, R., J. Hollenbeck, B. Gerhart, and P. Wright. 2016. *Human Resource Management: Gaining a Competitive Advantage,* 10th ed. Chicago: McGraw-Hill Higher Education.

Schawbel, D. 2017. "Workplace Trends You'll See in 2018." Published November 1. www.forbes.com/sites/danschawbel/2017/11/01/10-workplace-trends-youll-see-in-2018/#300c33e24bf2.

———. 2016. "Workplace Trends You'll See in 2017." Published November 1. www.forbes.com/sites/danschawbel/2016/11/01/workplace-trends-2017/.

Trustees of Boston College. 2016. "Diversity and Inclusion Definitions." Updated December 16. www.bc.edu/offices/diversity/diversity-and-inclusion-statement.html.

Wagner, K. 2017. "Harnessing the Strengths of a Multigenerational Workforce to Leverage Opportunities." *Healthcare Executive* 32 (6): 10–18.

White, K. R., and J. R. Griffith. 2019. *The Well-Managed Healthcare Organization*, 9th ed. Chicago: Health Administration Press.

CHAPTER 8

STAFFING: RETAINING EMPLOYEES

A company is only as good as the people it keeps.

Mary Kay Ash, entrepreneur and businesswoman

LEARNING OBJECTIVES

Studying this chapter will help you to

➤ explain how managers develop staff,

➤ understand how managers appraise staff performance,

➤ describe how managers compensate staff,

➤ explain how managers protect staff, and

➤ understand how onboarding improves staff retention.

HERE'S WHAT HAPPENED

When implementing their new strategic goals, managers at Partners HealthCare performed the staffing function. This function enabled Partners to obtain new workers and retain existing ones. An essential part of staffing was to determine the financial compensation for each position and employee. Compensation included base pay, incentives, and bonuses, as well as benefits such as paid vacation days, health insurance, and retirement plan contributions. In making compensation decisions, managers had to figure out what compensation would be needed to obtain and then retain the people Partners wanted. Managers had to understand and comply with dozens of laws regulating compensation and other aspects of employment. They also had to decide how to evaluate staff job performance and how performance evaluations would affect future compensation. Partners HealthCare's strategic goals were going to require innovation and change, so managers knew they would have to develop employees through training, coaching, and mentoring for changes in their jobs. Through these and other staffing processes, managers were able to achieve ambitious goals and the Partners HealthCare mission.

A s we see in the opening Here's What Happened, staffing a healthcare organization (HCO) is complex and requires much thought by managers. Staffing is another way managers make a difference and add value to their HCO. Chapter 7 identified seven staffing processes and explained the first three, which are used to obtain workers. This chapter builds on that discussion and studies the other four staffing processes, which help to retain workers: developing staff, appraising staff, compensating staff, and protecting staff. The processes overlap to some extent because they are interconnected and may support both obtaining and retaining workers. This chapter concludes with a discussion of onboarding, which combines several staffing processes to improve retention of new employees. If an HCO's managers perform these seven staffing processes well, they can obtain and retain the workforce needed to succeed. Employees will not wonder, "Should I stay or should I go?"

These seven processes can also improve employee engagement. Employees engage when they are emotionally committed and actively contribute to their work, workplace, and organization goals (Dye 2017). Employee engagement is an important challenge for organizations, including HCOs. Opinion surveys have shown that overall employee engagement in work is low and declining (Dye 2017). As a result, many concerned businesses are improving the "employee experience" by increasing training and development; expanding compensation and rewards; and improving employees' physical, mental, and financial well-being (Schawbel 2016). Learn to do the staffing processes well so you can engage your HCO's employees in their work, which will in turn help people in the community live healthier lives.

DEVELOPING STAFF

In chapter 7, we defined *developing staff* as helping employees acquire new knowledge, skills, attitudes, behaviors, and competencies for current and future jobs. (*Continuous learning, talent development*, and other terms are also used.) Staff development is done through training, coaching, mentoring, job rotation, formal education, and other methods. Managers must develop employees to motivate them, help them feel competent, enable them to succeed in their jobs, and give them opportunities to grow (McConnell 2018). Employees need development to continually perform their jobs well; some employees need it on their first day of work. Accreditation and professional licensure standards also require training and continuing education. Training, coaching, mentoring, and other approaches to developing staff enable HCOs and their workers to adapt to changes in the external environment (e.g., the changes described in chapter 1). If an HCO does not prepare workers for those changes, the organization and its workers will quickly fall behind because the half-life of learned skills is only five years (Schawbel 2017). Besides developing workers for current jobs, HCOs should also develop staff for future promotion and transfer to other jobs that help them grow and succeed. Do you see how this can improve staff retention?

Despite these reasons for staff development, some HCOs spend inadequate time and funds on it. White and Griffith (2019) urge managers to view training and development as an investment in the organization's workforce rather than a costly expense. Better HCOs invest to enable employees to perform work according to the HCO's preferred methods, meet service standards (e.g., empathy and responsiveness), and feel supported.

We will first study orientation of newly hired employees to help them successfully begin working. Then we will consider how to develop all employees so they can improve their performance and prepare for growth and promotion.

ORIENTATION OF NEW STAFF

After a manager hires a new employee to work in her department, she (and her HCO) then must orient the new employee to the department and the HCO. How well the orientation is done (or not done) will strongly shape the new employee's perceptions and feelings about her job, her coworkers, and the HCO, as well as her decision whether to stay in the job. **Orientation of new staff should focus on both the technical aspects of work (how to do the job well) and the social aspects of work (how to fit in and get along with coworkers).** Managers must orient new workers to help them succeed—which then helps the managers succeed.

HCOs differ in how they handle orientation of new staff (Kaye and Fottler 2015). At some HCOs, orientation may start online after workers have accepted a job but before they begin their first day of work. Smaller HCOs may provide a shorter, more casual, and less organized orientation than big HCOs do. New, start-up HCOs may not yet have a planned orientation, and new workers will become oriented day by day. In large HCOs, orientation might be part of a comprehensive, months-long onboarding process (described at the end of this chapter). Top managers orient all new employees to the HCO. Middle- and lower-level managers orient their new employees to their specific work departments. They might use videos, online tutorials, webinars, e-handbooks, online manuals, interactive meetings, mobile learning, buddies, mentors, and checklists.

Managers are likely to spread employee orientation over several days (or even weeks) so that new workers are not overloaded with information. For example, suppose Juan, the reimbursement manager at a healthcare system in Berkeley, hires Erin as a Medicare reimbursement specialist. Juan and the human resources (HR) department arrange for Erin to complete her payroll forms, enroll in the health insurance plan, and buy a company parking permit online, all before her first day of work. Juan then schedules time to orient Erin to the reimbursement department when she arrives there on her first day of work. Erin's department orientation includes

◆   a gracious, supportive, and enthusiastic welcome to the healthcare system and the department;

◆   introductions to her supervisor and a few immediate coworkers;

◆   a tour of the work area, department, and places such as restrooms and break room;

◆   specifics of the Medicare reimbursement specialist job—what, why, when, where, and how to do it the way Juan expects it to be done (which might differ from how Erin has done similar work elsewhere);

◆   information about work schedules, breaks, meals, and overtime;

◆   information about her workstation, equipment, and supplies;

◆   an explanation of essential policies, procedures, rules, and standards of behavior—especially those that pertain to the department (rather than to the entire HCO); and

◆   helpful, supportive answers to Erin's questions.

Juan and Erin then meet with Carla (an experienced reimbursement specialist), who will be Erin's mentor or buddy. Carla and Juan have already discussed this arrangement, and Carla has agreed to provide on-the-job guidance to Erin and help Erin socialize with others. Juan will talk with Erin at the end of her first day and during her first week to see how she is doing. He will gradually introduce her to further information to help her do her job well and become more engaged.

At some point Erin will participate in orientation to the whole organization. Whereas department orientation should begin the day an employee begins, organization orientation can be done later. Much of it is information that may be distributed via multimedia in small doses over a period of time. Most organizations include some "meet and greet" time with the HCO's senior leaders, perhaps on the first day of each month. Returning to the example in Berkeley, the HCO's top managers and HR staff may welcome Erin and 16 other new employees from 9 different departments who started the previous month. They may describe the healthcare system's mission, vision, values, and goals and give inspired messages about the HCO. Staff may describe or provide multimedia presentations on

◆ the organization chart and management team;

◆ essential policies, procedures, rules, and standards of behavior that pertain to all employees, such as those related to safety and customer interactions; and

◆ employee benefits, career-planning resources, and other support that is available to all workers.

After an hour of organization orientation, new employees should be better informed but often are restless. Break time! Snacks are provided, people chat informally, and new employees meet and socialize. Some HCOs may then include a brief tour of the facility.

In the real world, managers sometimes struggle for weeks or even months to keep a department going while a job is vacant. People work extra days to cover the job's tasks until a new employee begins. When a new employee finally arrives, everyone wants her to jump right in and get to work. The manager should resist a quick "Here's what I want you to do" orientation. A new employee will have questions and feel anxious about the new job, new place, new people, and so forth. She will feel supported—or not—depending on how her first day goes. The first day, first week, and first month will greatly affect how well the new employee does her job and how she feels about her job and the organization. Without an adequate, supportive orientation, she may soon be wondering, "Should I stay or should I go?" If she goes, then the manager, department, and HCO have to redo the hiring process. As a manager, remember: **Employee orientation improves employee engagement and satisfaction—which then improves employee performance and retention.** For the employee, manager, department, and organization, it's a win-win-win-win!

TRAINING STAFF

Although employees might have graduated with the latest knowledge and skills or might have years of experience, their knowledge will not be "best practice" forever. In fact, it can become outdated within months because of rapid changes in the external environment of HCOs. A manager must train and develop employees so that they can adapt to those changes and stay current. Partners HealthCare did this in the chapter's opening Here's What Happened. Many hospitals trained staff to better satisfy patients when Medicare began reimbursing hospitals based partly on patients' satisfaction scores. Many HCOs offer training to prepare workers for developments and challenges in healthcare (some of which we saw in chapter 1): patient engagement, patient experience, clinical care coordination, diverse cultures and multiple generations in the workforce, burnout, bullying, interactions with others, ethics, harassment, mobile health, population health, pay-for-performance, disaster readiness, safety, high-performing teams, embracing change, conflict resolution, and many others (Kaye and Fottler 2015; Ryan 2017). For example, Main Line Health in Philadelphia has been providing all managers with two days of experiential learning about diversity, respect, and inclusion. Similar training will be provided to all staff, including physicians (Lynch 2017).

When you are a manager, you will have to ensure your workers are trained for their jobs—the equipment, methods, processes, and so forth. Who provides the training? Who trained you for a job you once had? As manager, you will do some of the training. Experts in your department or in other departments such as information technology or infection control will provide training for their areas of expertise. Large HCOs are likely to have a department for education, training, and development. People in that department could help you plan and implement training for your staff. Many HCOs outsource some training to consultants with specific expertise, such as training in conflict resolution and teamwork. Vendors who sell products and equipment to HCOs are responsible for training the HCOs' employees in how to use the products and equipment.

Sometimes an HCO is in such a hurry to train staff that it does not take time to create effective training. Good training that has a lasting effect is not simple. How can managers prepare and provide effective training? They can use the training methods shown in exhibit 8.1 that are based on training models. To really stick, training must be done well—and be reinforced by leadership and organization culture, which will be studied in later chapters.

DEVELOPING STAFF

Managers should develop their staff for transfers, promotions, and career growth. This development goes beyond training for an existing job and prepares workers for other jobs in the HCO. Educational programs for workers, which are longer and more comprehensive than short-term training, can be planned by managers building on the methods listed in exhibit 8.1. Managers can provide internal or external coaches and mentors to help workers grow and develop for higher-level jobs and promotions. If an HCO does not provide development and opportunities for career growth, it will have trouble retaining younger workers. Further, many employees in clinical fields—such as nursing and therapy professions—seek career ladders that provide promotion into advanced clinical jobs rather than promotion into supervisory jobs. Offering promotions up clinical career ladders can help retain clinical workers.

EXHIBIT 8.1
Training Checklist

1. **Needs assessment:** Determine what training is needed (in the short term and long term) for the HCO and for specific employees. Examine prior planning for staff, employees' job performance appraisals, employees' career development plans, on-the-job safety reports, customer satisfaction data, employees' input, surveys, strategic plans, job redesign, and other relevant information. Needs may be prioritized and the most important ones addressed first.

2. **Purpose and objectives:** For each chosen training need, write the specific purpose, objectives, and desired outcomes. Which new knowledge, skills, attitudes, behaviors, and competencies should employees have as a result of the training?

3. **Content, methods, and instructors:** Decide appropriate curriculum, content, teaching and learning methods, instructors, and resources to achieve the desired purpose, objectives, and outcomes. Keep it simple, practical, and job related. Use appropriate methods, media, and technology, which may include videos, online apps, self-paced tutorials, teleconferences, webinars, games, assignments, simulations, lectures, interactive demonstrations, workshops, team-based learning, discussions, role-play, written materials, case studies, mobile learning, job shadowing, on-the-job training, behavior modeling, and mentoring. Allow time for trainers and facilitators to practice, revise the content and methods, and rehearse again before going live. If necessary, increase both organization support for the training and trainees' readiness (e.g., motivation) for the training.

4. **Implementation:** Make training as convenient as possible (e.g., schedule it on different days and times) for the trainees. Find out which days, times, and locations would avoid disrupting their usual work. Ensure all supplies and resources are available. Avoid trying to train too many employees at once. Be flexible and adjust as needed during the training. Deliver the training.

5. **Evaluation:** After the training is complete, evaluate all aspects of the training and monitor (initially and later on) how well it achieved its purpose. Consider how trainees feel about the training, what they learned, which behaviors changed (and for how long), whether the training objectives were achieved, and return on investment. Make notes on how to improve the next training.

Sources: Information from Cummings and Worley (2015); Kaye and Fottler (2015); McConnell (2018); Noe et al. (2016).

Often in HCOs, the "best" worker is promoted to supervisor when that position becomes vacant. If he is not properly prepared for the job, that new supervisor is likely to make mistakes and perhaps fail in this new job. He might maintain peer-to-peer relationships rather than shift to superior–subordinate relationships. He might hesitate to delegate tasks to other workers. A new supervisor might avoid giving necessary, critical feedback to the staff. Job development programs are essential to help workers prepare for promotion to a supervisory or management job. Ideally, prospective managers are developed for management prior to promotion into such a position. This preparation can be done in succession planning for the management team as a result of the first staffing process: planning for staff. Managers can identify employees for potential future promotion and then provide them with expanded mentoring, coaching, and other opportunities to develop needed competencies for promotion (White and Griffith 2019). Many large health systems have lengthy, comprehensive management development tracks to continually prepare their next managers and leaders.

In one important trend, more HCOs are seeking physicians for top management positions such as vice president of medical affairs, chief clinical quality officer, and even president and CEO. Because of the small supply of physicians who are ready for these jobs, some health systems are using management development, executive coaching, and other methods to prepare their own physicians for this work (Dye 2017).

APPRAISING PERFORMANCE OF STAFF

In chapter 7, we defined *appraising performance* as the process of evaluating the job performance of workers and discussing those evaluations with them. The appraisal process should develop an HCO's employees so they can help achieve the HCO's goals and their own career goals.

Top managers or HR staff design performance appraisal methods, procedures, schedules, and systems for the entire HCO. Supervisors and department managers then use those to appraise the workers for whom they are responsible. When done well, these appraisals can achieve many useful purposes, such as the following (Dunn 2016; Fried 2015; McConnell 2018):

◆   Enable manager and employee to openly discuss the employee's job, job performance, and related matters, including training and development, job transfer or promotion, and compensation

◆   Remind the employee what is expected based on the job analysis and job description

◆   Provide candid feedback to the employee regarding job performance, how well job expectations have been met, performance strengths, and needed performance improvement

◆   Coach the employee on how to improve specific aspects of performance

◆   Identify the employee's future developmental goals to support individual career plans and the HCO's succession planning

◆ Enable the HCO to maintain a skills inventory of each employee and of the HCO's workforce

◆ Guide and support future training and development for employees and the HCO as a whole

◆ Guide and support a manager's decisions about compensation

◆ Guide and support a manager's decisions about promotion, transfer, discipline, and termination

◆ Guide and support organization succession planning for critical jobs

◆ Support compliance with accreditation and legal requirements

Unfortunately, appraisals are not always done well (Dunn 2016; Fried 2015; McConnell 2018). They may be dreaded and considered a waste of time by both the appraiser (manager) and the appraisee (employee). What are barriers to effective appraisals?

The appraisal process must be well designed and based on clear, up-to-date job descriptions. Actual job performance must be measured, which takes a lot of time if appraisal apps and data collection systems are not available. Managers are human and may be influenced (consciously or unconsciously) by emotions, biases, favoritism, personalities, organization politics, time pressures, and factors that are not job related (Dunn 2016; Noe et al. 2016). Managers may inflate or deflate appraisals for reasons unrelated to job performance, such as wanting to get along with everyone. They may wish to avoid creating a realistic but negative appraisal that would remain in the employee's file for many years. Employees may perceive appraisals as demeaning, judgmental, condescending, punitive, or in other ways unpleasant and unfair (Fried 2015). An employee may not acknowledge performance problems (which should be discussed to guide future development goals) if doing so will affect future pay. Some people are uncomfortable judging or being judged by others. All these factors may cause managers and employees to superficially hurry through an appraisal or just skip it.

When appraisals are not done well, employees resent and distrust them, making the next appraisal even harder for both manager and employee. Many employees dislike annual evaluations because they don't think their boss knows how to do them (Fisher 2016). Managers can try to avoid problems by using the methods explained in the next section. However, some managers and organizations are abandoning annual appraisals and shifting to a faster, simpler, real-time approach. They feel the annual appraisal is too bureaucratic, time-consuming, and retrospective. They think it is not relevant when jobs, goals, and organizations change so often. Also, many younger employees want informal, frequent feedback. Methods for improving traditional evaluations are explained next, followed by the newer approach.

Appraisal Process and Methods

In many HCOs, managers formally appraise each employee once a year. In other HCOs, they do appraisals more often. New workers, such as a paramedic in Auburn, may be formally evaluated at 3 months, 6 months, and 12 months, and then annually thereafter. The same is often true for employees who have been transferred or promoted into a different job. If an appraisal identifies serious performance problems, the manager should appraise the employee again soon.

Even if a formal appraisal indicates acceptable performance, managers should regularly follow up with the employee to ensure satisfactory progress on annual performance goals. **Managers must continually monitor and talk with all employees about their job performance.** A medical assistant will benefit from receiving day-to-day feedback in short conversations during the week about specific aspects of job performance. Supervisors and managers should interact with their employees in their work setting often enough that this feedback happens easily and naturally. Newer, younger workers want frequent feedback—perhaps weekly or even daily—and companies have been changing their performance appraisal methods to provide it.

Who provides input for an employee's appraisal? The manager always does, and in some cases the employee may do a self-appraisal. Coworkers and team members who interact extensively with (and perhaps depend on) an employee may be invited to give input. Many HCOs use a multisource (or 360-degree) evaluation in which selected workers above, below, and at the same level as the employee all provide input for that employee's appraisal. Feedback and data from bosses, peers, subordinates, and team members assess an employee's performance from multiple perspectives. Depending on job requirements, input on performance may also be obtained from outside the HCO. For example, consider Priya, a hospice coordinator. Input may be obtained from employees in other organizations with whom Priya interacts for her job.

People can provide appraisal input by completing checklists, questionnaires, and surveys that involve marking their choices for prepared statements and factors. This input generally focuses on an employee's traits, behaviors, competencies, and results (Fried 2015). Larger HCOs with many employees invest in electronic performance management systems to collect and process this input for large workforces. Some managers use a less focused approach and ask people to write essays or answer open-ended questions about an employee. Conversations can provide more qualitative information. In all cases, managers should plan ahead and give people several weeks to respond with input. Information is usually recorded on standard forms—paper or electronic—although some HCOs are flexible and use customized appraisals (Fottler 2015).

HCOs often use forms with rating scales. These scales measure how well a worker performs (what he actually does) in relation to his job description and job standards. Some scales measure employees' skills, knowledge, behaviors, or traits. A current approach is to measure employees' results. Exhibit 8.2 shows a sample performance rating scale.

Unfortunately, these scales leave room for manager opinion and interpretation. Thus, HCOs often use more specific rating forms that define what each number rating means.

	(Low)				(High)	
1. Rate the employee's results on the job.	1	2	3	4	5	
2. Rate the employee's work quality.	1	2	3	4	5	
3. Rate the employee's quantity of work.	1	2	3	4	5	

EXHIBIT 8.2
Sample
Performance
Rating Scale

For example, a 1 might be defined as "results are often late and less than assigned." Yet, different managers still might interpret the rating scale differently. What does "often late" and "less than assigned" really mean? Managers should strive to use measurable standards and benchmarks to define what the ratings 1, 2, 3, 4, and 5 mean. Here are some measurable standards for a 5 rating:

◆   Number of patients treated per day is between 15 and 20.

◆   Average cost of supplies per week is less than $100.

Another useful approach is to design the rating scale with only three ratings to indicate that performance was below, met, or exceeded preset job standards (McConnell 2018).

Rate the employee's quantity of work:

1 = performance was below standards

2 = performance met standards

3 = performance exceeded standards

For each numerical rating, the manager should give specific examples to support the rating, especially for a low rating that the employee may challenge. A manager could keep track of and then identify specific examples of late work, such as "The monthly budget analysis was late in April, June, July, and October during the past year."

Although the rating scale method is common, a manager can use other appraisal methods. She may apply a comparative approach to all employees (or groups of employees) and rank them from best to worst. Or, she may use the forced distribution method that assigns (distributes) all employees to categories such as the top 20 percent, middle 60 percent, and bottom 20 percent (Fried 2015). However, these approaches are becoming less common.

After rating the performance of each essential job expectation, a manager should write about the worker's strengths and weaknesses and give recommendations for the coming year. The appraisal now becomes developmental to help the worker develop short-term and longer-term performance and career goals. This aspect of the appraisal takes careful thought and work and requires managers to pay attention to their employees throughout the year. The manager writes a performance appraisal to steer an employee's future efforts toward helping to achieve the HCO's goals and strategies. The next appraisal should then consider how well the previous recommendations were achieved.

In the final part of a performance appraisal, the manager must arrange and conduct a review meeting with the employee. This discussion may create anxiety for both of them, especially if performance was inadequate, they do not have a good working relationship, or the past review meeting was unpleasant. To ensure an effective review meeting, a manager can use the methods shown in exhibit 8.3.

As mentioned, some organizations and managers have been shifting from formal, annual appraisals to less formal, more frequent appraisals. Some are using frequent, continual, real-time feedback. Companies set expectations with employees and then give frequent, regular feedback without a formal annual appraisal (Schawbel 2016). With so much change in organizations, job expectations may change and be reset during a performance year to accommodate new goals and projects. Performance management software enables such changes, as well as continual monitoring and reporting of many aspects of each employee's performance and contributions to jobs, teams, projects, departments, and the organization. Attentive, engaged managers regularly (monthly or even weekly) make rounds in their departments to informally assess workers and give them frequent feedback. This approach uses informal conversations as things happen. Many managers and workers like this frequent feedback in small doses. It is more natural and doesn't require time for gathering input from stakeholders, checking boxes, and writing and reading commentary.

Texas Health Resources has 24,000 employees in 29 hospitals. It has been implementing an employee performance review process that provides ongoing, real-time feedback pertaining to work, goals, and outcomes. Texas Health Resources' CEO says it is like coaching a sports team as play happens. A vice president at Thomas Jefferson University Hospital in Philadelphia evaluates leadership team members using a one-page professional development plan. The plan includes personal and professional goals (short-term and long-term) and competencies to develop. He meets regularly with each team member to follow up on the plan (Wagner 2017).

In between the formal, annual approach and informal, frequent approach are many possible variations. Each HCO can determine its own process and decide who provides input, how input is gathered and presented, how the discussion occurs, and what documentation is prepared for follow-up.

WHEN JOB PERFORMANCE IS DEFICIENT

Sometimes an employee does not meet job performance expectations. The manager or supervisor should realize this deficiency long before an annual performance appraisal and

✓ Ensure that top management supports the performance appraisal process.
✓ Give feedback to the employee during the year to continually guide performance as needed and to avoid (unpleasant) surprises at the review meeting.
✓ Allow one month of lead time to schedule the review meeting, gather information from multiple sources, review the job description, and write the appraisal.
✓ Anticipate how the employee may react, and then plan how to respond.
✓ Arrange the review meeting to take place in a comfortable, private place at a convenient, uninterrupted time.
✓ Give performance feedback and recommendations, praise and reinforce good aspects of performance, honestly discuss unsatisfactory aspects of performance, and be specific and objective.
✓ Lead a discussion that is supportive, not punitive, and listen for content and feeling when the employee talks. Coach, inspire, and motivate.
✓ Focus on the employee's performance, behavior, and results (not personality), and then shift to future performance.
✓ Collaboratively plan future goals and expected outcomes; discuss the future more than the past.
✓ Document the appraisal review, developmental performance goals for the future, and plans for follow-up; sign the written appraisal and have the employee sign it.
✓ Give copies of the appraisal to the employee and the HR department; keep a copy to use for periodic follow-up. The appraisal is confidential, so do not share it with other employees.

Sources: Information from Dunn (2016); Fried (2015); McConnell (2018); Noe et al. (2016); Walston (2017).

EXHIBIT 8.3
Performance Appraisal Meeting Checklist

should manage it when it happens. This approach is one benefit of frequently assessing employee performance and frequently giving feedback throughout the year. If goals and standards are not being met or rules are not being followed, then the manager must discuss it with the employee promptly, privately, and professionally (Dunn 2016). Candid exploration of the problem with the employee may reveal factors such as lack of resources, training, or time; misunderstanding of goals and expectations; or other reasons beyond the employee's control that the manager must address.

Yet, in some cases, unsatisfactory job performance may result from the employee's lack of commitment, effort, or willingness. If this is the case, disciplinary action is appropriate.

Many HCOs use progressive discipline. The manager begins by mentioning the job performance problem in an informal, friendly discussion with the employee (Dunn 2016). If necessary, the manager follows up with a stern verbal warning. If the performance problem continues, a written warning is given and placed in the worker's employment file. The next step would be unpaid suspension from work (one or more days) to "think about your commitment." If the problem continues after suspension without pay, then termination is usually the final step. The manager should be prompt, fair, and consistent and document each step when it occurs. Some HCOs use an alternative, nonpunitive approach that forces the employee to take responsibility for the problem and solution. After counseling and discussion, the HCO pays the worker to stay home one day and make a decision: either return to work committed to fulfilling all job requirements, or do not return to work. This is called a decision-making paid leave, and the negligent employee must make a choice and live with it.

Each HCO can develop its own approach to progressive discipline. The HCO's managers must carefully follow the written policies and procedures for progressive discipline and document what was done at each step of the process.

The appraisal methods listed in exhibit 8.3 are useful for middle managers and supervisors who must evaluate their frontline workers. These methods can also be used by top managers to appraise middle managers, and to some extent by a CEO to appraise other C-suite managers and executives. Such appraisals may be done as a narrative explaining how well the manager has fulfilled the position's responsibilities, accomplished preset goals, and achieved outcome targets (White and Griffith 2019). These factors can pertain to finances, customer satisfaction, clinical outcomes, human resources, legal compliance, population health, and key organization-level outcomes under an executive's control. As much as possible,

 USING CHAPTER 8 IN THE REAL WORLD

When an HCO adopts a new vision and goals, it may have to modify its performance appraisals to drive achievement of those goals. A new CEO at Cooper University Health Care (CUHC) in Camden, New Jersey, was expected to improve patient service and experience. She stated a new vision for the HCO and set clear expectations for the staff to achieve it. A chief experience officer was hired as the conscience of the organization. An analytics system was developed to gather data—including patients' ratings—and to measure performance. Then CUHC started evaluating staff on values and behaviors as part of job performance. The evaluation closely looked at employees' emotional intelligence (EI), which is the "ability to recognize and understand emotions in yourself and others, and your ability to use this awareness to manage your behavior and relationships" (Kivland 2014, 72). Employees need appropriate EI to provide excellent patient experience. To achieve its patient experience vision, CUHC used performance evaluations to appraise its staff and, if necessary, to remove people who lacked the necessary values and behaviors (Radick 2016).

objective data should be used to measure goal achievement and outcomes. If an executive has an employment contract with the HCO, the appraiser must understand and comply with it.

As mentioned earlier, the performance appraisal process for an entire HCO interacts with other staffing processes. Appraisals uncover performance problems that must be addressed in future planning for staff. They may signal a need to redesign some jobs or show which type of training is needed. Appraisals also may reveal flaws in the hiring process. Finally, appraisals help a management team determine an employee's compensation. Compensation is the next staffing process we will consider.

COMPENSATING STAFF

In chapter 7, we defined *compensating staff* as the process of determining and giving wages, salaries, incentives, and benefits to workers. Compensation includes pay (e.g., wages, salaries, merit increases, cost-of-living increases, bonuses, shift differentials, cash incentives) and benefits (e.g., paid vacation, health insurance, child care, retirement contribution) given to workers (Noe et al. 2016). Pay and benefits vary according to several factors, including full-time or part-time status, salaried or nonsalaried status, and years worked at the HCO. Besides receiving financial compensation, employees may also receive other rewards for their work as part of a total rewards approach (Griffin, Phillips, and Gully 2017). Other rewards may include praise, recognition, and awards; special privileges and perquisites; promotion and advancement; and an organization culture and policies that enable workers to balance work lives and personal lives (McSweeney-Feld and Rubin 2014). Together, nonfinancial rewards and financial rewards make up total rewards to compensate employees for their work. This section focuses mostly on financial compensation, while nonmonetary rewards are discussed in the next section and in later chapters on leadership and organization culture.

Compensation strongly affects how well an HCO obtains and retains employees. Thus, it strongly affects an HCO's survival. Managers must "get it right." Yet, doing so is not easy because compensation is complex.

1. Compensation is an important and sensitive matter for each employee. (Today's management tip: Do not make a mistake with someone's paycheck!)

2. Dozens of laws and court decisions affect how HCOs compensate workers.

3. Compensation differences among employees arise because of differences in the value of jobs, individual human motivations, the generations in the workforce, required licensures and certifications, chronic shortages of available workers for essential jobs, and other factors.

4. Differences in pay must occur, yet employees may feel that the differences (real or assumed) are unfair.

Top managers and HR staff are responsible for developing their HCO's compensation system. In large HCOs, someone in the HR department will have compensation expertise to help managers. Some HCOs outsource compensation work to consultants who design and administer effective, legal plans for pay and benefits. Before developing the compensation details, top executives make broad organization decisions about how competitive their HCO will be in their labor market. Will the HCO pay above-average, average, or below-average wages? How will the wages affect spending on other forms of compensation (e.g., employee benefits) and spending on other needs (e.g., medical equipment)? How will it affect staffing recruitment and retention?

Managers play several important roles in compensating employees (McConnell 2018). First, they must work with HR and payroll staff to apply the HCO's overall compensation program to their own department. They might determine merit pay or bonuses for their direct-report employees. Second, managers must be familiar with the HCO's compensation methods and benefits to answer questions from their employees (perhaps after checking the HCO's compensation policies or with HR). Detailed questions may be referred to HR and payroll staff. Third, managers must be attentive to employees' complaints about pay and compensation, and strive to resolve issues with help from HR staff and higher managers when necessary.

How Is Pay Determined?

How do an HCO's managers determine pay? Base pay, wages, and salaries are set for each job based on (1) the value of each job to the HCO, (2) prevailing pay in the community for jobs, and (3) the HCO's approach to compensation competitiveness.

Large HCOs have more than a hundred unique jobs. Managers assign each job a value indicating how much it is worth and should be paid. In doing so, they must strive to ensure fair pay for each job in relation to all other jobs. This valuation is not easy. When managers determine the value of a job, they depend on accurate position descriptions to analyze jobs.

A common approach to figuring job values is the **point-factor system** (Fried and Smith 2015; Noe et al. 2016). The basic method is explained in this section, and HCOs can create their own variation of it. The point-factor system may be implemented by a committee of selected HR staff and managers. The committee chooses a group of compensable factors that the organization values and will pay for, such as skill, effort, responsibility, and working conditions. These factors may all have the same weight, or they may be weighted differently if one or more factors (e.g., skill) are felt to be more important than others. Each factor (e.g., skill) has several levels (e.g., levels 1, 2, 3, 4, and 5) worth increasingly more points (e.g., 20, 40, 60, 80, and 100). The committee uses job descriptions and other information to evaluate each job based on that same set of factors. The committee assigns points to each job (e.g., accountant) for each factor (e.g., skill) by judging which level is

point-factor system
A system for determining a job's value, in which points are assigned to each job based on how each job rates on a common set of factors used to evaluate all jobs; total points for a job determine pay for that job.

required (e.g., skill level 4, worth 80 points). Then for each job (e.g., accountant), the points for *all* factors (e.g., skill, effort, responsibility, and working conditions) are added together. The sum is the total point value of that job. This calculation is done for each job so that each job has a total point value or worth.

Let's consider the computer programmer job. Managers evaluate it and assign points for all four factors as follows.

- ◆ Skill = 80 points

- ◆ Effort = 60 points

- ◆ Responsibility = 40 points

- ◆ Working conditions = 20 points

The programmer job is worth 200 points. All jobs are similarly evaluated and assigned their total point value.

Then the committee gathers market research data for competitive prevailing pay rates for common key jobs such as computer programmer, pharmacist, accountant, chef, and nurse. This helps create competitive wages. As a result of the programmer's point value, the prevailing competitive salary data for programmers, and the HCO's overall organization decisions about compensation, the HCO's managers set the programmer's annual base pay. From the data gathered for other key jobs, such as pharmacist, accountant, chef, and nurse, annual base pay is set for these key jobs. A spreadsheet program is used to plot a regression line for all key jobs to find the best fit between job value points and job base pay. The point value of each job can then be individually entered into the regression equation to determine the annual base pay for each job. If managers feel it is necessary for a specific job, they can adjust pay up or down from what is indicated by the regression curve.

Sometimes jobs are grouped (classified) into job grades (classes) based on how they rate for the compensable factors. For example, the federal government uses a classification system that groups most jobs into 15 different job grades. A pay rate is set for each grade, and the pay rate for a given grade applies to all jobs in that grade. Using job grades greatly reduces the amount of work required to set pay. However, jobs that would have different point values are grouped together and paid the same. This weakens **internal equity.**

Sometimes compensation becomes more complicated. Suppose a manager later finds that the base pay rate is not high enough to obtain and retain workers because of higher prevailing pay in the community. If the average local base pay for a job has increased, the HCO may have to set its own base pay close to that higher local pay rate (or else offer a much richer benefit package). Raising programmer pay to meet the prevailing pay in the community helps create **external equity** of the programmer's pay compared to pay for similar jobs *outside* the HCO. However, this pay raise causes the job to be paid more than

internal equity
Fairness in compensation for a job compared to compensation for other jobs inside the organization.

external equity
Fairness in compensation for a job compared to compensation for other similar jobs outside the organization.

when its pay was based on the internal point value. Thus, the programmer job pay increase to achieve external equity upsets the internal equity of programmer pay. Managers often face this dilemma and must balance internal and external equity.

Once the base rate of pay for a job has been set, the base rate of pay for *a specific person* in that job might be increased because that person has extra education or years of experience beyond the minimum required. Suppose Samantha is a programmer with five more years of experience than the minimum required. Managers may decide to pay her $5,000 more annually because she is more experienced.

The base pay rate of all jobs in an HCO usually increases each year. However, if funds are not available, base pay might be held constant. If an HCO is struggling financially, base pay might even be reduced. Top-level managers make these compensation decisions each year. Sometimes they make further adjustments midyear to adapt to internal and external changes.

Workers in lower-valued jobs receive hourly wages generally based on *how many hours they work* times their *hourly rate of pay*. Workers in higher-level jobs, such as managers and professional staff, receive a salary regardless of how many hours they work. Beyond their base pay, some workers may be eligible for additional pay, such as

- ◆ sign-on bonuses for newly hired workers;
- ◆ retention bonuses for those who reach longevity targets;
- ◆ overtime pay for nonsalaried workers;
- ◆ differential pay for working second shift, third shift, weekends, and holidays;
- ◆ profit sharing (in for-profit HCOs); and
- ◆ various forms of incentive pay, including pay-for-performance bonuses.

HCOs have been increasing their use of performance-based pay and incentives (Fried and Smith 2015). This kind of pay is earned for achieving preset goals, standards, and other performance targets. Driven by payers reimbursing HCOs more for value (rather than volume) of care, incentive targets often reflect quality of care, clinical outcomes, and patient experience and satisfaction (rather than traditional volume of services and procedures). Pay for productivity performance is also common. These incentives may include bonuses and merit pay. Another trend shows HCOs offering compensation and incentives based on performance of teams, departments, and entire organizations. This trend creates challenges in deciding how much to base pay on individual performance versus group performance. Top managers will have to decide how much to decentralize incentive pay decisions throughout an HCO.

HOW ARE BENEFITS DETERMINED?

In addition to paying workers, managers must compensate them with benefits. To properly manage benefits and compensation, managers must obtain clear advice from experts, such as labor attorneys or compensation consultants. Managers may check the US Department of Labor website to learn how laws affect benefits. A few benefits are required by federal and state laws, such as the HCO's contributions to employees' social security (for retirement) and workers' compensation (for on-the-job injuries).

Most benefits are voluntary, although some are expected by most workers and thus essential for staffing an HCO. Everyone expects paid personal time off for holidays, sickness, vacation, and other purposes. There are dozens of possible benefits, and employees differ in which ones they prefer. Younger employees may want day care for children, whereas older workers often prefer contributions to a retirement plan. Therapists like payment for continuing education, whereas housekeeping staff might like another paid day off. Other possible benefits are numerous: fitness facilities, tuition reimbursement, life insurance, disability insurance, subsidized meals, dues for professional associations, and many others. Managers often create flexible benefits plans that allow each employee to choose from a variety of benefits up to a specified dollar value. Although this "cafeteria" approach is more complicated to administer, it increases employees' satisfaction and retention because they can pick the benefits they want. Many larger HCOs have a secure employee compensation management system that enables managers to administer and monitor pay and benefits for all employees. These systems may also enable employees to monitor and (to some extent) control their own benefits selection and use.

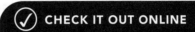 **CHECK IT OUT ONLINE**

The **US Department of Labor** offers much information about federal laws for pay and benefits. Its wages webpage (www.dol.gov/general/topic/wages) provides a wealth of information for employees and employers. Topics covered include labor laws related to wages, overtime pay, educational level and pay, record keeping and reporting, and more. This resource can help you be better informed as both an employee and a manager. Check it out online and see what you discover.

The value of employees' benefit packages in many HCOs exceeds 25 percent or even 30 percent of base pay (Clement, Curran, and Jahn 2015). Because employees often underestimate the value of their benefits, managers should provide data to staff showing the value of their benefits.

PROTECTING STAFF

Imagine how hard it would be for an HCO to achieve its mission and goals if employees stayed home because of an on-the-job accident, uncontrolled infection, job stress, low

⊖ **TRY IT, APPLY IT**

Suppose both you and one of your parents began working this year at a large for-profit pharmaceutical company. It offers a flexible cafeteria approach to employee benefits. List the top seven benefits you would choose. Then list the top seven benefits you think your parent would choose. How are the lists similar? Different? (Discuss this exercise with your parent if possible.)

morale, an abusive coworker, or an uncaring supervisor. In chapter 7, we defined *protecting staff* as the process of ensuring that employees have proper and safe working conditions, their rights are protected, and their opinions are considered by managers. When staffing an HCO, a manager must protect staff, which is the last of the seven staffing processes. Similar to other staffing processes, protecting workers helps an HCO maintain the workforce needed to achieve its mission and goals. The importance of this process is reflected in the shift toward protecting *employees* rather than *employers* (Fottler 2015).

Protection is especially important for a diverse workforce because employees and managers may have different beliefs, cultures, and behaviors. Thus, managers must set clear policies and model behaviors that will ensure appropriate working conditions, rights, and consideration of all workers. Some businesses have formed employee resource groups to support diverse groups of workers who have different cultures and lifestyles. The methods described in this chapter, and in later chapters on leadership and communication, can help you provide such support.

Employee protection is good for business for several reasons. First, it is required by the Occupational Safety and Health Act, by other laws, and by The Joint Commission, which accredits HCOs. Second, it can improve employee morale, productivity, and retention. Third, it helps an HCO become known as a safe place to work. Fourth, safety and health violations can become costly because of lost business, lawsuits, overtime wages to cover absent staff, employee resignations (and subsequent staff shortages, vacancies, and hiring expenses), and higher costs for liability insurance and employee health insurance.

Yet, in general, employee protection in HCOs is inadequate. They have high levels of workplace violence, burnout, bullying, and safety hazards (Fried 2015; McConnell 2018). Pause and think of the dangers in HCOs, especially large ones. They present physical hazards such as radiation, biological waste, potential for fires, injuries from lifting patients, infectious diseases, noise, dangerous equipment, repetitive motions, needle sticks, slippery floors, and workplace violence. Mental and emotional hazards include stress, hostility, privacy violations, and harassment (which can be based on race, gender, religion, age, disability, and other factors). Increasingly, workers bring their depression, anxiety, and stress to work with them. Some of it is caused by employers expecting workers to respond to after-hours e-mail and text messages. No wonder some HCOs have high turnover and vacancies.

Violence and burnout in HCOs require more discussion. "The healthcare field experiences higher rates of workplace violence than any other industry, according to the Occupational Safety and Health Administration" (Blouin 2017, 76). Patients—and their relatives and visitors—cause the most violence in HCOs; healthcare employees are the second most common cause (McConnell 2018). Managers must work to prevent such violence. The following actions can help (Blouin 2017; McConnell 2018):

- Having (and enforcing) a zero-tolerance policy

- Ensuring an organization culture of civility, respect for others, and inclusion

- Carefully assessing and screening job applicants

- Investigating and acting on warnings of violence

- Modifying buildings and work areas to increase security and prevent, detect, and control violence

- Training staff to prevent, recognize, and de-escalate violence

- Providing counseling and employee assistance programs to employees struggling with mental and behavioral health, substance abuse, and life crises

- Providing staff and others with a hotline to report threats, bullying, harassment, and potential violence

According to Swensen (2018), burnout of healthcare providers has become much too common and affects about half of the nurses and physicians in HCOs. Burned-out employees feel emotionally exhausted, cynical, detached, and isolated. They struggle to perform their jobs well. Managers can reduce burnout by addressing working conditions and human needs for camaraderie, trust, and passion for work (Swensen 2018). They can

- design organizations to support human needs,

- use participative management and servant leadership,

- remove obstacles that frustrate clinical staff who are trying to care for patients,

- be fair with and care for staff involved in an adverse patient event,

- sponsor inclusive staff gatherings and meals, and

- make wellness opportunities easily available.

Perlo and Feeley (2018, 85) go further and argue that HCOs must create more joy in work. An absence of burnout is not enough: "When people experience joy on the job, they have an intellectual, emotional, and behavioral commitment to meaningful and satisfying work." That enables HCOs to improve patient experience, customer satisfaction, safety, employee engagement, teamwork, productivity, and other goals.

Department managers and frontline supervisors are responsible for safety in their departments and work areas. Suppose Trevon manages an ambulatory surgery facility in Springfield that is owned by a healthcare system. He should monitor working conditions, lighting, ventilation, comfort, and security; arrange repair of broken equipment; report workplace accidents and injuries; arrange training on workplace safety; orient employees to policies needed for safety and protection; and include safety as part of annual performance appraisals. Trevon may be assisted when necessary by specialists from the healthcare system. They would have expertise in safety, security, infection control, employee health, plant engineering, human resources, maintenance, housekeeping, and other specialties. Smaller HCOs have fewer of these staff specialists and contract with consultants and external businesses for expertise when needed.

Working conditions include the workplace culture, and managers must not let it become toxic. Bullying behavior often is enabled by a very competitive culture that allows and even encourages rivalry to the point of bullying coworkers, subordinates, and others (Fried 2015). Managers can create a culture that safeguards employees and their rights and safety. Chapter 11 explores how to develop culture.

Employees in HCOs have rights at work determined by laws and court decisions that managers must follow (McConnell 2018). They have rights that pertain to speech, privacy, justice, nondiscrimination, and due process. These rights are limited in the workplace, however, just as rights are limited outside the workplace in society. **Managers (and employees) must try to balance the rights of one or more employees with the rights of others (e.g., patients, visitors, suppliers, other employees, and the HCO itself).** Thus, HCOs use electronic surveillance to deter and detect narcotics theft and to ensure handwashing technique is followed, even though this surveillance infringes on workers' privacy. Employers monitor internet use and e-mail at work (and sometimes social media outside of work). For some jobs in HCOs, managers require drug testing. Some businesses and HCOs apply surveillance, biometrics, and big-data analytics to workers to improve workplace safety, productivity, and proper use of supplies and equipment. Federal and state laws are struggling to keep up with rapidly evolving technology that affects the rights of employees, employers, and others.

An important right of workers is the opportunity to present work-related problems and grievances to managers and then have managers respond to those concerns. Effective managers make sure to do this. How? **Managers and the HR staff should establish multiple ways that workers can be heard and have their concerns addressed** (McConnell 2018; White and Griffith 2019). These may include

◆ policies supporting employees' rights;

◆ communication via open-door policies, suggestion boxes, and town hall meetings;

◆ formal written grievance procedures with prompt follow-up and resolution;

◆ visits by top managers to all departments, including on weekends and during second and third shifts if HCOs are staffed then;

◆ a disciplinary review board through which an employee may seek a review of disciplinary action;

◆ HR managers who present employees' views and concerns at management staff meetings and help managers consider how their potential decisions would affect the workforce;

◆ HR staff who assist employees in voicing individual concerns to management;

◆ sensitivity to and respect for people of diverse cultures and backgrounds;

◆ an employee ombudsman to investigate and resolve employees' complaints;

◆ an employee advisory council that meets regularly with managers; and

◆ supervisors and managers who genuinely care about their workers and manage that way.

What happens when employees believe managers have mistreated them, feel their rights are being violated, or think their concerns are being ignored? What happens when other staffing processes are not done well? Recall the discussion of labor unions in chapter 4. Employees might vote to join a labor union through which they will seek better jobs, work, rules, schedules, compensation, and other terms of employment. Their concerns will be heard. The union enables workers to join together and gain power as a group to collectively present concerns to managers and negotiate demands. Some people think workers join unions to gain better compensation. That is only part of the story. Workers also join unions for protection against perceived unfairness, humiliation, harassment, anxiety, insecurity, dangers, and managers who do not seem to care.

ONBOARDING

Onboarding is the process of "helping new hires adjust to social and performance aspects of their new jobs" (Noe et al. 2016, 307). The methods discussed throughout this chapter are used to onboard staff. Recall what you learned earlier about orientation of new employees, mentoring, training, feedback and performance appraisals, HR support, and managers listening to employees. All of those actions help to onboard new employees.

onboarding
The process of helping new hires adjust to social and performance aspects of their new jobs.

Onboarding goes beyond traditional orientation (Noe et al. 2016). It involves activities, learning, and interactions that should make a new employee feel more confident, engaged, and accepted by peers and supervisors. Suppose Georgina joins a physician group in Shreveport as a new medical biller. After onboarding, Georgina should better understand and fit in with her new roles, responsibilities, organization culture, and performance expectations at that physician group. Managers spread onboarding activities over several months (sometimes even a full year). Resources are provided, such as mentors, toolkits, tours, videos, meetings, social events, online discussion boards, social media, workshops, webinars, newsletters, and other materials. When done well, onboarding improves employee satisfaction, commitment, performance, and retention.

To make onboarding effective, managers should do it proactively and systematically. They should intentionally address four levels of onboarding (Noe et al. 2016, 307) from basic to complex:

1. *Compliance* is the most basic level and teaches employees the organization's basic rules, policies, and regulations.

2. *Clarification* ensures that employees fully understand their new job and all performance expectations.

3. *Culture* helps employees understand the organization's history, mission, values, and expected behaviors (formal and informal).

4. *Connection* helps employees develop interpersonal and work relationships.

Notice that these four levels of onboarding, combined, help new employees adjust to their new job and organization so they can perform their job well and fit in socially with coworkers.

ONE MORE TIME

Managers must staff their HCO to perform the HCO's work and achieve its mission and goals. They must obtain and retain people to perform jobs. While managers are responsible for these tasks, HR specialists often assist in staffing the HCO. The four staffing processes studied in this chapter are especially helpful for retaining employees: training and developing staff, appraising performance, compensating staff, and protecting staff. These processes affect each other and the three staffing processes discussed in chapter 7.

Training and developing staff enables employees to acquire new knowledge, skills, attitudes, behaviors, and competencies for current and future jobs. All employees in a manager's department need ongoing training and development, which begins with orientation and onboarding of new employees. To achieve lasting results, managers should follow a structured approach that addresses prioritized needs; has a clear purpose and objectives; uses appropriate content, methods, and instructors; is implemented effectively; and includes evaluation.

Appraising performance evaluates the job performance of workers and discusses those evaluations with the workers. In some HCOs, managers do an annual, formal, written appraisal for each employee. In other HCOs, more frequent, shorter appraisals are used. Throughout the year, all managers should informally monitor and give feedback to their workers. For the annual evaluation, a manager should obtain input from multiple sources during the year using valid questionnaires, checklists, interviews, and other sources of information. The appraisal must be discussed with the employee to share results and plan future goals. This discussion should focus on performance of the job (not personality) and on future performance (more than past performance). Managers and employees may feel uncomfortable about appraisals, so managers should prepare properly to make them more effective. Results guide future goals, training, compensation, and other aspects of staffing.

Compensating staff determines and gives wages, salaries, incentives, and benefits to workers. Managers decide on the compensation, and payroll and HR specialists help managers administer pay and benefits. Pay is largely based on the value of a job and prevailing rates of pay in labor markets. HCOs offer legally mandated benefits and a variety of voluntary benefits. Employees of different generations and backgrounds prefer different types of benefits. Many HCOs offer flexible benefit plans so that individual employees have some choice of benefits up to a preset dollar value. Managers and staff must carefully design pay and benefits to achieve internal and external equity.

Protecting staff ensures that workers have proper and safe working conditions, their rights are protected, and their opinions are considered by managers. Safety includes both physical and emotional safety. Workplace violence and bullying have become serious problems in HCOs, along with many other dangers. Employees should have their rights protected and be able to present concerns to managers. Without that, and without all the other staffing processes, managers may be unable to obtain and then retain sufficient workers. Further, workers may join a labor union and collectively bargain for better working conditions and employment.

Onboarding for new employees goes beyond traditional orientation to help them adjust to social and performance aspects of their new jobs. Over an extended period of time, onboarding combines elements of training, appraising, and protecting workers to improve their commitment, satisfaction, performance, and retention.

(T) **FOR YOUR TOOLBOX**

- Training checklist
- 360-degree evaluation
- Performance rating scales
- Performance appraisal meeting checklist
- Progressive discipline

- Point-factor system
- Internal equity and external equity
- Methods to ensure employees' concerns are heard
- Onboarding

FOR DISCUSSION

1. Discuss reasons that employees' training might not have lasting effects. How can managers ensure that training lasts?

2. Explain the pros and cons of 360-degree appraisals of employees.

3. Review exhibit 8.3, Performance Appraisal Meeting Checklist. Which items do you think would be most important for the person who is being appraised? Why?

4. Compare and contrast internal equity and external equity for employees' pay.

5. Describe the benefits you think would be preferred by workers in different generations. How do cafeteria benefit plans enable HCOs to satisfy workers with different benefit preferences?

6. Discuss rights that employees should have at work. What can managers do to ensure employees' rights are not ignored?

CASE STUDY QUESTIONS

These questions refer to the Integrative Case Studies at the back of this book.

1. Disparities in Care at Southern Regional Health System (SRHS) case: Using this chapter, explain how training, appraising, compensating, and protecting staff could be used to reduce disparities in care at SRHS.

2. "I Can't Do It All!" case: Using this chapter, explain how Mr. Brice could use the training, appraising, and compensating processes to increase and improve decision making by his vice presidents.

3. Increasing the Focus on Patient Safety at First Medical Center case: Using this chapter, explain how training, appraising, compensating, and protecting staff could support patient safety at First Medical Center.

4. Hospice Goes Hollywood case: In this case, Dr. Frank complained that the staff was not given adequate training. Use this chapter to describe how to train the clinicians to follow the new protocols for accreditation.

 RIVERBEND ORTHOPEDICS MINI CASE STUDY

Riverbend Orthopedics is a busy group practice with expanded services for orthopedic care. It has seven physicians and a podiatrist, plus about 70 other employees. At its big, new clinic building, Riverbend provides extensive orthopedic care. Several technicians provide diagnostic medical imaging, from basic X-rays to magnetic resonance images. The physicians perform surgery in their own outpatient surgery center with Riverbend's own operating nurses and technicians. Therapy is provided by three physical therapists and one part-time contracted occupational therapist. In addition to staff providing actual patient care, the clinic has staff for financial management, medical records, human resources, information systems/technology, building maintenance, and other administrative matters. Occasional marketing work is done by an advertising company. Legal work is outsourced to a law firm. Riverbend is managed by a new president, Ms. Garcia. She and Riverbend have set a goal of achieving "Excellent" ratings for patient experience from at least 90 percent of Riverbend's patients this year.

(continued)

RIVERBEND ORTHOPEDICS MINI CASE STUDY *(continued)*

Ms. Garcia believes in accountability. She thinks Riverbend should do more to hold employees accountable for their performance—especially as it pertains to patient experience. Yet, she also believes Riverbend Orthopedics must be accountable to employees for ensuring their safety and rights.

MINI CASE STUDY QUESTIONS

1. To help Riverbend achieve its goal, explain in detail how Ms. Garcia could apply performance appraisal methods from this chapter to evaluate the performance of all employees who have direct interaction with patients.

2. Based on information in this chapter, suggest at least five ways in which the Riverbend workplace might be unsafe or employees' rights might not be ensured. What could Ms. Garcia do to protect employees' safety and rights?

REFERENCES

Blouin, A. S. 2017. "Taking a Stand Against Workplace Violence." *Healthcare Executive* 32 (2): 76–79.

Clement, D. G., M. A. Curran, and S. L. Jahn. 2015. "Employee Benefits." In *Human Resources in Healthcare*, 4th ed., edited by B. J. Fried and M. D. Fottler, 321–49. Chicago: Health Administration Press.

Cummings, T. G., and C. G. Worley. 2015. *Organization Development and Change*, 10th ed. Stamford, CT: Cengage Learning.

Dunn, R. T. 2016. *Dunn and Haimann's Healthcare Management*, 10th ed. Chicago: Health Administration Press.

Dye, C. F. 2017. *Leadership in Healthcare,* 3rd ed. Chicago: Health Administration Press.

Fisher, A. 2016. "How to Give an Annual Performance Review (If You Must)." *Fortune.* Published December 19. http://fortune.com/2016/12/19/annual-performance-review/.

Fottler, M. D. 2015. "Strategic Human Resources Management." In *Human Resources in Healthcare*, 4th ed., edited by B. J. Fried and M. D. Fottler, 1–34. Chicago: Health Administration Press.

Fried, B. J. 2015. "Performance Management." In *Human Resources in Healthcare*, 4th ed., edited by B. J. Fried and M. D. Fottler, 235–73. Chicago: Health Administration Press.

Fried, B. J., and H. L. Smith. 2015. "Compensation Practices, Planning, and Challenges." In *Human Resources in Healthcare*, 4th ed., edited by B. J. Fried and M. D. Fottler, 275–320. Chicago: Health Administration Press.

Griffin, R. W., J. M. Phillips, and S. M. Gully. 2017. *Organizational Behavior: Managing People and Organizations*, 12th ed. Boston: Cengage Learning.

Kaye, D. L., and M. D. Fottler. 2015. "Organizational Development and Learning." In *Human Resources in Healthcare*, 4th ed., edited by B. J. Fried and M. D. Fottler, 351–88. Chicago: Health Administration Press.

Kivland, C. 2014. "Your Future Gets Brighter with Emotional Intelligence." *Healthcare Executive* 29 (1): 72–75.

Lynch, J. 2017. "The Three-Legged Stool: Why Safety, Quality, and Equity Depend on Each Other." *Journal of Healthcare Management* 62 (5): 298–301.

McConnell, C. R. 2018. *Umiker's Management Skills for the New Health Care Supervisor*, 7th ed. Burlington, MA: Jones & Bartlett Learning.

McSweeney-Feld, M. H., and N. Rubin. 2014. "Human Resource Considerations at the Top." In *New Leadership for Today's Health Care Professionals: Concepts and Cases,* edited by L. G. Rubino, S. J. Esparza, and Y. S. Reid-Chassiakos, 95–109. Burlington, MA: Jones & Bartlett Learning.

Noe, R., J. Hollenbeck, B. Gerhart, and P. Wright. 2016. *Human Resource Management: Gaining a Competitive Advantage,* 10th ed. Chicago: McGraw-Hill Higher Education.

Perlo, J., and D. Feeley 2018. "Why Focusing on Professional Burnout Is Not Enough." *Journal of Healthcare Management* 63 (2): 85–89.

Radick, L. E. 2016. "Improving the Patient Experience: Every Interaction Matters." *Healthcare Executive* 29 (1): 32–38.

Ryan, C. 2017. "Sustaining and Growing a Winning Culture." *Journal of Healthcare Management* 62 (6): 361–65.

Schawbel, D. 2017. "Workplace Trends You'll See in 2018." *Forbes*. Published November 1. www.forbes.com/sites/danschawbel/2017/11/01/10-workplace-trends-youll-see-in-2018/.

———. 2016. "Workplace Trends You'll See in 2017." *Forbes*. Published November 1. www.forbes.com/sites/danschawbel/2016/11/01/workplace-trends-2017/.

Swensen, S. J. 2018. "Esprit de Corps and Quality: Making the Case for Eradicating Burnout." *Journal of Healthcare Management* 63 (1): 7–11.

Wagner, K. 2017. "Harnessing the Strengths of a Multigenerational Workforce to Leverage Opportunities." *Healthcare Executive* 32 (6): 10–18.

Walston, S. L. 2017. *Organizational Behavior and Leadership in Healthcare: Leadership Perspectives and Management Applications*. Chicago: Health Administration Press.

White, K. R., and J. R. Griffith. 2019. *The Well-Managed Healthcare Organization*, 9th ed. Chicago: Health Administration Press.

CHAPTER 9

LEADING: THEORIES AND MODELS

The key to successful leadership today is influence, not authority.

Ken Blanchard, management author,
speaker, and consultant

LEARNING OBJECTIVES

Studying this chapter will help you to

➤ define leading and explain its relation to other management functions;

➤ examine, compare, and contrast leadership theories and models;

➤ identify practical tools and approaches for leading workers in organizations; and

➤ describe methods for leading physicians.

HERE'S WHAT HAPPENED

The Partners HealthCare board of directors hired a CEO to lead the organization. The board looked for someone with the necessary leadership traits, skills, and behaviors. The CEO then led thousands of employees to achieve the organization's vision and mission. Yet, the CEO was not the only manager who led. People in other top management jobs, such as executive vice president and chief information officer, also were leaders who used leadership theories, models, and methods to lead employees. So, too, did managers in middle and lower levels of the organization who led their own departments and workers. Throughout the organization—at all levels—managers influenced people to accomplish work, tasks, goals, mission, and vision. For example, achievement of one goal required staff to implement telehealth technology to monitor discharged hospital patients at home. Telehealth would help patients stay healthy and not have to be readmitted to the hospital. But some nurses resisted the "high-tech" approach because they favored their "high-touch" approach to patient care. Managers used leadership methods to influence the nurses and gain their support for telehealth. Leading was an essential part of what managers at all levels of Partners HealthCare did to achieve the organization's goals.

The opening Here's What Happened presents an example of leading in a healthcare organization (HCO). You know there are leaders at the top of an HCO, such as the CEO at Partners HealthCare. But did you know there are leaders in middle and lower levels of an HCO? As we learned in chapter 2, directing (also called leading) is one of the five main management functions, so it is something that all managers do. Management is the process of getting things done through and with people, and leading is part of that process. In chapter 2, we also learned about ten roles performed by managers. One of the roles is leader, in which the manager creates a vision and motivates others to work toward it.

Leading is part of being a manager, and all managers lead—that is the view this book takes. However, there are other points of view. Scholars, managers, and leaders have debated what *leadership* and *management* mean, how they are related, and who leads and manages. Considering many writings about leading and leadership, this book defines **leading** to be a process by which a person tries to influence someone else to voluntarily accomplish a task, goal, or vision.

Managers lead, and other people sometimes do, too. An occupational therapist may lead a nervous client in trying adaptive equipment after an accident. A health administration student may lead several other students to complete their group project.

This chapter is the first of three chapters on leading. It focuses on leading as part of management. Leading is defined and related to other management functions. We examine

leading
A process by which a person tries to influence someone else to voluntarily accomplish a task, goal, or vision.

various perspectives of leading, including trait theory; skill theory; behavior theory; contingency and situational theory; and theories X, Y, and Z. The chapter also explains how managers use other practical leadership theories and methods, including transactional, transformational, servant, collaborative, and competency-based leadership. Managers should lead physicians somewhat differently from the way they lead many other workers; this chapter suggests how to do that. In chapter 10, we will examine how managers motivate people, which is essential for leading. Then, in chapter 11, we will study how managers use organization culture and ethics to lead people in HCOs. Together, these three chapters will help you learn to lead others in HCOs. You can add the leadership tools from these chapters to your healthcare management toolbox.

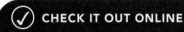

CHECK IT OUT ONLINE

Many ideas exist about what leadership is. Try Googling "what is leadership" and you'll get millions of results! You can find leadership definitions from leaders, scholars, famous people, and many others. Perhaps you will want to form your own definition. Check it out online and see what you discover.

How does leading connect to what we have already learned in this book? To sum up the book so far in 50 words or less: **First, managers *plan* the HCO's mission, vision, and goals. Second, they *organize* the HCO's tasks, jobs, and resources to achieve the plans. Third, they *staff* the HCO with people to do the jobs to achieve the plans. Fourth, they *lead* the people who staff the jobs to achieve the plans.** We see how the fourth management function—leading—connects to three other management functions. (Stay tuned, because in chapter 12 we will connect those to the fifth and final management function.)

THEORIES AND MODELS FOR LEADING

Scholars and managers have developed useful theories and models of leadership and leading. These help us understand how managers lead people. Consider some leaders throughout world history, business, government, sports, and society. No single theory fully explains all leaders or all aspects of leading. By examining multiple theories, we can more fully learn how to lead in organizations.

TRAIT THEORY AND SKILL THEORY

Research in the early part of the twentieth century examined traits and characteristics of leaders. Think about effective leaders you know from a job, club, sports team, or other activities. Which personal traits do you think enabled these people to lead? Early leadership *trait theory* suggested that effective leadership was associated with traits such as intelligence, extroversion, confidence, and energy (Griffin, Phillips, and Gully 2017). Later studies emphasized ambition, sociability, assertiveness, and adaptability. Hundreds of studies were done, but that research revealed inconsistent results and identified so many traits that little practical advice on leading could be found. Research shifted to other aspects of leadership. However, in recent years, leadership trait studies have reemerged, now focusing on emotional intelligence, integrity, self-confidence, and other traits.

Some traits (e.g., "Justine is decisive") can also be viewed from a skills perspective (e.g., "Justine has good decision-making skills"). Thus, skill theory emerged from trait theory to study skills and abilities for leading. Which skills do you think leaders need to influence others? Robert Katz determined that leaders need three types of skills (Dunn 2016):

1. Technical skills for working with things (e.g., making health products and services)

2. Conceptual skills for working with ideas (e.g., thinking of new goals)

3. Human skills for working with people (e.g., mentoring employees)

Do some leaders rely on one kind of skill more than another? Katz found that leading in high-level management positions requires more use of conceptual skills than technical skills. The opposite is true for leading in low-level positions. For leading in middle-level management jobs, both technical and conceptual skills are moderately important. Human skills (i.e., "people skills"), needed to influence others to achieve goals, are important for leading at all levels of management. In the Partners HealthCare case, conceptual skills would be especially important for the new CEO to conceive mission, vision, values, and long-range goals for the system. Technical, hands-on skills would be especially important for lower-level leaders, such as a pharmacy shift supervisor, to ensure that technical tasks are properly done. Human skills would be important at all levels of Partners HealthCare to influence others.

BEHAVIOR THEORY

Researchers next looked beyond leaders' traits and skills and studied their behaviors, actions, and conduct. Behavior theory examines leadership behavior (sometimes called *leadership style*) and how it influences leadership effectiveness. Rather than study the traits and skills a leader *has*, this theory looks at what a leader *does*—how she behaves or how she conducts herself. When you are a leader in healthcare, which behaviors will you use? How will you conduct yourself? Suppose you are a middle-level manager at a health information technology company in St. Paul. Your management team decides it must relocate to a bigger office building. Which behaviors would you use to lead (influence) your employees to support relocation?

Leadership studies at Ohio State in the mid-1900s helped to develop behavior theory (Griffin, Phillips, and Gully 2017). This research examined two dimensions of leader behavior:

1. *Consideration behavior:* A leader considers the workers and their concerns, ideas, and feelings. The leader–worker relationship is characterized by mutual trust, communication, and respect.

2. *Initiating structure behavior:* A leader initiates work, tasks, and structure to complete jobs and achieve goals. The leader establishes clear roles, expectations, and communication channels for the leader and the workers.

The Ohio State studies rated leaders as *high* or *low* for each dimension, which created four types of leaders:

◆   Low initiating structure / Low consideration

◆   Low initiating structure / High consideration

◆   High initiating structure / Low consideration

◆   High initiating structure / High consideration

Behavior theory was further developed by similar studies that investigated which leadership behaviors were associated with the greatest employee satisfaction, job performance, goal achievement, and other effectiveness outcomes.

Pop quiz: In leadership behavior studies, which leadership style do you think was most effective?

a.   Low initiating structure / Low consideration

b.   Low initiating structure / High consideration

c.   High initiating structure / Low consideration

d.   High initiating structure / High consideration

It seems like High initiating structure / High consideration would be a good approach. But recall contingency theory from chapter 2. Maybe we need to add another answer choice: "It depends"!

Further research on leaders' behavior was done by Blake and Mouton (1964). This research, like the Ohio State studies, used two dimensions: *production orientation* and

EXHIBIT 9.1

The Managerial Grid

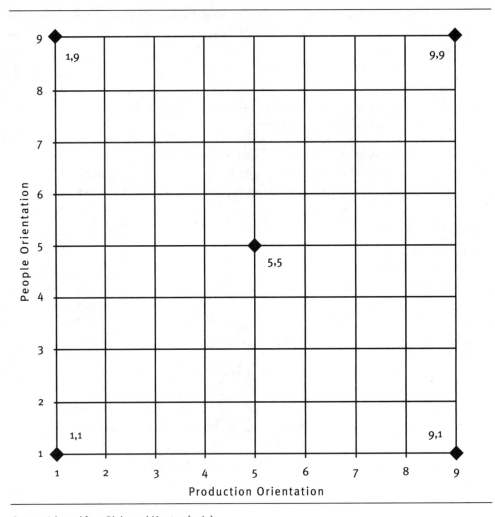

Source: Adapted from Blake and Mouton (1964).

people orientation (Griffin, Phillips, and Gully 2017). Leaders were rated from 1 (low) to 9 (high) for each dimension. These orientations (leadership styles) created a managerial (or leadership) grid as shown in exhibit 9.1.

The researchers who developed the managerial grid conceived the same four leadership styles as the Ohio State studies, and they added a fifth style in the middle:

◆ Low production orientation / Low people orientation (1,1): Impoverished style

◆ Low production orientation / High people orientation (1,9): Country club style

◆ High production orientation / Low people orientation (9,1): Authoritarian style

- High production orientation / High people orientation (9,9): Team leader style

- Middle production orientation / Middle people orientation (5,5): Middle-of-the-road style

Leaders who use one of the four corner styles in exhibit 9.1 would lead as follows (Esparza and Rubino 2014, 10):

- (1,1) *Impoverished style*—is detached and uncommitted to work or workers, lets workers do whatever, "delegates and disappears"

- (1,9) *Country club style*—uses rewards and recognition to encourage workers, avoids authority and discipline, maintains positive relationships with workers

- (9,1) *Authoritarian style*—is tough on workers, expects workers to get work done no matter what, not interested in workers' input, doesn't want dissent, expects loyalty

- (9,9) *Team leader style*—leads by example, helps workers achieve their highest potential, promotes goal achievement, develops close relationships among workers

The (5,5) middle-of-the-road style is in between the four corner styles—it includes some characteristics of each.

The managerial grid model was developed long ago, and organizations today still use it to guide leaders' behavior. Many managers seem to like it and think it works well. Leaders do not have to exactly fit one of the five styles—they can be anywhere on the grid. The team leader style is often considered to be the best way to lead. However, while behavioral studies show the importance of leaders' behaviors, the studies are not complete enough to provide universal recommendations for how to lead (Griffin, Phillips, and Gully 2017). As is true for the Ohio State studies, no single style always leads to the best outcomes. Apparently, something else affects the results. What could it be? Read on.

SITUATIONAL THEORY

By the early 1960s, scholars and leaders realized that the trait, skill, and behavior theories of leadership did not fully explain leadership effectiveness (Griffin, Phillips, and Gully 2017). Furthermore, they realized there was no universal best way to lead. Organizations and people are too complicated for that. The best leadership approach seemed to vary from situation to situation and from person to person. That is, the best approach was **contingent**—it depended on something.

contingent
Dependent on something.

This realization led to situational leadership research and a variety of situational theories of leadership. Different situations (contingencies) need different leadership styles. According to researchers, these contingencies included the following (Dye 2017; Griffin, Phillips, and Gully 2017; Walston 2017):

1. Characteristics of the leader (e.g., skills, traits, behaviors, earned trust, power to reward)

2. Characteristics of the followers (e.g., skills, traits, behaviors, motivation, relationship with leader)

3. Characteristics of the situation (e.g., clarity of goals, work to be done, urgency)

As an example, imagine an extroverted leader in a primary care patient-centered medical home in Aurora. The leader likes to chat with the employees (followers). This sounds like a good idea; after all, leaders should be friendly and get to know their employees (followers). However, such a style might not work equally well with all employees. Why? Because the best style is contingent on characteristics of the followers. An extroverted style would likely work well with extroverted followers. It would not work as well with introverted followers; with them, the leader could adjust to a less chatty style.

How about a contingency example based on the situation? A personal care home leader might ordinarily prefer thoughtful group discussions to lead staff to collaboratively make team decisions. However, if the building is on fire and the fire alarm is blaring, the leader will likely use a more direct, take-charge style.

Several situational leadership models are available to guide managers when they lead employees. One is the Hersey and Blanchard situational model. It was created as a consulting tool and is popular with practicing managers (Griffin, Phillips, and Gully 2017). The model calls for a leader to adjust behavior to fit with a subordinate worker's readiness to work. "Readiness refers to the subordinate's degree of motivation, competence, experience, and interest in accepting responsibility" (Griffin, Phillips, and Gully 2017, 437). Readiness can also be described as "the ability and willingness to accomplish a specific task" (Ledlow and Johnson 2019, 69). As a worker's readiness for a task increases, the manager should adjust the leadership style. If a subordinate worker has low readiness for a task, then the manager's *task-oriented behavior* (i.e., task direction, production orientation) should start high. As the worker's readiness increases, the leader can reduce task behavior and follow an inverse relationship with readiness. Simultaneously, the manager should adjust *relationship behavior* (i.e., support, people orientation) toward the subordinate as readiness to perform the task increases (Dye 2017; Griffin, Phillips, and Gully 2017):

◆ If a subordinate has *low readiness*, the manager uses a "telling style" of high task emphasis and low relationship emphasis, stating a clear, firm direction and defined roles.

◆ If a subordinate has *low to moderate readiness*, the manager uses a "selling style" of high task emphasis and high relationship emphasis, giving the subordinate direction and identifying roles, plus offering information and explanation for persuasion.

◆ If a subordinate has *moderate to high readiness*, the manager uses a "participating style" of low task emphasis and high relationship emphasis, giving little direction and allowing the subordinate to join in making decisions.

◆ If a subordinate has *high readiness*, the manager uses a "delegating style" of low task emphasis and low relationship emphasis, enabling the subordinate to work independently without much supervision.

The bottom line: "People in leadership and management positions become more effective when they use a leadership style that is appropriate to the developmental level of the individual or group they want to influence" (Ledlow and Johnson 2019, 70). One size does not fit all! Each of the four styles is useful and appropriate for a particular set of contingencies.

Research and practice indicate that managers should develop a mix of leadership styles, such as those in the managerial (leadership) grid and those in the Hersey and Blanchard situational model. You can also develop the ability to assess yourself, your followers, and situations. Emotional intelligence will help with that; it is discussed in chapter 15. Based on those assessments, you can decide which style of leading to use with specific followers and situations. Returning to the grid in exhibit 9.1, perhaps leaders like this tool because it helps them deliberately ask themselves, For the leadership situation I now face, where should I be on the grid? How much should I use a people orientation and how much should I use a production orientation? This approach to leading cannot be developed in a semester of study or a year of work. Experience and trial-and-error are necessary. Everyone makes mistakes,

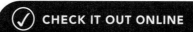 **CHECK IT OUT ONLINE**

Employers sometimes use personality tests to learn more about their employees. These tests also can help you assess yourself, which is needed for the situational theory approach to leading. A commonly used assessment is DiSC, which measures a person's levels of dominance, influence, steadiness, and conscientiousness. Another popular test is the Myers-Briggs Type Indicator, which measures attitudes, functions, and lifestyles. You can learn more about these assessments at www.discprofile.com and www.myersbriggs.org. Check it out online and see what you discover.

and we can learn from them. Good role models and mentors can help too, so choose role models and find mentors to help you develop your leadership styles.

Theory X, Theory Y, and Theory Z

Research by Douglas McGregor led him to believe that leaders hold one of two different views of people and workers. These two contrasting views—known as **Theory X** and **Theory Y**—are summarized in exhibit 9.2.

Theory X
Leader assumes people dislike work, are lazy and stupid, are motivated by rewards from others, lack self-discipline, want security, and do not want responsibility.

These two views are important for contingencies, leadership, and how managers influence workers. A biotech genetics company manager who views people from a Theory X perspective would influence employees (followers) with an *autocratic* style of close oversight, distrust, coercion, monetary rewards, minimal communication, and unilateral decision making. In the same company (situation) with the same employees (followers), a manager with a Theory Y perspective would influence employees with a *consultative/participative* style of loose oversight, trust, open communication, shared decisions, freedom, self-direction, and personal development rewards. The two leadership styles depend on the leader's view (Theory X or Theory Y) and are summarized in exhibit 9.3.

Theory Y
Leader assumes people like meaningful work, are creative and capable, are motivated by rewards from within themselves, have self-control, can direct themselves, and want responsibility.

Theory Y managers assess contingencies that may affect how they manage, lead, and influence workers (Ledlow and Johnson 2019). Based on particular contingencies, these managers might alter their usual approach to influencing workers. For example, previously we learned that time urgency and a worker's low readiness are contingencies that affect how managers influence workers. After considering contingencies, a Theory Y manager may shift to a more authoritarian style for a particular situation or worker. In contrast, Theory

Exhibit 9.2
Theory X and Theory Y Assumptions

Theory X assumes people	Theory Y assumes people
• dislike work	• like meaningful work
• are lazy and stupid	• are creative and capable
• are motivated extrinsically (by rewards from other people)	• are motivated intrinsically (by rewards from within themselves)
• lack self-discipline and must be directed	• have self-control and can direct themselves
• want security and do not want change	• want to contribute and participate
• do not want (and avoid) responsibility	• want (and seek) responsibility

Sources: Dunn (2016); Ledlow and Johnson (2019); Walston (2017).

EXHIBIT 9.3
Leadership Style
Based on Theory X
and Theory Y

Autocratic Leadership Based on Theory X	Consultative/Participative Leadership Based on Theory Y
• Tight supervision, close oversight	• Loose general supervision, self-direction
• Distrust	• Trust
• Decisions made unilaterally by manager	• Decisions shared by manager and workers
• Minimal involvement of workers	• Extensive involvement of workers
• Limited, top-down communication	• Open, frequent, two-way communication
• Coercion, externally controlled rewards	• Internal rewards from the work and job

Sources: Dunn (2016); Ledlow and Johnson (2019); Walston (2017).

X managers are more rigid and thus are unlikely to consider contingencies or adjust their leadership style (Ledlow and Johnson 2019).

Theory Z emerged in the late 1970s and was further developed through the work of William Ouchi in the 1980s. This approach emphasizes concern for workers and strives to develop long-term, cooperative relationships among workers, peers, and the organization (Dunn 2016). It assumes that workers want close, supportive working relationships with other workers, including supervisors and subordinates. Supervisors influence workers using trust and teamwork while avoiding fear and reprisal. Growth opportunities for workers are important but are developed more slowly and deeply in Theory Z than in Theory Y. Individual responsibility is important, as is collective responsibility for coworkers and the organization. Theory Z seeks lasting employment and relationships with workers, which discourages the short-term job-hopping common among some workers and organizations.

Theory Z
Leader emphasizes concern for workers, develops long-term cooperative relationships, provides slow yet steady long-term growth opportunities for workers, and promotes individual and collective responsibility.

TRANSACTIONAL AND TRANSFORMATIONAL LEADERSHIP

Leadership has commonly been viewed from a transactional perspective, in which the leader transacts a deal with the followers: You perform tasks and comply with rules to help achieve the organization's goals, and I will give you pay, benefits, and other rewards. That's the deal, and it can be a win–win situation for everyone. Did you experience this type of leadership when you were young, with a parent transacting deals with you for home chores and compliance with rules? Managers often make these types of deals, influencing workers by giving or withholding rewards. Many organizations have **transactional leadership**, and followers go along with it. But the deals tend to maintain the status quo. This way of leading is not inspirational for achieving great change and excellence.

An alternative is **transformational leadership**, which was begun by James Burns in the late 1970s and further developed by Bernard Bass. Leaders who use this approach do not transact deals with followers (employees) based on self-interests. Instead, leaders strive to inspire and influence workers by appealing to higher-level human needs of self-actualization and fulfillment (Walston 2017). Whereas transactional leaders tend to maintain the existing way of doing things, transformational leaders challenge the existing way and influence workers to change and revitalize the organization—sometimes radically!

Earlier, we learned about the trait, skill, and behavior theories of leadership. Which traits, skills, and behaviors do you think are needed for transformational leadership? What would a leader need to inspire others, challenge the status quo, and lead followers to transform an HCO to higher levels of performance? Take a few minutes to brainstorm and jot down your ideas. Then read what several writers emphasize (Elkins, Melton, and Hall 2014; Ledlow and Johnson 2019; Walston 2017):

- ◆ *Charisma*—provides a vision and purpose, develops pride, earns respect and trust

- ◆ *Inspiration*—clearly and simply communicates purpose and expectations, focuses efforts

- ◆ *Intelligence*—promotes rational thinking, careful problem solving, and use of intellect

- ◆ *Individual consideration*—coaches, advises, gives personal attention to each employee

Transformational leaders are guided by their organization's mission, vision, and values, and they communicate those often to workers. Influence comes from a transformational leader's charismatic emotional appeal, intellectual stimulation, and supportive concern for individual workers. Walston (2017) emphasizes that influence comes from creating a vision that inspires others. People who follow transformational leaders admire, respect, and trust the leader. As a result, the workers transcend their own self-interests in favor of their group's interests, goals, and "the greater good." Transformational leaders know their employees as unique individuals, interact with them in their work settings, teach and mentor them individually, share the future vision with them and explain how to achieve it, and look for ways to enable each of them to become more self-fulfilled and satisfied. With so much support, workers develop loyalty, respect, and admiration for the transformational

transactional leadership
Leadership based on transactions; workers perform tasks to achieve goals and then the leader gives workers pay and other rewards.

transformational leadership
Leadership that uses a compelling vision, inspiration, charisma, intelligence, and attention to employees' individual needs to revitalize an organization with change for the greater good of all.

leaders and the organization. Workers want to help the organization succeed because they feel they are contributing to something important. All of this motivates employees to work hard to achieve the organization's mission, vision, and values, which in turn leads them to feel more fulfilled.

Transformational leadership has the potential to influence each employee (and an entire HCO) to grow and achieve great (rather than merely good) performance. "Healthcare today requires strong transformational leaders" to advance HCOs amid rapid change and uncertainty (Walston 2017, 145). This kind of leading does not happen easily—it takes dedicated hard work!

SERVANT LEADERSHIP

The **servant leadership** style emerged in the 1970s and has gained many advocates (Dye 2017). It is similar to transformational leadership because both are concerned with followers. However, servant leadership emphasizes that a leader should *serve* the followers (not just be concerned about them). A servant leader empowers workers (followers) by sharing power, information, and autonomy with them. Then the servant leader unselfishly respects, listens to, responds to, helps, reassures, teaches, supports, connects with, celebrates, and is a role model for the workers (followers). The servant leader serves followers by understanding and respecting their views, giving them necessary resources, meeting their needs, providing nonblaming performance feedback, and helping them grow with opportunities to succeed (Dye 2017; Ledlow and Johnson 2019; White and Griffith 2019). This approach requires humility, and many organizations are searching for humble leaders (Kaissi 2017). Servant leaders create a bottom-up approach that delegates more power and control to followers than top-down leaders would delegate. These leaders expect their approach to favorably influence workers' morale, goal achievement, and development for future management positions.

Dye (2017) believes that servant leadership is needed in healthcare, which is supposed to be altruistic. Walston (2017), on the other hand, feels it may be hard to practice servant leadership because rewards and incentives (from traditional leadership styles) may motivate leaders toward self-interest and self-promotion instead of selfless service. Yet, servant leadership is in fact practiced in HCOs and can be effective, as shown in the Using Chapter 9 in the Real World sidebar. Both of the HCOs in the sidebar have earned the prestigious Malcolm Baldrige National Quality Award.

COLLABORATIVE LEADERSHIP

Collaborative leadership is used to form alliances, partnerships, and other forms of interorganization relationships. This type of leadership has become—and will continue to be—essential for healthcare managers. Recall from chapter 1 the trend of hospitals, medical

> **servant leadership**
> Leadership style that emphasizes that a leader should serve the followers by respecting, empowering, hearing, teaching, and supporting workers and helping them succeed.

> **collaborative leadership**
> Leadership used to form alliances, partnerships, and other forms of interorganization relationships.

USING CHAPTER 9 IN THE REAL WORLD

Senior leaders of Mercy Health System (now part of Mercy/Rockford Health System in Wisconsin and Illinois) adopted a servant leadership philosophy. The leaders believe that when they give excellent service to Mercy's partners (workers), those partners give excellent service to Mercy's customers. The leaders inverted a top-down management style and instead became facilitators, serving those who serve patients (White and Griffith 2019).

Jayne E. Pope, FACHE, a registered nurse and CEO of Hill Country Memorial Hospital in Fredericksburg, Texas, leads by serving and empowering staff and patients. "We need to remove any obstacles standing in the way of medical staff, nurses, and other care providers so that those at the point of service can provide the highest-quality care," she says (Kash 2016, 308). "My mantra is to make heroes out of others" and "highlight the work of team members" (Kash 2016, 308). She communicates with team members so they have the information they need to make their own decisions. The hospital's vision is "empower others, create healthy," and Pope does that as a leader. This leadership approach has helped the hospital consistently deliver exceptional patient experience that rated in the 97th percentile of the Hospital Consumer Assessment of Healthcare Providers and Systems survey (Kash 2016).

groups, insurers, ambulatory clinics, long-term care companies, community agencies, and other HCOs forming more mergers, alliances, networks, integrated delivery systems, accountable care organizations, patient-centered medical homes, and other collaborative structures.

Collaborative leadership is complex because it involves influencing people from multiple organizations toward a common purpose. For example, to improve population health in a community, many organizations (including public schools and government agencies) may try to form a community health alliance to work together to reduce health risks in the community. Someone who leads the formation of the alliance would not have direct control or authority over all the organizations and people. A collaborative leader must influence people from other organizations who are likely to have different goals, cultures, management styles, attitudes, assumptions, knowledge, constraints, awareness of problems, and commitments (Borkowski and Deppman 2014). Some of these organizations may be competitors vying for each other's resources, customers, market share, and revenue. Can somebody lead this group toward a common purpose?

Yes, it can be done—by using the collaborative leadership style. A leader needs specific skills, traits, and competencies for collaborative leading. The transformational leadership and servant leadership styles are often equated with the collaborative leadership style because they use similar skills and behaviors. Additional competencies are also important for collaborative leadership. These leaders must be able to manage conflict, coordinate teams, create trust, share power, share credit, work with people over whom they do not have authority, apply political skills, and use emotional intelligence. Patience is a virtue because life in the collaboration lane is usually slow.

AUTHENTIC LEADERSHIP AND ETHICAL LEADERSHIP

In the early part of the twenty-first century, two approaches to leading emerged that include much of transformational leadership and servant leadership. In these two new approaches—authentic leadership and ethical leadership—leading is based on values, morals, and the fair and trustworthy personal actions and interactions that leaders demonstrate (Walston 2017). Leaders, managers, and scholars are likely to continue developing these two approaches.

LEADERSHIP COMPETENCY MODELS

A final approach to leading, based on competencies, also emerged early in the twenty-first century and has gained support. "Leadership competencies are a set of professional and personal skills, knowledge, values, and traits that guide a leader's performance, behavior, interaction, and decisions" (Dye and Garman 2015, xiii). This approach may remind you of the earlier research on leadership traits, skills, and behaviors. Today, the healthcare management profession uses several competency models to lead healthcare organizations.

The Healthcare Leadership Alliance (HLA), comprising the American College of Healthcare Executives (ACHE) and several other healthcare professional associations, developed a competency model of leadership with five broad domains. "When it was first published in 2005, the HLA Competency Directory was a landmark effort to identify the competencies that were important across diverse professional roles within healthcare management. It contained 232 competencies that were common to all the professions participating in its development as well as another 68 competencies that were specific to certain disciplines within healthcare management" (HLA 2010).

From this, ACHE developed its Healthcare Executive Competencies Assessment Tool, which is used to assess expertise in a subset of common management and leadership competencies. This tool includes competencies in five domains: communication and relationship management, leadership, professionalism, knowledge of the healthcare environment, and business skills and knowledge (HLA and ACHE 2018).

TRY IT, APPLY IT

Use what you have learned in this chapter to describe your usual leadership style (which might change sometimes because of contingencies). Apply the leadership theories and models to yourself while you reflect on your past experiences with leading. Think about how you led a club, team, or group of students. Which skills, traits, and behaviors did you use? Which theories and models of leadership did your leadership style seem to follow? After some thought, write a paragraph or two describing your usual leadership style.

Another healthcare management competency model is the Dye–Garman model. It uses 16 competencies in four domains—self-awareness, vision, execution, and people—that are essential for exceptional leadership (Dye and Garman 2015). Finally, the National Center for Healthcare Leadership (NCHL 2018) health leadership competency model 3.0 includes 28 core competencies. These are grouped into four action competency domains (transformation, execution, relations, and boundary spanning) and three enabling competency domains (health system awareness and business literacy, self-awareness and self-development, and values).

LEADING PHYSICIANS

Do you remember (from chapters 4 and 5) that managing physicians involves special considerations and approaches? Physicians, and some other highly professional workers, expect a great degree of autonomy without managerial oversight. Physicians expect managers to respect and defer to their professional medical expertise. This expectation is one way physicians (and some other patient care professionals) think and behave differently from managers. These differences arise from differences in education, professional norms, job purpose, and other factors. Exhibit 9.4 examines managers and physicians in relation to several important factors. The information reflects broad generalities that do not apply to every manager, physician, and HCO. However, it does offer useful insights for managers who lead physicians.

As exhibit 9.4 shows, in general **physicians think and behave differently than managers do.** This understanding is important because physicians and HCO managers are interdependent. Contingency theory reminds us that the best style for leading depends on the leader, followers, and situation. When the followers are physicians, managers should adjust their style of leading to what works well with physicians. (This can be taken a step further by adjusting to specific physicians because they are not all alike.) Some managers

Factor	Managers	Physicians
Authority	Organizational, legitimate, expert; shared or individual	Professional, expert; individual
Responsibility	Individual and group	Mostly individual
Work relationships	Hierarchical, bureaucratic, group	Peer, collegial
Allegiance, loyalty	To the organization	To patients and clients
Decisions	Deliberative, uses input from others, based on consensus	Quick, based on own judgment
Resources	Viewed as limited, must be used wisely	Assume resources will be available
Patient focus	Groups and populations of patients	Usually one patient at a time
Time frame	Ranges from now to years in the future	Now, today, this week, short-term
Dealing with uncertainty	Accepted as part of the job	Expects more certainty
Feedback received	Sporadic, vague	Specific, frequent
Responsiveness	To patients, families, physicians, board members, employees, accreditors, other stakeholders	To patients, families, physicians, other patient care team members
Compensation	Salary	Shifting from pay per patient/procedure to value-based payment

Exhibit 9.4
Differences Between Managers and Physicians

Sources: Data from Dunn (2016); Dye (2017); Walston (2017); Welch (2010); White and Griffith (2019).

have created problems (and even derailed careers) by trying to lead physicians the same way they lead the general workforce. Here are suggestions for managers who are trying to lead physicians. (These ideas may also be useful when leading other types of professional healthcare workers.)

◆   Realize how your view of healthcare and your HCO may differ from that of physicians. Work to understand their views, concerns, language, culture, and behaviors.

◆ Create structures and opportunities for physicians to be heard (formally and informally). Be a good listener.

◆ Minimize the use of formal authority based on position, bureaucratic rules, and organization hierarchy.

◆ When appropriate, let physician leaders and the physician peer review process lead physicians.

◆ Develop and maintain contact with physicians. Be known by them and accessible to them.

◆ Understand and strive to meet physicians' professional needs.

◆ Respect physicians' time; avoid scheduling unnecessary meetings.

◆ Show how your ideas will help physicians and their patients, but avoid simply claiming everything you want is "good for patient care."

◆ Develop trusting relationships with a few key physicians who can help you understand other physicians, explain your ideas to other physicians, and help you work with specific physicians.

◆ Use data that can be easily understood and easily judged as valid and reliable.

◆ Acknowledge and respect physicians' medical expertise in medical matters; point out your managerial expertise in management matters.

◆ Explain yourself to physicians who may misinterpret your ideas and actions.

In recent years, healthcare systems and hospitals have increasingly hired physicians for high-level management and administrative leadership positions. Demand for them has greatly expanded and exceeds supply. This is a result of developments described in chapter 1, such as clinical integration, payment based on clinical outcomes, and population health. Although some of these jobs are directly responsible for medical affairs, others are more generally administrative—including CEO positions. After someone has studied, trained, and practiced as a physician for years, management development and executive coaching can help that person shift focus and prepare for a high-level management position such as CEO or chief operating officer. When physicians understand and embrace managerial thinking and behaviors, they can help managers and physicians throughout an HCO understand each other and collaborate toward the HCO's goals. Physicians in management jobs help other managers understand physicians and vice versa.

ONE MORE TIME

Leading is influencing. It is a process by which a person tries to influence someone else to voluntarily accomplish a task, goal, or vision. Leading is one of the five management functions, and thus it is performed at all management levels in an HCO. It has been studied for more than a century by examining traits, skills, and behaviors of leaders.

A common behavioral approach to leading looks at how much leaders focus on getting tasks and goals done and how much they focus on employees and their needs. Managers may use a managerial grid to judge how much their leadership should focus on completing tasks and on employees' needs. When managers have to lead, they may apply the Hersey and Blanchard situational model of leading to assess the situation and assess the people to be led (followers). Based on those contingencies, managers choose a style of leading that puts the appropriate amount of focus on tasks and on employees' needs. Therefore, managers should develop a range of styles for leading, assess contingencies (people and situation), and then adjust their leadership style to fit the people and situation.

Other perspectives further explain how managers lead. Managers tend to use a style of leading that fits their assumptions about people—Theory X or Theory Y. Theory Z emphasizes concern for workers and strives to develop long-term, cooperative relationships among workers, peers, and the organization. Transactional behavior by leaders tends to maintain the status quo. With healthcare in a constant state of change, healthcare managers often must lead change. Transformational leadership is effective for leading change, and it is done through a compelling vision, inspiration, charisma, intelligence, and attention to employees' individual needs. This type of leadership enables leaders to revitalize an organization with change for the greater good of all. Managers may also use servant leadership, by which a leader serves workers by respecting, empowering, hearing, teaching, and supporting them and helping them succeed. Collaborative leadership is used to form alliances, partnerships, and other interorganization relationships. Authentic leadership, ethical leadership, and competency-based leadership have emerged in the twenty-first century as new approaches for leading people in healthcare and HCOs. When leading physicians, managers must realize they think differently from physicians about important work-related factors. Physicians expect professional autonomy based on their extensive medical education and training.

People can learn, develop, and improve their leadership. During their careers, leaders should develop a mix of leadership styles and be flexible. Then they can assess contingencies and use the style that is best for themselves, their followers, and their situations.

FOR YOUR TOOLBOX

- Trait theory
- Skills theory
- Behavior theory
- Managerial (leadership) grid
- Situational leadership
- Hersey Blanchard model
- Theory X and Theory Y
- Theory Z

- Transactional and transformational leadership
- Servant leadership
- Collaborative leadership
- Leadership competency models
- Differences between managers and physicians

FOR DISCUSSION

1. How did your understanding of leading and leadership evolve while reading this chapter?

2. This chapter explained trait theory, skill theory, behavior theory, situational (contingency) theory, Theory X, Theory Y, Theory Z, transactional leadership, transformational leadership, servant leadership, and collaborative leadership. Which of these theories and approaches do you think you will most likely use in your career? Why?

3. How do contingencies affect leading? Give examples to illustrate your answer.

4. Describe how physicians and managers differ in their work-related perspectives. Considering these differences, what steps could managers use to lead physicians?

CASE STUDY QUESTIONS

These questions refer to the Integrative Case Studies at the back of this book.

1. Disparities in Care at Southern Regional Health System case: Mr. Hank wants to reduce disparities in care at Southern Regional. To do this, should he use situational

theory, transformational theory, or some other approach to leading? Justify your answer using information from the case study and this chapter.

2. Hospice Goes Hollywood case: Using information from this chapter and the case study, explain how Ms. Thurmond should lead Dr. Frank to help achieve Joint Commission accreditation. Which leadership theories or models should she use?

3. I Can't Do It All case: Use leadership theories, concepts, and models from this chapter to describe Mr. Brice's leadership style.

4. Increasing the Focus on Patient Safety at First Medical Center case: Why might the transformational leadership approach be appropriate for Dr. Frame to use? Using information from this chapter and the case study, describe specific steps and actions she should take while using transformational leadership.

5. Rocky Road to Patient Satisfaction at Leonard-Griggs case: Ms. Ratcliff wants to implement patient satisfaction surveys at the five physician practice sites. Refer to the managerial grid in exhibit 9.1. Where on the grid (i.e., how production oriented and how people oriented) should she be to lead the clinics' employees to perform the survey work? Justify your answer.

🔍 RIVERBEND ORTHOPEDICS MINI CASE STUDY

Riverbend Orthopedics is a busy group practice with expanded services for orthopedic care. It has seven physicians and a podiatrist, plus about 70 other employees. At its big, new clinic building, Riverbend provides extensive orthopedic care. Several technicians provide diagnostic medical imaging, from basic X-rays to magnetic resonance images. The physicians perform surgery in their own outpatient surgery center with Riverbend's own operating nurses and technicians. Therapy is provided by three physical therapists and one part-time contracted occupational therapist. In addition to staff providing actual patient care, the clinic has staff for financial management, medical records, human resources, information systems/technology, building maintenance, and other administrative matters. Occasional marketing work is done by an advertising company. Legal work is outsourced to a law firm. Riverbend is managed by a new president, Ms. Garcia. She and Riverbend have set a goal of achieving "Excellent" ratings for patient experience from at least 90 percent of Riverbend's patients this year.

(continued)

RIVERBEND ORTHOPEDICS MINI CASE STUDY *(continued)*

Ms. Garcia knows that merely setting the goal will not achieve it—she must lead the staff to achieve it. The board has told her that funds will be available to support what is needed to reach the goal. She begins to think about various leadership theories and models.

MINI CASE STUDY QUESTION

1. Using information from this case and chapter, describe how Ms. Garcia should lead to achieve the patient experience goal. How should she lead Dr. Barr, Dr. Chen, and other physicians? How should she lead other staff? Which leadership theories and models should she use? Why? You may make (and state) additional reasonable assumptions about Riverbend Orthopedics.

REFERENCES

Blake, R. R., and J. S. Mouton. 1964. *The Managerial Grid: The Key to Leadership Excellence.* Houston, TX: Gulf Publishing.

Borkowski, N., and B. P. Deppman. 2014. "Collaborative Leadership." In *New Leadership for Today's Health Care Professionals: Concepts and Cases,* edited by L. G. Rubino, S. J. Esparza, and Y. S. R. Chassiakos, 193–203. Burlington, MA: Jones & Bartlett Learning.

Dunn, R. T. 2016. *Dunn and Haimann's Healthcare Management,* 10th ed. Chicago: Health Administration Press.

Dye, C. F. 2017. *Leadership in Healthcare,* 3rd ed. Chicago: Health Administration Press.

Dye, C. F., and A. N. Garman. 2015. *Exceptional Leadership: 16 Critical Competencies for Healthcare Executives,* 2nd ed. Chicago: Health Administration Press.

Elkins, E., J. Melton, and M. Hall. 2014. "Transformational Leadership." In *New Leadership for Today's Health Care Professionals: Concepts and Cases,* edited by L. G. Rubino, S. J. Esparza, and Y. S. R. Chassiakos, 209–21. Burlington, MA: Jones & Bartlett Learning.

Esparza, S., and L. Rubino. 2014. "A Call for New Leadership in Health Care." In *New Leadership for Today's Health Care Professionals: Concepts and Cases,* edited by L. G. Rubino, S. J. Esparza, and Y. S. R. Chassiakos, 1–19. Burlington, MA: Jones & Bartlett Learning.

Griffin, R. W., J. M. Phillips, and S. M. Gully. 2017. *Organizational Behavior: Managing People and Organizations*, 12th ed. Boston: Cengage Learning.

Healthcare Leadership Alliance (HLA). 2010. "Overview of the HLA Competency Directory." Accessed August 22, 2018. www.healthcareleadershipalliance.org/Overview%20of%20 the%20HLA%20Competency%20Directory.pdf.

Healthcare Leadership Alliance (HLA) and American College of Healthcare Executives (ACHE). 2018. *ACHE Healthcare Executive 2018 Competencies Assessment Tool.* Accessed August 31. www.ache.org/-/media/ache/career-resource-center/competencies_booklet.pdf.

Kaissi, A. 2017. "How to Be a 'Humbitious' Leader." *Healthcare Executive* 32 (6): 54–57.

Kash, B. A. 2016. "Interview with Jayne E. Pope, RN, FACHE, CEO of Hill Country Memorial Hospital." *Journal of Healthcare Management* 61 (5): 307–10.

Ledlow, G. R., and J. A. Johnson. 2019. "Organizational Leadership Theory." In *Health Organizations: Theory, Behavior, and Development*, 2nd ed., edited by J. A. Johnson and C. C. Rossow, 59–81. Sudbury, MA: Jones & Bartlett.

National Center for Healthcare Leadership (NCHL). 2018. "Health Leadership Competency Model 3.0." Accessed August 21. http://nchl.org/static.asp?hyperlinkId=8357.

Walston, S. L. 2017. *Organizational Behavior and Leadership in Healthcare: Leadership Perspectives and Management Applications*. Chicago: Health Administration Press.

Welch, S. 2010. "Understand Physician Culture to Facilitate Change." *Healthcare Executive* 25 (3): 92–95.

White, K. R., and J. R. Griffith. 2019. *The Well-Managed Healthcare Organization,* 9th ed. Chicago: Health Administration Press.

CHAPTER 10

LEADING: MOTIVATING AND INFLUENCING

Pleasure in the job puts perfection in the work.

Aristotle

Studying this chapter will help you to

➤ define motivation,

➤ describe theories of and methods for motivation,

➤ explain how managers motivate employees in organizations,

➤ define and describe power in organizations,

➤ identify types of power managers use in organizations, and

➤ explain how managers use politics to influence people in organizations.

HERE'S WHAT HAPPENED

In Boston (and the entire nation), external forces were changing the way healthcare would be organized, delivered, and paid for in the future. Stakeholders were demanding patient-centered care, fewer hospital readmissions, and payment based on the value (rather than volume) of services. Managers at Partners HealthCare planned how to adapt to—and fit with—these external changes. They planned new strategic initiatives and goals that, if achieved, would enable Partners to survive and thrive in its changing external environment. Then managers had to lead thousands of employees to carry out these plans, which included creating the cardiac telehealth program. Leading required influencing and motivating people. Managers throughout Partners had to motivate employees to accept new goals and, in some cases, change how they worked. Employees were unlikely to be motivated by the same methods, so managers had to figure out which motivational approaches to use with which employees. They understood that some employees might be motivated by feelings of achievement whereas others would be motivated by financial rewards or opportunities for professional growth. Managers also considered the various sources and kinds of power they had. They used appropriate power to influence and motivate employees to implement the cardiac telehealth program.

A s evident in the opening Here's What Happened, managers must lead others to accomplish the mission and goals of a healthcare organization (HCO). They can do this by influencing and motivating people. Managers at all levels of an HCO influence and motivate others, usually beginning at the top and flowing down through the organization. Top executives motivate their management team and the organization as a whole. Middle managers motivate staff in their departments. Lower-level supervisors motivate staff in their work units.

This chapter describes how managers influence and motivate others to accomplish an HCO's goals and desired outcomes. It builds on ideas discussed in chapter 9 and adds to our managerial toolbox of tools, methods, theories, and techniques for managing HCOs. Chapter 9 explained that leading is a process by which a person tries to influence someone. Well, how do managers influence someone? Chapter 10 answers that question.

Perhaps you already have some answers. You probably have influenced people—a sibling, a roommate, or a coworker—to do things. How did you try to influence them? Did you try the same approach with everyone or try different methods with different people? Which methods worked best?

This chapter explains what motivation is and then presents eight motivation theories. Each has strengths and weaknesses, and each is used in HCOs. **The best motivation approach depends on the situation and the people involved.** Managers must understand their employees well enough to judge which motivation approach to use for which employees in which situations. Motivation and influence involve the use of power and politics, which are also discussed in this chapter. We learn the kinds of power that leaders use and when power and political tactics are likely to be used (and sometimes abused).

MOTIVATION THEORY AND MODELS

Motivation is the "set of forces that leads people to behave in particular ways" (Griffin, Phillips, and Gully 2017, 170). Reading this definition carefully, we realize that motivation is not the act of doing something; it is the forces that lead people to do something. When managers motivate employees, they apply forces to create workers' desire and willingness to behave a certain way. However, managers must realize that motivation is not enough to ensure a worker actually behaves as desired. For example, Matt may be motivated to shampoo the waiting room carpet at a medical group practice in Albany. But if the carpet-cleaning equipment is broken, Matt will be unable to do that task despite his motivation. The same would happen if his boss reassigned him to some other task that was more urgent.

motivation
The set of forces that leads people to behave in particular ways.

This chapter examines motivation theories (sometimes referred to as *motivation approaches* or *motivation perspectives*). Some might not technically fulfill all the requirements of a true *theory*, so that word is used loosely. First we consider four theories based on human needs, after which we consider four theories that are based on other factors:

1. Maslow's hierarchy of needs theory (based on physiological survival, safety and security, belongingness, esteem, self-actualization)

2. Alderfer's ERG theory (based on existence, relatedness, growth)

3. Herzberg's two-factor theory (based on hygiene factors and motivators)

4. McClelland's acquired (learned) needs theory (based on achievement, affiliation, power)

5. Adams's equity theory (based on fairness of outcomes relative to inputs)

6. Vroom's expectancy theory (based on effort, performance, outcome)

7. Locke's goal-setting theory (based on goals)

8. Skinner's reinforcement theory (based on rewards and punishments)

Use of human needs theories is challenging because workers belong to four or even five generations that have different values, motivators, interests, and feelings about work. So which of these theories or approaches should a leader use? Like many other aspects of management, it depends. We know that in HCOs today, workers are very diverse regarding their generations, ethnicities, and other characteristics. These differences cause differences in values, preferences about work, and motivators. For example, the American culture values achievement, and Eastern cultures value harmony. Further, a person's motivators may change over time. When Adrianna graduates from college with loans to repay, she will be motivated by money. After she repays her loans, she may be more motivated by opportunities for professional growth. When it comes to motivation, one size does not fit all.

So as a manager, what should you do? First, assess the situation and people. Second, choose appropriate motivation methods to fit the situation and people. Think about the quote at the beginning of the chapter. Figure out what brings pleasure to each of your employees. If you can provide that through their work, it may help motivate them to work. If an employee gains pleasure from being with other people and forming friendships, then be sure the job provides opportunities for social interaction. Think about this advice as you study each motivation theory.

To strengthen your understanding of each theory, consider how leaders at Partners HealthCare could apply each theory. Think, too, about how these theories could be used to motivate you—in your college studies, a volunteer service role, a part-time job, or a club or sport activity.

MASLOW'S HIERARCHY OF NEEDS THEORY

Abraham Maslow theorized in the 1950s that human motivation comes from five basic human needs that have a hierarchical order—from the lowest, most basic need for physiological survival to the highest need for self-fulfillment (Griffin, Phillips, and Gully 2017). He thought people had to fulfill their lowest unsatisfied need before they would be motivated by higher needs. Thus, they would have to fulfill their physiological survival need before the safety need would motivate them. The needs are shown in exhibits 10.1 and 10.2.

EXHIBIT 10.1
Maslow's Hierarchy
of Needs

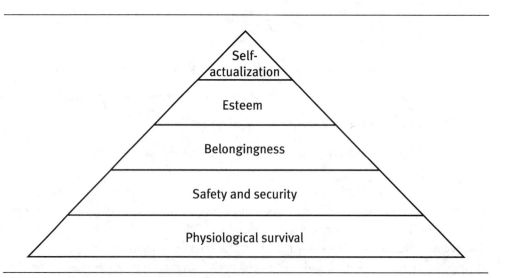

Sources: Information from Griffin, Phillips, and Gully (2017); Johnson and Rossow (2019); Walston (2017).

Maslow's Need	Examples from Daily Life	Examples for HCO Worker
Self-actualization	Accomplishing personal goals, fulfilling one's potential	Accomplishing professional goals, fulfilling one's career
Esteem	Self-respect, respect from others, status, competence	Recognition, respect from boss, performance awards
Belongingness	Friendship, love, affection	Friendly coworkers, informal work group
Safety and security	Warm housing, protection from crime, no worries	Job security, health insurance, protection from harassment, safe workplace
Physiological survival	Food, water, air	Clean indoor air, income to buy food

EXHIBIT 10.2
Examples of Maslow's Five Needs

Sources: Information from Griffin, Phillips, and Gully (2017); Johnson and Rossow (2019); Walston (2017).

How do HCOs satisfy employees' five needs as theorized by Maslow? Take a few minutes to jot down your ideas, and then confer with a classmate. Maslow's approach to motivating employees is used in many organizations, including HCOs. However, managers should consider several current views about this hierarchy of needs (Griffin, Phillips, and Gully 2017; Johnson and Rossow 2019):

1. The five types of needs can overlap; a single need can fit in more than one category.

2. The hierarchy is culturally biased because it is based on American values.

3. People do not always fully satisfy the lowest unmet need before seeking to satisfy higher needs.

4. A manager can motivate employees by enabling them in their jobs to meet their most urgent needs.

ALDERFER'S ERG THEORY

To overcome criticism of Maslow's theory, Clayton Alderfer later theorized that people could be motivated to seek three needs in varying order and while seeking more than one need at the same time (Griffin, Phillips, and Gully 2017; Johnson and Rossow 2019; Walston

2017). His approach seems more realistic than Maslow's. Sometimes we are simultaneously motivated by more than one need or by a need that does not follow a set sequence.

Alderfer's needs are shown in exhibit 10.3. These needs are similar to Maslow's, but they are more distinct, overlap less, and are not rigidly hierarchical:

1. Existence (similar to Maslow's physiological and safety needs)

2. Relatedness (similar to Maslow's belongingness and esteem needs)

3. Growth (similar to Maslow's self-actualization needs)

Managers can use Alderfer's needs to motivate employees. Consider a medical clinic in Oshawa where managers are trying to motivate workers to improve patient care. For workers with basic existence needs, managers could explain that if the workers help implement the patient care goal, the clinic will attract patients and earn revenue. As a result, the workers will keep their jobs and have money to buy things to satisfy their basic existence needs. Without enough patients and revenue, the clinic might have to lay off workers, which would threaten the workers' existence needs.

HERZBERG'S TWO-FACTOR THEORY

In the late 1950s and early 1960s, Frederick Herzberg studied workers and concluded that they are motivated by things that increase feelings of satisfaction. Herzberg's research led him to conclude that satisfaction and dissatisfaction are caused by different factors (Griffin,

EXHIBIT 10.3
Examples of Alderfer's Three Needs

Alderfer's Need	Examples from Daily Life	Examples for HCO Worker
Existence	Food, water, air, housing, protection from crime	Job security, protection from harassment, clean indoor air, income to buy food
Relatedness	Self-respect, respect from others, status, competence, affection, friendship, love	Recognition, respect from boss, performance awards, friendly coworkers, informal group
Growth	Accomplishing personal goals, fulfilling one's potential	Accomplishing professional goals, fulfilling one's career

Sources: Information from Griffin, Phillips, and Gully (2017); Johnson and Rossow (2019).

Phillips, and Gully 2017; Walston 2017). One group of factors, which he labeled *hygiene*, is associated with dissatisfaction. Hygiene (maintenance) factors are extrinsic—external to the work itself—and would generally fit with Maslow's three lower needs (Johnson and Rossow 2019). Hygiene factors include company policies, pay, supervision, coworkers, and other work conditions. If these are adequate, they prevent workers from feeling dissatisfied. If workers are dissatisfied, improving the hygiene factors reduces their dissatisfaction. Herzberg argued that better hygiene factors would make workers feel less dissatisfied but would not make them feel more satisfied.

So what would satisfy workers? A second group of factors, which Herzberg labeled *motivators*, come from the work itself and include achievement, growth, recognition, challenge, autonomy, and responsibility. Herzberg believed motivators are intrinsic—internal to the work—and arise from the content of the work itself and how it makes a worker feel. Motivators could be viewed as equivalent to Maslow's two higher needs (Johnson and Rossow 2019). For example, feeling achievement and fulfillment after completing a new, challenging project comes from the work itself. Herzberg argued that workers are motivated to do work that includes more motivators, which would enable the workers to realize more satisfaction. These motivators would not reduce or affect dissatisfaction, however.

Dissatisfaction and satisfaction are *not* opposite ends of one scale, as shown here:

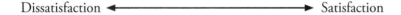

Dissatisfaction ◄———————————————► Satisfaction

Instead, dissatisfaction and satisfaction are separate concepts. Each may be present in varying degrees, such as on a scale of 0 to 10:

Dissatisfaction   0 ——————————————————— 10
Satisfaction   0 ——————————————————— 10

Herzberg advised managers to first use hygiene factors to reduce workers' dissatisfaction (Griffin, Phillips, and Gully 2017). Managers should ensure adequate pay, supervision, policies, and coworker relationships and provide safe, secure jobs and working conditions. When workers do not feel dissatisfied, managers should then design jobs and work to enable workers to experience motivators and satisfaction. Managers should organize their employees' work for achievement, recognition, autonomy, responsibility, fulfillment, growth, and respect.

This two-factor theory became popular, but it has weaknesses (Griffin, Phillips, and Gully 2017; Walston 2017). For example, some hygiene factors can affect both dissatisfaction and satisfaction. Sometimes both hygiene and motivator factors can motivate workers to higher levels of performance. Workers may perform better because a hygiene factor (e.g., a big pay raise) also provides a form of recognition and thus is a motivator.

Limitations arise when culturally diverse workers grow up with different feelings about hygiene factors (e.g., following rules, interacting with supervisors, accepting a job's working conditions) and about motivators (e.g., desire for achievement, challenge, autonomy). Research findings are mixed and seem to depend on other factors, such as an employee's organization level and age.

Despite its limitations, managers often use the two-factor theory. As a manager, pay attention to both dissatisfaction and satisfaction and realize that different factors might be needed to *reduce dissatisfaction* and to *increase satisfaction*. When applying the two-factor motivation theory, you might first have to improve hygiene factors such as working conditions and rules so that workers do not feel dissatisfied. Then, you can increase motivators to increase job satisfaction—and work motivation. This step may require redesigning jobs to give workers more opportunities for achievement, recognition, growth, responsibility, and self-accountability. To do so, you can follow Hackman and Oldham's job characteristics model (Griffin, Phillips, and Gully 2017, 213; Walston 2017, 65):

1. Increase workers' *work variety* with different activities and skills.

2. Increase workers' *work identity* with responsibility to complete a whole piece of work.

3. Increase workers' *work significance* with awareness of how work affects other people.

4. Increase workers' *work autonomy* with freedom and choice regarding work decisions.

5. Increase workers' *work feedback* with clear information about job performance.

Think about how job redesign connects to organizing work and staffing, discussed in earlier chapters. Repetitive data-entry keyboard jobs could be redesigned to include more task variety with different equipment. Clinical career ladders could be developed for nurses (as discussed in chapter 8) to motivate them with potential job-growth opportunities. A maintenance worker could be given more responsibility for scheduling preventive maintenance or selecting supplies. However, managers must ensure that workers have the ability to perform the increased job duties; training might be necessary. Further, extrinsic dissatisfiers must be minimized so they do not interfere with intrinsic satisfiers (motivators).

Managers should periodically survey employees as a group and also ask them individually about their job satisfaction and dissatisfaction. The responses will help managers plan what to do. Leaders need to understand their employees well enough to know how to satisfy them. Otherwise, at Employee Karaoke Night, someone might sing the Rolling Stones song "(I Can't Get No) Satisfaction."

McClelland's Acquired Needs Theory

In the late 1980s, David McClelland developed an approach to motivation based on learned human needs. McClelland's theory argues that people grow up learning and acquiring (from family and society) three culturally rooted needs (Griffin, Phillips, and Gully 2017; Hellriegel and Slocum 2011; Walston 2017):

1. *Achievement.* The need to effectively accomplish tasks, responsibilities, meaningful work, high standards, competitive goals, and challenges

2. *Affiliation.* The need for social interaction, approval, participation, friendships, and other supportive relationships with people

3. *Power.* The need for control and influence over people, resources, and one's environment

CHECK IT OUT ONLINE

Have you heard of online leadership style tests? They include short questions, such as "Do you tend to rally for a cause at work?" and "Do you accept input from group members?" These interactive tests immediately analyze your answers and explain your leadership style. The tests are fun, easy, and give some insight into your leadership style. They may lead you to think more about leadership. Two examples may be found at www. verywellmind.com/whats-your-leadership-style-3866929 and www.yourleadershiplegacy.com/assessment/assessment.php. If you search online for "leadership style test," you will find others. Check it out online and see what you discover.

An important component of the acquired needs theory is that needs are learned and can be learned throughout one's life. People differ in how much they desire to fulfill each need because of differences in their life experiences (especially while growing up). In their work lives, people tend to pursue jobs that enable them to fulfill their desired amount of these three needs. For example, many allied health jobs (e.g., therapist, nurse, pharmacist) involve much individual work, personal responsibility, and self-sufficiency—all of which enable workers to experience individual achievement. People with a high need for achievement often are found in these jobs, and managers can motivate them by appealing to their need for achievement. Millennial workers tend to have a high need for affiliation. Managers may motivate them by creating opportunities to work in teams and interact with others.

To apply McClelland's theory, you as a manager can do two things. First, for each job, consider how much the job would enable someone to experience achievement, affiliation, and power—and then hire someone who has similar needs for achievement, affiliation, and power. As mentioned, jobs vary in how much they enable someone to fulfill each of these three needs. It would not make sense to hire someone with high affiliation needs to fill an isolated job located in a basement cubicle. (As a manager, you can use what you learned about staffing in chapter 7 to hire people with motivational needs that fit the job.) Second, while someone is working in a job, pay attention to the worker's needs (which may change over time), and adjust the job, if possible, so that it enables the worker to fulfill unmet needs. For example, to motivate Henrik, his manager might be guided by the acquired needs theory and adjust Henrik's job to include more challenging goals, more opportunity for affiliation, or more autonomy and control.

The four theories discussed so far focus on human needs as a way to motivate workers. Managers who use these theories should understand which workers have which unmet needs. These needs are likely to vary among the four to five generations in the workplace. Baby boomers may be motivated by achievement, whereas millennials prefer work–life balance. We now turn to motivation theories that use approaches other than human needs.

ADAMS'S EQUITY THEORY

John Stacey Adams developed equity theory in the 1960s. It is based on people's desire to be treated fairly (equitably). The theory has two main elements: inputs and outcomes (Griffin, Phillips, and Gully 2017; Walston 2017). A worker's inputs are the education, experience, skills, knowledge, time, efforts, and so forth given to the job. Outcomes are the pay, benefits, recognition, and other rewards received for performing the job. A worker compares her outcomes received to her inputs given to the job and then judges whether it seems fair. She also compares her inputs and outcomes to those of other workers and judges whether everything seems fair. Have you ever gone through this mental process? Here is an example:

1. Sean, a health insurance sales representative, considers his education, years of experience, sales ability, knowledge of the healthcare market, and effort that he brings to his job. He considers his pay, benefits package, and other rewards received for doing the job.

2. Sean knows the background of some other sales reps at his company. From conversations and other sources, he has a pretty good idea what Megan, Brandon, and Danielle are earning. He mentally sizes up the outcomes-to-inputs ratio of each sales rep:

$$\frac{\text{Sean's outcomes}}{\text{Sean's inputs}} \quad \frac{\text{Megan's outcomes}}{\text{Megan's inputs}} \quad \frac{\text{Brandon's outcomes}}{\text{Brandon's inputs}} \quad \frac{\text{Danielle's outcomes}}{\text{Danielle's inputs}}$$

3. Sean figures he compares fairly (equitably) with Megan and Brandon. Sure, Brandon makes more money, but he has much more experience than the others, so it seems fair. But Sean is annoyed to think that Danielle's ratio is higher than his and everyone else's. In his opinion, she is getting about the

same pay despite having a lot less education, experience, and sales ability. He feels it is unfair, and he becomes dissatisfied. Of course, this feeling is based on Sean's perceptions and judgments, which might not be accurate. The secondhand information might be incorrect. He might not know the full story about his coworkers. Nonetheless, he makes his judgments. This manner of judging fairness is not ideal, but workers often do it.

Inequity causes a worker to feel tension and become motivated to resolve the inequity. If Sean feels underpaid, he becomes motivated to seek increased rewards (e.g., pay, time off, work schedule) or reduces his work effort to match (in his mind) his rewards. He might slack off and take long breaks. Some workers will leave the organization if they cannot achieve equity with their current employer. Some employees deviously increase their rewards by stealing supplies from their company. Inequity can also work in the other direction. If Danielle becomes aware of this information, she may feel overpaid. Perhaps she will feel tension (guilt) about the inequity and work extra hard to feel she really does deserve her pay.

Inequitable situations arise in HCOs, especially when workers compare themselves to similar workers in other organizations. Labor markets for some jobs are unstable, and pay scales are moving targets. (Recall chapters 7 and 8 on staffing, recruitment, and compensation.) A nurse or pharmacist might know a peer who is getting much higher pay somewhere else because that employer was frantic and paid a high starting salary for an essential position. Paying a higher salary upsets the outcomes-to-inputs ratio for the position.

Managers should pay attention to equity theory and realize that workers compare themselves with others. **A challenge for managers is to get workers to consider all of their rewards rather than just pay.** Sometimes, a worker feels her lower pay is unfair when compared with someone else's pay, not realizing that she gets better health insurance than the other person. Managers should remind employees about their total compensation. Managers must also realize that workers compare their work effort with other workers' efforts. Good workers quickly become frustrated and feel tension from inequity if they have to work with slackers. If HCO leaders do not motivate (or replace) low performers, high performers may leave the organization to relieve their tension. Then the HCO loses good workers and is left with lousy ones. Hmmm, what's wrong with this picture?

VROOM'S EXPECTANCY THEORY

The expectancy theory of motivation was developed by Victor Vroom and others, also in the 1960s. Work effort, performance, and outcomes are the main components of this theory. It "suggests that people are motivated by how much they want something and the likelihood they perceive of getting it" (Griffin, Phillips, and Gully 2017, 187). Let's imagine

Latasha is an associate in a healthcare consulting company in St. Louis. She could improve her work to earn a year-end pay bonus.

1.   Latasha considers whether her improved *work effort* would be likely to produce good enough job performance. Does she expect that her better effort will be enough to create the necessary level of performance? Or will other factors (e.g., lazy coworkers, broken equipment) interfere with her improved work effort and prevent achieving sufficiently improved performance?

2.   Latasha considers to what extent improved work *performance* would obtain the desired outcome. Is the outcome tightly connected to her job performance? If she improves her work and produces better job performance, will she really get that pay bonus? Or will the bonus depend on other factors, such as the company's overall financial situation?

3.   Latasha considers how strongly she wants the *outcome*. How much does she really want the bonus pay? The extra money would be great, but how about the added stress and having to work late some days? Would it all really be worth it?

Taken together, this approach argues that Latasha will wonder if her *effort* will produce the *performance* needed to obtain a valued *outcome*. The more she really wants the pay bonus—and expects that her improved work effort will produce the performance needed to obtain that bonus—then the more motivated she will be to improve her work effort.

Research generally supports this theory, although it has weaknesses (Griffin, Phillips, and Gully 2017). Expectancy theory assumes that workers (e.g., Latasha) rationally and logically do the mental calculations, yet in reality they might not. Also, even if workers try to rationally calculate the value of rewards, they might easily misjudge the connection between effort and performance or between performance and outcome. Finally, some workers feel outcomes are not within their control and instead are mostly influenced by other forces and events, so why bother? If workers perceive favoritism or a biased boss, applying expectancy theory will be less effective. Expectancy theory, like others, is culturally biased and thus works better in some countries and cultures (e.g., the United States) than in others (e.g., Brazil, China) depending on the extent to which workers feel they can control their work, performance, and outcomes.

As a manager, you can use this approach to motivate workers as long as you realize its limitations. Workers may put forth the effort you want *if* they expect their work will lead to the performance level that will earn them the rewards they desire. Realize that the value of rewards (outcomes) varies according to people's unique needs. Suppose two workers—Ricardo and Ahmad—work in a hospital's information systems department in Northridge. Ricardo wants professional growth and new experiences, whereas Ahmad prefers more vacation days. As an incentive to improve job performance, the hospital offers to send one worker to the Healthcare Information and Management Systems Society conference. Ricardo would value (and be motivated by) that reward more than Ahmad would.

Students sometimes are motivated to study based on expectancy theory. Consider a student who attended college on a scholarship and had to maintain a B average (performance level) to keep her scholarship (valued outcome). She wondered how much she had to study for a final exam. After thinking about it, she expected that if she studied five hours (effort), that would be enough to earn at least a B on the exam (performance), which would be enough to maintain her scholarship (valued outcome).

LOCKE'S GOAL-SETTING THEORY

Edwin Locke in the 1960s theorized that goals would motivate people. Research has confirmed his theory—under certain conditions (Griffin, Phillips, and Gully 2017; Hellriegel and Slocum 2011). Motivation from a goal increases under the following conditions:

◆ The goal is specific, not general.

◆ The goal is challenging yet attainable; it is of manageable size and complexity.

◆ People know the goal.

◆ People accept and are committed to the goal.

◆ People have the knowledge, ability, and resources to attain the goal.

◆ People receive enough feedback on progress toward the goal.

Goal-setting theory can be effective if managers apply it based on careful thought and planning. A leader must take three steps to set this theory into action (Borkowski 2011):

1. *Set the goal.* The goal may be set by the manager, by the worker, or by both (cooperatively). The goal's specificity and degree of difficulty require careful judgment. If the goal is too easy to achieve, it will not motivate the worker. If it is too hard to achieve, it will *de*motivate the worker and create negative feelings toward the manager. Each employee is unique, and managers must know their employees well. Highly confident workers respond better to a harder goal than do workers with low self-confidence. Internal and external factors—such as laws, accreditation standards, consumers' demands, and community standards—may have to be considered in setting a goal.

2. *Obtain the employee's acceptance of the goal and commitment to accomplish it.* If the employee helped set the goal or provided input for it, acceptance and

commitment are more likely. Employees' prior success in achieving goals also contributes to acceptance of new goals.

3. *Provide ongoing support and resources to enable achievement of the goal.* This support could include training; help with breaking a goal into smaller steps and activities; and providing supplies, equipment, time, information, and so forth. The manager must support the employee by giving regular feedback regarding goal progress.

This approach to motivation is used in many organizations, including HCOs. Some use it as part of a management-by-objectives approach to goal setting throughout the organization.

Let's consider a government-funded behavioral health clinic. As a result of changes in policy and priorities, the state government reduced funding for the clinic by 10 percent. Meanwhile, more people are experiencing stress, depression, and behavioral health problems. Lori, the clinic supervisor, meets with her three counselors to set goals for the number of clients each counselor will see per week. After discussion, they set a goal of increasing client visits per counselor by four visits per week for the next six months (after which the goal will be reevaluated). All counselors accept and commit to this goal, although Lori senses hesitation by one of them.

The counselors brainstorm ideas that could help achieve this goal, and Lori ensures resources are available. She arranges for the clinic's scheduling coordinator to provide a weekly report to each counselor so they can monitor progress. Later that week and then monthly, she meets individually with each counselor to give feedback (and seek feedback) on progress toward the goal.

SKINNER'S REINFORCEMENT THEORY

The final motivation theory discussed here comes from B. F. Skinner's work in the mid-1900s. Skinner thought that people learn from and become motivated by the consequences of their behavior (Griffin, Phillips, and Gully 2017). (More recently, social learning theory has shown that people also learn from and become motivated by observing other people's behavior and consequences.) Let's examine reinforcement theory and how a leader can use it:

1. The theory begins with a *stimulus*—a leader's policy, instruction, or goal that informs a worker what should be done. This stimulates the employee to behave (or not behave) a certain way. The leader can also state which consequences will occur if the employee does (or does not) behave the desired way.

2. The stimulus is followed by a *response*, which is the worker's behavior or action.

3.   That response is followed by a *consequence*, which is one of four kinds of reinforcement by the leader (described later). Depending on what the consequence (reinforcement) is, it might increase or decrease the frequency of that response (behavior) in the future. The consequence motivates the employee to respond a certain way.

Sports coaches often use this method with players and teams. Duke University men's basketball coach Mike Krzyzewski has won five National Collegiate Athletic Association championships and more than one thousand games. Coach K (as he is known) is a master motivator who uses reinforcement theory with players. Parents also use this method with children and teenagers. Can you recall examples from your life? Managers use reinforcement theory with employees in HCOs. **Managers can increase or decrease the frequency of a specific work behavior by using positive or negative consequences.**

1.   A leader *gives something positive* (e.g., verbal praise) as a consequence of behavior. This action reinforces desired behavior and makes it *more likely* to reoccur.

2.   A leader *removes something negative* (e.g., having to work every third weekend) as a consequence of behavior. This action reinforces desired behavior and makes it *more likely* to reoccur.

3.   A leader *gives something negative* (e.g., a verbal warning) as a consequence of behavior. This action makes unwanted behavior *less likely* to reoccur.

4.   A leader *removes something positive* (e.g., catered lunch each Friday) as a consequence of behavior. This action makes unwanted behavior *less likely* to reoccur.

Leaders must think carefully about which behaviors are reinforced or not reinforced, intentionally or unintentionally. Sometimes a leader unintentionally gives something positive to a worker and thereby reinforces unwanted behavior. For example, in a meeting the leader gives time and attention to a disruptive person, which reinforces disruptive behavior. The leader should avoid the positive reinforcement—time and attention—so that the undesired behavior decreases and stops. Further, in the meeting the leader might forget to commend a helpful person who contributes good ideas. Because he does not positively reinforce that desired behavior, that person might not contribute as much in the future. During the meeting, the leader should thank someone who contributes good ideas—then that behavior will more likely be repeated.

Reinforcement theory works best when there is a clear relationship between someone's response to a stimulus and the consequence of that response (Griffin, Phillips, and

Gully 2017). Although big consequences are more noticeable than small consequences, even small, symbolic consequences may be effective. Prompt consequences to behavior are more effective than delayed consequences. However, the consequence does not have to occur for every response. The relationship may vary, such as an immediate reward for every response initially and then, after some improvement, a reward for every third or fourth response. What really matters is that employees know how consequences relate to their behaviors.

Managers should be cautious about removing a positive consequence that employees have become used to because, after a while, employees assume it is permanent. Managers should also be cautious about punishments as consequences and clearly explain the reason for them. If employees perceive those consequences as unfair or undeserved, they will feel resentment, anger, and hostility that can jeopardize future working relationships or make the worker try to secretly "get back at" the boss. Managers should strive to reinforce good behavior, ensure they do not reinforce bad behavior, and avoid punishing bad behavior too often. Finally, managers must know their employees as individuals to properly apply motivational theory.

Reinforcement theory is common in HCOs. Let's consider a radiologic technology school in Detroit. The instructor teaches students to "get it right the first time" to avoid repeat scans that require more time and discomfort for patients. The students must ensure the patient is properly positioned so scans and images fully capture the area of interest and do not have to be repeated. The instructor's statement is a *stimulus*. It stimulates a *response* from student Sofia, who has been careless and had to repeat scans. After receiving the stimulus, she works more accurately. In the next week, Sofia has fewer repeats than usual and only has to redo one procedure. Her teacher rewards her with verbal praise for this specific

---

→ TRY IT, APPLY IT

Suppose you are a summer intern in a company that does website design and social media work for HCOs. More than a hundred employees work there in different jobs, teams, and departments. The company president wants to reduce energy use by 12 percent during the next two years. Employees submit suggestions for how they could reduce their energy use. But these ideas would require people to change behaviors and be inconvenienced. Who wants that? Using this chapter, explain how managers could apply three different theories of motivation to influence workers, teams, and departments to reduce their energy use. What are the pros and cons of your motivation approaches? Discuss your ideas with classmates.

improvement. The praise is a *consequence* of fewer repeat scans, and it feels good to Sofia. It motivates her to keep improving to continue getting the praise. Meanwhile, Jason, another radiologic technology student, has had to repeat many scans and has not improved. The teacher talks privately with Jason, emphasizes why his careless work is not acceptable, and advises him that he might not pass the course. To avoid this negative consequence, Jason improves his work. The next week, he "gets it right the first time" for all but one of his patients—a big improvement! The instructor praises Jason, and that positive consequence further motivates him to behave as desired.

POWER AND POLITICS

The use of power is important for leading, influencing, directing, and motivating. For example, although not stated explicitly, reinforcement theory involves the use of power to create consequences (e.g., rewards and punishments). In management, we can think of **power** as "the ability of one person or department in an organization to influence other people to bring about desired outcomes" (Daft 2016, 523). To be more concise, power is the ability to influence others to achieve outcomes. Some people think power and authority are the same, but authority is just one type of power. What are other types of power? Read on.

power
The ability to influence others to achieve outcomes.

SOURCES AND TYPES OF POWER

People and managers use multiple sources and types of power. Some are tied to a specific *person*, and others are tied to a specific *position* in an organization. A person in an HCO can have certain personal powers based on her character, behavior, abilities, values, and so forth. A person can develop a range of personal powers, and these can change over time. A position in an HCO—such as quality manager in a hospice—can have certain positional powers based on the position itself: its responsibilities, authority, place in the organization structure, and so forth. Whoever is appointed to the position is granted and may use the position's powers. When that person leaves the position, she no longer can use that position's powers. In an organization's vertical hierarchy, higher-level managers establish and may change positional powers of lower-level positions, such as by decentralizing more authority to a lower position.

The early work of John French and Bertram Raven in the mid-1900s identified five types of power: legitimate, reward, coercive, expert, and referent. Further study of power in organizations has identified others (Daft 2016). Exhibit 10.4 defines various personal powers and positional powers and gives examples of each. Note that types of power may overlap and are not entirely independent of each other. Returning to the Here's What Happened at the beginning of this chapter, which types of power do you think people used at Partners HealthCare?

In their jobs, managers use **personal power** and **positional power** to motivate and influence others to achieve goals. Of course, other HCO workers also have power to

personal power
Power based on a person.

positional power
Power based on a position in an organization.

EXHIBIT 10.4	**Personal Power**		
Types of Power	**Type**	**Definition**	**Examples**
	Reward	Give something that is valued	Give praise, money, friendship, a ride to work
	Coercive	Punish, penalize, reprimand	Ignore, insult, withdraw friendship
	Expertise	Provide needed knowledge, skill, ability	Set up a new tech device, explain history of the community
	Referent	Inspire through charisma, trust, respect, emotion, admiration	Give an emotionally compelling speech about children

	Positional Power		
	Type	**Definition**	**Examples**
	Legitimate	Authorize decisions, take actions, direct subordinates and expect obedience from them	Assign a subordinate to work Saturday, sign an e-health contract, hire a new chaplain
	Reward	Give something that is valued	Give praise, promotion, pay raise, bigger office, reserved parking
	Coercive	Punish, penalize, reprimand	Scold, reduce pay, deny requested time off
	Resource control	Give, remove, use, or assign valued resources that others need or want	Give equipment, approve funds, restrict use of space
	Information control	Give (or not give) selected information to others to affect their perceptions and knowledge	Serve as information gatekeeper; decide who gets which information about a possible merger
	Network centrality	Be in the flow of information ("in the loop") and connected to key people to know what is going on	Serve on key committees, network with others, exchange information with a friend in the mayor's office

Sources: Information from Daft (2016); Griffin, Phillips, and Gully (2017); Johnson and Rossow (2019); Walston (2017).

USING CHAPTER 10 IN THE REAL WORLD

In 2017, Philip Newbold retired after a total of 30 years as the CEO of Memorial Hospital of South Bend, Indiana, and later as the CEO of its parent Beacon Health System. He is widely known for—and has received national awards for—innovation in healthcare. As a manager and leader, he used referent power to motivate and influence.

Newbold's deep commitment to improving his community and its health inspired him and many others. He initiated "community plunges" by hospital and community leaders to visit and directly witness local populations with difficult health problems. Newbold took employees from all levels of his HCO on dozens of "inno-visits" to non-HCOs, including Whirlpool, John Deere, The Hershey Company, and Nike Inc., to discover new ideas to improve work. "Good Try" awards were given to employees for good ideas that were tried, did not work, and were examined for lessons to guide the next try. During his career, Newbold mentored younger employees, taking a personal interest in them to help them grow.

His inspirational vision of what Memorial Hospital and Beacon Health System could (and did) become inspired the board, medical staff, employees, volunteers, and other stakeholders. They respected and trusted Newbold, were excited by him and his vision, and followed both. Newbold's example as a role model for innovation, service, and success inspired others. His actions exemplified the use of referent power to motivate and influence the thousands of people he worked with. His influence continues as Beacon innovates with virtual healthcare to fit millennials' extensive use of smartphones and social media (Bailey 2017; Radick 2016).

motivate and influence others. Many healthcare workers, especially physicians, have power based on their expertise in a specific type of healthcare work. The Using Chapter 10 in the Real World sidebar describes a CEO who used referent power while leading his health system to become nationally known for innovation.

ORGANIZATION POLITICS

Managers and others who have power may use it by engaging in politics to influence decisions and resolve conflicts. Politics enables their organization to move forward to achieve its goals. **Politics** is "the use of power to influence decisions" to achieve desired outcomes (Daft 2016, 536). Politics involves using force other than one's job performance

politics
The use of power to influence decisions.

and professional competence to increase one's stature, gain advantage, and influence others (McConnell 2018). Politics is a normal part of organization life and can be helpful or harmful to an organization.

Politics and political behavior arise from conflicts and disagreement about goals, scarce resources, task interdependence, and other aspects of organizations. However, the intensity and manner of politics may vary depending on each organization's culture and the behavior it considers acceptable. Managers may use politics as an appropriate positive force to resolve disagreements and reach decisions so the organization can proceed with a course of action. Sometimes stubborn conflict paralyzes an organization for months or longer until someone uses power and politics to influence enough stakeholders to reach a decision.

When managers use power in self-serving ways that are contrary to the organization's goals, policies, values, and rules, then politics is negative. A manager who wants the big office that became available may engage in politics by spreading false rumors to discredit someone else vying for the office. In these situations, people feel "playing politics" is bad—or nasty, dishonest, manipulative, unfair, deceptive, unethical, and self-serving. This is a common view of organization politics, and it hurts employee morale, satisfaction, and job performance.

The following list contains political tactics managers, groups, and other people use to influence others and gain their support (Griffin, Phillips, and Gully 2017, 472):

- ◆ Appeal—ask for a favor or support "because we are friends"

- ◆ Coalition—build a group of supporters and loyal followers

- ◆ Consultation—consult others for advice or about decisions and goals

- ◆ Exchange—give others something they want in return for a favor

- ◆ Ingratiation—flatter and praise others

- ◆ Inspiration—appeal to others' ideals, hopes, values, and aspirations

- ◆ Legitimacy—refer to authority, official documents, formal rules, and precedents

- ◆ Pressure—coerce, harass, or persistently remind

- ◆ Reason—persuade using facts, logic, and rational thinking

Other methods involve controlling who has access to which information, which conflicts and decisions get attention, who provides input on decisions, and how one looks in the organization. Unprofessional tactics include starting deceptive rumors and sabotaging a rival's work (McConnell 2018).

A person engages in politics to influence other people. Those people may respond to political tactics by actively supporting the person and her requests, actively opposing the person and her requests, or offering passive support or passive resistance. Multiple political tactics might be used over an extended period of time to try to influence people—perhaps succeeding and perhaps not. The effectiveness of politics varies depending on the people and situation. Daft (2016) asserts that effective managers use "soft power" (personal traits and relationships) more often than "hard power" (based on job authority).

Unfortunately, managers and others who have power sometimes abuse it. Power is more likely to be abused in the following situations. Managers should try to prevent abuse of power by minimizing these situations in their HCOs (McConnell 2018; Walston 2017):

◆ Scarcity of resources (e.g., budgets, staff, promotions, space, opportunities)

◆ Unclear or unknown organization goals

◆ Many layers of management in the vertical hierarchy

◆ No information or fuzzy, unclear information; rumors and gossip rather than clear, hard data

◆ Power consolidated in one person or only a few people

◆ Unequal dependencies among people

◆ Complacent organization culture that does not care

Note that new managers often focus on the technical parts of their job while overlooking the political aspects. They focus on tasks to complete a project without realizing the politics of the project. New managers can benefit by understanding organization politics in their HCO. As a manager, you should watch how people practice politics and develop your ability to use it appropriately.

ONE MORE TIME

Management involves leading, and leading involves motivating (influencing). Motivation must happen at all levels of an HCO, beginning at the top and flowing down through the organization. People are different and do not respond equally to the same motivators. Thus, a manager should first assess the situation and people. Then, a manager should choose appropriate motivation methods to fit the situation and people. Leaders can apply theories of motivation that focus on the human needs that people have. These approaches include Maslow's hierarchy of needs theory, Alderfer's ERG theory, Herzberg's two-factor theory, and McClelland's acquired needs theory. Leaders can also apply Adams's equity theory, Vroom's expectancy theory, Locke's goal-setting theory, and Skinner's reinforcement theory.

Managers and leaders should use power and organization politics to help their HCO achieve its goals. They may use different sources of power in organizations, and these sources may change as circumstances change. Individual people have power, and individual positions (jobs) in organizations have power. Managers should understand and use their personal power and the power of their positions to influence, motivate, and lead others. They can become more effective by paying attention to which workers have which types of power and how they use those powers. People and groups in organizations engage in politics to increase power and influence for their preferred goals, which might or might not support organization goals.

 FOR YOUR TOOLBOX

- Maslow's hierarchy of needs theory
- Alderfer's ERG theory
- Herzberg's two-factor theory
- McClelland's acquired needs theory
- Adams's equity theory
- Vroom's expectancy theory

- Locke's goal-setting theory
- Skinner's reinforcement theory
- Personal power
- Positional power
- Politics and political tactics

FOR DISCUSSION

1. Which of the motivation theories do you like best? Why?

2. What are some difficulties managers may face when applying motivation theories in an HCO?

3. Compare and contrast the sources of power discussed in this chapter.

4. Which types of power do you prefer? Which would you feel least comfortable using?

5. How do you feel about people using politics and political tactics in HCOs? How can this be helpful? Harmful?

CASE STUDY QUESTIONS

These questions refer to the Integrative Case Studies at the back of this book.

1. Hospice Goes Hollywood case: Using at least two of the motivation theories discussed in this chapter, explain how Ms. Thurmond could motivate the medical director and nurse to support implementation of new policies and procedures for accreditation.

2. How Can an ACO Improve the Health of Its Population? case: Using at least two of the motivation theories discussed in this chapter, explain how Ms. Dillow could motivate the patients, consumers, and community members to care about and improve their health.

3. "I Can't Do It All!" case: Using at least two of the motivation theories discussed in this chapter, explain how Mr. Brice could motivate his vice presidents to make decisions in their areas of responsibility.

4. "I Can't Do It All!" case: Referring to the types of power in exhibit 10.4, describe which types of power you think Mr. Brice could use to achieve his desired outcomes.

5. Increasing the Focus on Patient Safety at First Medical Center case: Based on what you learned in this chapter, do you think Dr. Frame should use politics and political tactics to achieve her desired outcomes? If so, explain how she could use specific tactics.

6. Managing the Patient Experience case: Based on what you learned in this chapter, do you think Mr. Jackson should use politics and political tactics to achieve his desired outcomes? If so, explain how he could use specific tactics.

 RIVERBEND ORTHOPEDICS MINI CASE STUDY

Riverbend Orthopedics is a busy group practice with expanded services for orthopedic care. It has seven physicians and a podiatrist, plus about 70 other employees. At its big, new clinic building, Riverbend provides extensive orthopedic care. Several technicians provide diagnostic medical imaging, from basic X-rays to magnetic resonance images. The physicians perform surgery in their own outpatient surgery center with Riverbend's own operating nurses and technicians. Therapy is provided by three physical

(continued)

RIVERBEND ORTHOPEDICS MINI CASE STUDY *(continued)*

therapists and one part-time contracted occupational therapist. In addition to staff providing actual patient care, the clinic has staff for financial management, medical records, human resources, information systems/technology, building maintenance, and other administrative matters. Occasional marketing work is done by an advertising company. Legal work is outsourced to a law firm. Riverbend is managed by a new president, Ms. Garcia. She and Riverbend have set a goal of achieving "Excellent" ratings for patient experience from at least 90 percent of Riverbend's patients this year.

Ms. Garcia knows that to lead staff, she must motivate staff. To do this, she usually has relied on reinforcement theory and legitimate, reward, and coercive powers.

MINI CASE STUDY QUESTIONS

1. Using information from this case and the chapter, suggest to Ms. Garcia how she could use other motivation theories to motivate the employees to achieve the quality goal. Then do the same for physicians.

2. Using information from this case and the chapter, describe how Ms. Garcia could use other types of power to achieve the quality goal.

REFERENCES

Bailey, L. 2017. "Phil Newbold: Innovator, Leader and Trusted Mentor." *The Beam*. Published September 19. https://beam.beaconhealthsystem.org/phil-newbold-innovator-leader-trusted-mentor/.

Borkowski, N. 2011. *Organizational Behavior in Health Care,* 2nd ed. Sudbury, MA: Jones & Bartlett.

Daft, R. L. 2016. *Organization Theory and Design,* 12th ed. Mason, OH: South-Western Cengage.

Griffin, R. W., J. M. Phillips, and S. M. Gully. 2017. *Organizational Behavior: Managing People and Organizations*, 12th ed. Boston: Cengage Learning.

Hellriegel, D., and J. W. Slocum. 2011. *Organizational Behavior,* 13th ed. Mason, OH: South-Western Cengage Learning.

Johnson, J. A., and C. C. Rossow. 2019. *Health Organizations: Theory, Behavior, and Development,* 2nd ed. Sudbury, MA: Jones & Bartlett.

McConnell, C. R. 2018. *Umiker's Management Skills for the New Health Care Supervisor,* 7th ed. Burlington, MA: Jones & Bartlett Learning.

Radick, L. E. 2016. "The Virtual Delivery of Care." *Healthcare Executive* 31 (5): 21–30.

Walston, S. L. 2017. *Organizational Behavior and Leadership in Healthcare: Leadership Perspectives and Management Applications.* Chicago: Health Administration Press.

CHAPTER 11

LEADING: CULTURE AND ETHICS

Clarifying the value system and breathing life into it are the greatest contributions a leader can make.

Thomas Peters and Robert Waterman,
management consultants

LEARNING OBJECTIVES

Studying this chapter will help you to

➤ define culture and subculture in an organization;

➤ explain why culture is important for management;

➤ identify factors that create and shape culture;

➤ learn how to interpret culture in an organization;

➤ define ethics;

➤ describe four types of ethics and four ethical principles important for healthcare; and

➤ explain how to lead, create, and maintain desired cultures and ethics.

HERE'S WHAT HAPPENED

Changes outside Partners HealthCare (in its external environment) forced changes inside the healthcare organization (HCO). Thus, managers had to lead thousands of employees to change. In the process, managers were helped by their organization culture—the values, norms, and guiding beliefs that were considered correct at Partners. The HCO had developed a culture that valued technology, innovation, openness, preparedness, and adaptiveness. This culture had evolved over the years because of leaders who emphasized and rewarded these values. Also, past success with technological innovations and adaptation had reinforced innovation and adaptation as "the way we do things around here." When employees tried to figure out what really mattered at work and how to succeed in their jobs, they were influenced by the organization's cultural emphasis on technology, innovation, and adaptation. This shared set of values, norms, and beliefs was appropriate for an HCO that had to adapt to frequent changes in its external environment. It enabled managers to lead employees in developing an innovative Connected Cardiac Care program that uses telehealth for remote patients with heart disease. If Partners' culture had not valued technology and innovation, managers would have struggled to lead employees toward this goal.

Learning what happened at Partners HealthCare helps us realize that leading HCOs requires careful management of organization culture and ethics. It is among the most important work leaders do *at all levels* of an HCO. This idea might surprise people who view culture and ethics as the "soft side" of management. Yet, experienced managers know that the culture and ethics of an organization determine what employees actually do, how the organization performs, how satisfied stakeholders are, and whether the organization thrives or even survives. Culture and ethics are especially important for HCOs. In a 2016 national survey of hospital CEOs and other senior staff, 83 percent of respondents said they think their HCO will invest more resources in changing their organization culture (Kaufman 2017).

This chapter explains what organization culture and subcultures are and how to interpret them. It also discusses the factors that create and influence culture in HCOs. The chapter explains how to use that knowledge to change culture to achieve new plans and goals. Next, it focuses on ethics (which is part of culture) and four types of ethics that guide behavior and decisions in HCOs. The chapter explores how managers can create and maintain the ethics they feel are needed. Top-level managers in an HCO create and maintain the culture and ethics for the overall HCO. Then managers and supervisors in departments, teams, and other organization units create and maintain the right culture and ethics in their specific areas. When you are a manager, you will do this work. The tools and methods presented in this chapter will help you successfully manage culture and ethics.

What Is Culture?

You have probably heard of culture, such as "the Chinese culture" or "the culture of professional sports." We talk about the culture of a group of people, such as the Chinese or professional athletes. Similarly, an HCO comprises a group of people and has a culture. Smaller subgroups of people within an HCO may have subcultures.

Culture in an organization is "the set of values, norms, guiding beliefs, and understandings that is shared by members of an organization and taught to new members as the correct way to think, feel, and behave" (Daft 2016, 386). The norms and values that make up culture can be *espoused* or *enacted* (Griffin, Phillips, and Gully 2017, 527). The espoused values and norms are those that the organization explicitly states on its website, in employee orientation videos, on posters in the cafeteria, and in public relations speeches. However, enacted values and norms are what employees actually do based on what they observe in their organization. Sometimes espoused values differ from observed values, and when they do, "actions speak louder than words." Therefore, leaders must be role models who demonstrate their espoused (stated) culture.

As we saw earlier in the Here's What Happened, culture helps people understand what matters and how things are done in an organization. Suppose Kathy takes a job with a home health care agency in Framingham. She might wonder what it takes to get along in this HCO: How formal should I be? Is it OK to speak up if I see a problem? Does efficiency matter here? Do diversity and inclusion matter here? What does matter here? The organization culture will help her answer these questions.

Here are some other important points about culture:

- Culture is shared and learned.

- Culture evolves gradually and does not change quickly.

- Culture is mostly invisible, so it is interpreted by observing and listening to what can be seen and heard.

- Culture guides behavior and is powerful in doing that.

Managers should never forget this last point. In fact, some managers feel that "culture beats strategy" because culture is so powerful. For example, the executive director of an HCO tried to implement a new strategy of innovation that conflicted with the long-term culture that "we do not like mistakes." Innovation requires trying new ideas, some of which might not succeed. So what happened? The culture prevailed. The strategy failed. Culture beat strategy. People were afraid to try new ideas that might not work and would be viewed as mistakes. Managers soon realized they first had to change the organization's culture so that employees would feel it was acceptable (and safe) to try new ideas that might not succeed.

culture
The values, norms, guiding beliefs, and understandings shared by members of an organization and taught to new members as the correct way to think, feel, and behave.

The power of culture is evident in the fact that 30 percent of failed mergers are the result of culture clashes (Walston 2017). To avoid failure, what did Baylor Health Care System and Scott & White (a multispecialty academic medical center) do when they considered merging? Did they first examine the balance sheets, income statements, and financial status of each HCO (as is often done for proposed mergers)? Nope. They first examined the culture of each HCO to decide if the two cultures could fit together and work as one (Jacob 2013). That lesson is important when we recall from chapter 1 that many hospitals, medical groups, health insurers, ambulatory clinics, long-term care facilities, and other HCOs have been joining in mergers, alliances, networks, integrated delivery systems, accountable care organizations, and other collaborations. If their cultures clash, their strategy will not succeed. **Culture beats strategy.**

WHAT CAUSES AND CREATES CULTURE?

How do organizations—such as your college, your favorite store, and HCOs—end up with the cultures they have? What causes and creates culture? Why does culture differ among HCOs? For example, some HCOs have a cautious, risk-averse culture whereas others have an innovative, risk-taking culture. Organization culture is partly a result of leaders deciding which norms, behaviors, and values they want in the HCO. But there is more to it than leaders deciding which culture they *want*. Strong forces and factors determine what the culture actually *will be*, and as we learned earlier, that might be different from what managers want it to be! Many forces and factors—some external and others internal—influence an HCO's cultural values, norms, and beliefs (Daft 2016). A model of these forces and factors is shown in exhibit 11.1; the forces and factors (Daft 2016; Griffin, Phillips, and Gully 2017; Walston 2017) are listed here, with relevant healthcare-related examples. The Using Chapter 11 in the Real World sidebar has additional real-world examples from HCOs.

◆ *External laws, standards, demands* (e.g., nondiscrimination laws, accreditation standards, public demands for diversity and inclusion)

◆ *Organization mission* (e.g., mission to improve the population health status of all people in the local community)

◆ *Organization structure* (e.g., decentralized structure giving lower-level employees more autonomy in their work)

◆ *Rewards and punishments* (e.g., praise for improving clinical integration throughout the continuum of care)

◆ *Training and education* (e.g., an online video tutorial that demonstrates how to use active listening to improve the patient experience)

◆ *Physical work setting* (e.g., remodeling and redecorating work spaces to support creativity)

◆ *Beliefs, values, and norms of formal leaders* (e.g., the vice president believes that too much competition among staff might cause unethical behavior)

◆ *Beliefs, values, and norms of informal leaders* (e.g., a longtime employee telling new employees during lunch that honesty is what really matters in the HCO)

◆ *Beliefs, values, and norms of employees* (e.g., a dental hygienist values cleanliness)

◆ *Ceremonies, symbols, rituals, and activities* (e.g., the daily morning huddle celebrates yesterday's handling of an emergency and then prepares the team for today's priorities)

◆ *Stories and legends* (e.g., the story about how Andrea made it to work despite three feet of snow—or was it four?—back in 2007 because her patients needed her)

◆ *Language* (e.g., the way the supervisor talked enthusiastically about teamwork and collaboration)

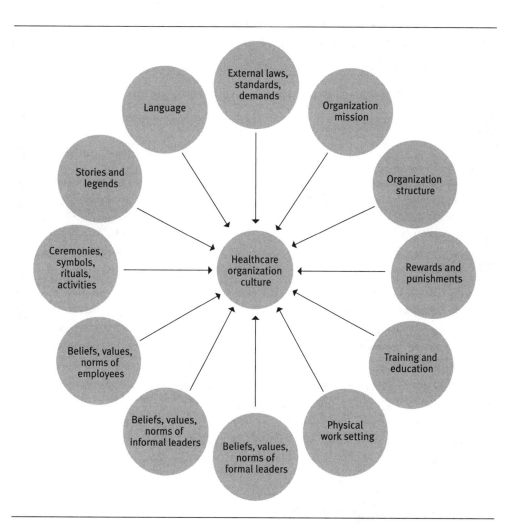

EXHIBIT 11.1
Model of Forces and Factors That Influence HCO Culture

Sources: Information from Daft (2016); Griffin, Phillips, and Gully (2017); Walston (2017).

Purpose and Benefits of Culture

Culture influences employees to work, act, think, feel, and behave a certain way. When managers develop the right culture for their organization, employees are more likely to know what to do to achieve the mission and goals (Daft 2016). In the Here's What Happened at the beginning of this chapter, managers developed a culture that guided staff to support and

 USING CHAPTER 11 IN THE REAL WORLD

Nemours Children's Health System based in Talleyville, Delaware, created an organization culture that guides staff toward performance improvement. Reflecting this chapter's definition of culture, this "set of values, norms, guiding beliefs, and understandings that is shared by members" of Nemours Children's Health System includes some interesting values-based behaviors needed to improve performance (Van Dyke 2017):

- Be in the moment

- Be authentic

- Have courageous conversations

- Be curious

- Be accountable

At Baptist Medical Center South in Jacksonville, Florida, the beliefs, values, and norms of formal leaders have been a powerful force in creating the HCO's "caring and caregiving culture." Nicole B. Thomas, FACHE, became the organization's CEO in 2016 and has continued to instill that culture by living and demonstrating those values. She explains, "I set the example of the hospital experience that ultimately will become our reputation" (Thomas 2017, 80). Ms. Thomas strives to remove barriers for physicians and to empower them to achieve the HCO's patient experience goals. She makes rounds among frontline workers and emphasizes that patients judge the hospital by their interactions with the staff. While rounding, she expresses her gratitude to volunteers. With leaders who directly report to her, she takes time to get to know them professionally and personally so she can help them succeed. Her engagement with the larger leadership team of about 40 department managers supports them in ways that show she cares. Thomas says, "When we support our leadership team, we nurture better leaders. And they, in turn, are sensitive to their teams. Ideally, compassion flows down to where it impacts our patients and families. If I care about my team, they're going to care about their team and so on" (Thomas 2017, 81).

achieve Partners HealthCare's mission and goals. Culture also helps employees figure out what to do in situations that are not covered by specific rules and policies. Finally, organization culture helps workers understand how to adapt to and "fit in" at their organization.

Healthcare has been learning from other fields just how important culture is to achieve safety. Consider this frequently cited example: In a tragic, stunning accident, the space shuttle *Columbia* exploded as it returned to Earth and disintegrated, killing all seven crew members. The shuttle accident investigation concluded that "no specific individual was at fault, but many individuals were influenced by the culture of the organization as a whole" (Haraden and Frankel 2004, 21). In its early years, the National Aeronautics and Space Administration (NASA) had a safety-first culture, but then NASA moved to a low-cost, high-productivity culture in which safety was given less attention. Think about that. Then think about safety in HCOs, where there have been too many medical errors (e.g., wrong amputations), burns from unsafe equipment, accidents, and other patient safety problems. Some of these errors happened because, like NASA, some HCOs moved to a low-cost, high-productivity culture in which safety was given less attention. Now, because of pressure from stakeholders, the culture of HCOs has been changing so that safety is valued more. Top executives in HCOs are making rounds in patient care areas to talk directly with frontline workers about patient safety, develop more trust with them, and solve safety problems (Jarrett 2017).

INTERPRETING CULTURE

An HCO's workers figure out its culture based on what they see and hear. Although underlying cultural beliefs, values, and norms (e.g., "Honesty matters" and "You have to be creative to get ahead") cannot actually be seen, employees might infer that honesty matters and feel that they have to be creative to get ahead. Because people interpret an organization's culture based on what they can see and hear, they may be confused by conflicting signs or mixed signals.

For example, suppose managers want a culture of competence. The written dress code explains how employees should dress to convey competence. But a new employee sees that workers often do not follow the written code. The enacted culture does not match the espoused culture. So employees look, listen, wonder, ask, infer, think, and learn by trial and error to determine what the culture *really* is and "what really matters around here." Some factors that influence culture (see exhibit 11.1) can be seen and heard and thus offer useful sources of information for interpreting the culture. The following list provides examples for some of these factors (see also the model for interpreting culture in exhibit 11.2):

1. Organization structure (e.g., management's official standards, rules, policies, and scripted procedures for how employees should interact with patients for excellent patient experience)

2. Rewards and punishments (e.g., an award for zero medical errors in the intensive care unit last month)

3. Physical work setting (e.g., open office doors in the C-suite that suggest managers are open to hearing from employees)

4. Actions, words, and behaviors of informal leaders (e.g., Jenna, an informal leader on the third shift, tells a new employee, "We're from four generations, yet we're all on the same team")

5. Actions, words, and behaviors of formal leaders (e.g., each day for lunch the director of human resources sits with different employees in the cafeteria)

6. Actions, words, and behaviors of employees (e.g., a nurse calls, "Time out!" and asks the surgical team to verify which leg is to be operated on)

7. Ceremonies, symbols, rituals, and activities (e.g., the medical school dean presents diplomas at commencement)

8. Stories and legends (e.g., a favorite story in the maintenance department about how Rick planned ahead and thereby prevented flooding in the building when a hurricane struck)

9. Language (e.g., the sincere caring words used in the "Annual Report to Our Community")

SUBCULTURES

When everyone in the organization interprets the culture the same way and describes the culture in similar terms, the culture is strong and consistent. That culture creates the

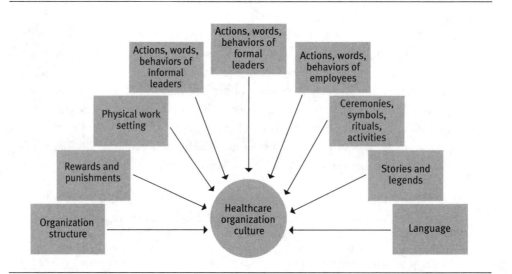

EXHIBIT 11.2
Model for Interpreting an HCO's Culture

advantages of employee harmony, working in the same direction, and presenting a consistent image to customers. However, a rigidly strong and consistent culture may have disadvantages and impede the performance of some individual parts of the organization. An individual department or team may need its own values, norms, guiding beliefs, and understandings that differ somewhat from the organization culture. This creates a **subculture**, which is the culture of a distinct part of an organization (e.g., a team or department) that exists within the organization's overall culture.

> **subculture**
> Culture of a distinct part of an organization (e.g., a team or department) that exists within the organization's overall culture.

Consider a large organization with many departments that have different purposes and functions. In chapter 4, we learned that because of the kind of work they do, some departments should be mechanistic whereas other departments should be organic. Thus, within the same organization, different departments may need different cultures. An accounting department may have a bureaucratic, rule-driven culture, while the marketing department may have a loose, creative culture. Yet, both of these subcultures must fit with the overall organization culture as much as possible. **Leaders should strive for the HCO to have a strong overall culture yet also allow for some varied subcultures.** Managers will have to decide how much a subculture can vary from the overall culture. For example, how much informality will be allowed in the marketing department of a hospital that strongly values a formal professional image?

In one healthcare trend, many hospital systems have been buying, owning, and operating physician practices. These medical groups often have different cultures than hospital systems do. The culture of medical groups is a subculture within the larger hospital system's overall culture. Executives have to decide to what extent the culture of medical practices can differ from the system's organization culture. Top managers and leaders must balance between (1) developing a strong, consistent, overall organization culture and (2) letting individual facilities, subunits, departments, and teams develop their own subcultures to fit their own distinct goals and needs. When you are a department manager, team captain, group leader, shift supervisor, or work unit coordinator, you will have to develop the right subculture for your unique area of responsibility (without moving too far from the HCO's overall culture). The next section explains how to develop culture.

SHAPING AND MANAGING CULTURE

To successfully lead an HCO, managers must deliberately shape and influence the culture so that it guides employees to achieve the HCO's goals and mission. This is a social process. Managers must use **organizational socialization**—the process by which employees learn (and share with others) their organization's culture, including what is and is not acceptable behavior (Griffin, Phillips, and Gully 2017). Just as Partners HealthCare had to socialize employees, so do other HCOs.

> **organizational socialization**
> The process by which employees learn (and share with others) their organization's culture, including what is and is not acceptable behavior.

We can connect this concept with strategic planning, which we studied in chapter 3. Let's consider a group of primary care physicians that has a traditional, physician-centered practice in which physicians decide what to do for patients. The group analyzes its environment and realizes that stakeholders and external forces favor patient-centered medical practices rather than physician-centered practices. In their strategic planning process, the physicians and their group practice manager decide to implement the patient-centered medical home (PCMH) model of primary care. Doing so will require much change, including changes to the group's organization culture. The physicians, manager, and other employees will think, feel, and behave differently than they do in their current, traditional approach. They will engage patients to partner with clinicians in deciding how to treat their own medical problems. Staff will communicate more openly and completely with patients. Active listening will be practiced and valued more. Employees will work more as a team, and the team will be less hierarchical. These changes will require a different culture—a different "correct way to think, feel, and behave." If a group practice in West Chester wants to become a PCMH, it will need a PCMH culture to guide physicians and others to behave that way.

Which tools and methods can managers use to change a traditional group practice culture to a PCMH culture? (Hint: Look at exhibit 11.1.) By managing the forces and factors that create culture, managers can re-create the culture to reflect a different set of beliefs, norms, and values:

◆ State the new patient-centered values in the group's mission, vision, and values

◆ Redesign the vertical, hierarchical structure to a more horizontal, team-based structure

◆ Reward employees who accept and demonstrate the new organization culture; withhold rewards from those who cling to the old approach (Does this sound like motivation theory, discussed in chapter 10?)

◆ Train staff on how to communicate more openly with patients by sharing clinical information that previously was kept from them

◆ Redesign the facility and physical setting for patients' comfort and convenience

◆ Ensure that the physicians, group practice manager, and other leaders consistently demonstrate (as role models) the new cultural norms, values, and behaviors

◆ Help informal leaders among the staff to demonstrate the new cultural norms, values, and behaviors

◆ Help employees demonstrate to each other the new cultural norms, values, and behaviors

◆ Celebrate the new cultural norms, values, and behaviors in morning staff huddles and other activities

◆ Share stories among staff that make the new culture come alive

◆ Revise documents, signs, e-forms, webpages, and other materials to use the language of PCMHs

In addition to trying to socialize existing staff to the new organization culture, an HCO should try to hire new people who already fit the desired organization culture. You may recall this approach from chapter 7 on staffing. For example, one HCO evaluates job applicants for how well they fit with the HCO's culture *before* evaluating them for job skills (Kash 2016).

Chapter 9 explained that values-based leadership is evident in some leadership theories. That approach to leadership is essential for culture change. "Clarifying the value system and breathing life into it are the greatest contributions a leader can make. Moreover, that's what the top people in the excellent companies seem to worry about most." Those words come from the classic book *In Search of Excellence* (Peters and Waterman 1982, 291). They are still true today—for HCOs as well (Dye 2017; Walston 2017).

What Is Ethics?

We now turn to ethics, which is part of values. We learned that values are part of culture, so ethics is also part of culture. **Ethics** is a code of values and moral principles regarding what is right and wrong (Daft 2016). Like other aspects of culture, ethics influences someone's

ethics
Values and moral principles regarding what is right and wrong.

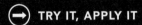 **TRY IT, APPLY IT**

Suppose you work for a large, nonprofit voluntary organization that advocates for children's health. The organization's 50 employees range in age from 18 to 67 and come from several different generations. Unfortunately, they don't always work well together. There seem to be many small groups of workers who stick together. Some workers disrespect older or younger workers. Some don't cooperate. Some have different attitudes and methods for advocating for their cause. Now suppose that after donations, grant funding, and service all decline, a new director takes over the organization. He feels that if employees work *with* others rather than *against* others, performance will improve. Describe in detail at least five suggestions for how this advocacy organization could change its culture to better achieve its purpose. Then, discuss your ideas with classmates.

behavior. Four ethical principles have long guided healthcare services (Johnson and Rossow 2019; Walston 2017):

1. *Autonomy* includes individual privacy, freedom of choice, self-control, and making one's own informed decisions.

2. *Beneficence* includes doing good and acting for the benefit of others.

3. *Justice* includes fairness and equality.

4. *Nonmaleficence* includes doing no harm, or at least avoiding unnecessary harm.

In HCOs, ethical situations and questions arise often. Some are obvious (e.g., informed consent is required for a medical procedure) and some are subtler (e.g., how much should he tell the supervisor about a problem?). Leaders and managers of HCOs must be concerned with **medical ethics**, **professional ethics**, **managerial ethics**, and **social responsibility**. Examples of these types of ethics are listed in exhibit 11.3. Some types may overlap.

medical ethics
Ethics that guide right and wrong in the practice of medicine.

professional ethics
Ethics that guide right and wrong for a profession, such as the nursing profession.

managerial ethics
Ethics that guide right and wrong in the practice of management.

social responsibility
Ethics that guide right and wrong for the good of society.

ETHICS PROBLEMS

Every day, all types of organizations deal with a wide range of situations involving ethical behavior and judgment. Managers do not always handle these situations well, as evident in news headlines. Some of the biggest ethical problems in HCOs have been financial, such as HealthSouth's and Columbia/HCA's extensive fraud, illegal billing for services, and false financial statements. Executives were jailed and fines exceeded $1.5 billion (Walston 2017). Here are other examples of ethical situations that arise in HCOs:

◆ A medical director at a health insurance company must decide whether to cover experimental treatment for a cancer patient.

◆ A president, director of finance, and director of human resources at a medical supply company discuss which employees will be laid off after a merger.

◆ A physician worries that if she is employed by a healthcare system, she might be pressured to place profits above patient care.

◆ A hospital executive realizes that more emphasis on population health would reduce needed revenue from a very profitable inpatient service.

◆ A personal care home resident tries to "friend" several nurses on Facebook.

Type of Ethics	Examples
Medical ethics guides right and wrong in the practice of medicine and clinical care.	• Remove life support equipment from a terminally ill patient • Conduct experimental medical research on humans in an academic medical center
Professional ethics guides right and wrong for a profession.	• Maintain confidentiality of private information obtained in professional work • Avoid exploiting professional relationships for personal benefit
Managerial ethics guides right and wrong in the practice of management.	• Allocate scarce resources in a way that will best fulfill the mission of the medical group practice • Avoid deceptive advertisements for a clinic
Social responsibility ethics guides right and wrong for the good of society.	• Reduce the amount of toxic waste produced by a hospital • Provide unprofitable health services that the community needs

EXHIBIT 11.3

Types of Ethics in HCOs

♦ A scientist from the Middle East wonders if the medical school lab will be inclusive and supportive of her culture.

♦ A surgeon considers what to tell a man whose spouse was seriously harmed by a medical error.

♦ A clinic's marketing director avoids exaggerating the benefits of a new treatment for stress.

♦ A healthcare management professor reviews community data and sees wide disparities in access to care and in health status.

♦ A woman asks if patient-centered care means she can request to be seen by a physician of her own ethnicity.

♦ An indigent care safety-net manager must decide how to use limited funds, staff, and facilities to care for more patients.

♦ Two teenagers bring their friend, a 16-year-old opioid abuser, to the emergency department and plead with the staff not to call his parents.

conflict of interest
A situation in which a person's self-interest interferes with that person's obligation to another person, organization, profession, or purpose.

ethical dilemma
A situation in which any decision or course of action will have an undesirable ethical outcome.

moral distress
A situation in which an organization's constraints prevent someone from doing what the person thinks is ethically right.

As the list shows, HCOs' clinicians, managers, employees, and others can face serious ethical problems, questions, and uncertainty. Some involve a **conflict of interest**, in which a person's (e.g., a physician's) self-interests (e.g., an extravagant meal from a pharmaceutical company) interfere with an obligation (deciding which medication to order) to someone else (a sick patient). Others involve an **ethical dilemma**, which is especially troubling because no matter what is decided, someone will suffer. For example, some HCOs consider requiring all workers to get a flu shot to help protect patients. But some employees believe that mandatory flu shots violate their autonomy and self-determination. Other employees may struggle with **moral distress**, in which an organization's constraints (e.g., rules and available resources) prevent them from doing what they think is ethically right (Hamric, Epstein, and White 2014). For example, DeAndre is often told to care for so many patients that he feels he cannot give them all the care they need.

Managers and leaders in HCOs must strive to ensure that employees, physicians, volunteers, and others understand (and follow) appropriate ethics. In addition, managers should ensure that their HCO has resources, structures, and processes to help people handle difficult ethical situations. These resources are needed to enable the HCO to achieve its mission, vision, values, and goals. The next section discusses how managers can do this.

SOURCES OF ETHICS

In broad terms, the ethics of an HCO comes from three general sources:

1. The people in the organization

2. The organization itself

3. The organization's external environment

Ethics starts to develop early in people's lives. Take a few minutes to think of where your own ethics and morality came from. Perhaps they came from people who influenced you as you grew up—parents, relatives, peers, teachers, leaders of youth organizations, and religious and faith leaders. Even fictional characters in novels, movies, and TV shows can influence what we view as right and wrong. How about laws and legal requirements? Yes, those shape our ethics as well. Maybe you thought of the social norms and cultural values in the community where you grew up. Perhaps you sensed what was considered right and wrong based on who got in trouble at school. Some current events and news headlines also make us think about right and wrong.

Personal ethics and morals formed while growing up become part of a person's ethics at work. Thus, to create an ethical HCO, managers should try to hire people who already have the desired ethics. As discussed in chapters 7 and 8, careful interviewing can help detect who is likely (or unlikely) to respect a patient's confidential information and how someone would respond to a salesman's offer of free tickets to a Dallas Cowboys game.

Another source of ethics is the HCO itself. Think back to the earlier part of this chapter. We learned that an organization's culture includes values, and values include ethics. The organization's **ethical climate** is the "shared perceptions of how ethical issues should be addressed and what is ethically correct behavior for the organization" (Rorty 2014, 12). This part of the culture can strongly influence HCO employees and shape their sense of right and wrong. An HCO will decide on certain ethics—such as justice and privacy—and emphasize them. However, an HCO faces barriers when developing, maintaining, and actually behaving according to an appropriate ethical climate. Employees are culturally diverse and may have differing views of what is moral and ethical (Walston 2017). Also, stakeholders exert pressures and demands on HCOs that push and pull in different directions.

Some HCOs develop codes of conduct as part of their ethical climate and organization culture. The ethical principles in these codes may be determined at a strategic planning retreat, approved in a staff meeting, or declared by the CEO following a crisis. They may be advocated by an employee. Ethical principles may also be identified when developing organization culture, resolving ethics problems, or in other ways. For example, employers are creating social media codes of conduct to guide employees regarding the ethical use of social media.

Sources outside the HCO also affect what is deemed ethical in the organization. These sources include laws, regulations, court decisions, and Joint Commission accreditation standards, to name a few. External professional codes of ethics guide members of many professions, such as nursing, engineering, pharmacy, accounting, occupational therapy, law, teaching, healthcare management, and other fields. Professional codes of ethical conduct may override an HCO's policies and guidelines when members of a profession feel more allegiance to their profession and its guidelines than to the HCO and its guidelines.

The American College of Healthcare Executives (ACHE) is the largest professional association for healthcare managers. Like many other professional organizations, ACHE has carefully prepared a code of ethics for its members. This *Code of Ethics* (see exhibit 11.4) lists the healthcare manager's ethical responsibilities to the profession, patients, organization, employees, and society. Take time to study the code to better understand managers' ethics in healthcare. Managers use this code to guide appropriate managerial conduct for a wide range of ethical situations. Other professional associations, such as the Medical Group Management Association, the Healthcare Financial Management Association, and the Association of University Programs in Health Administration, also provide ethical guidance related to healthcare management.

ethical climate
The shared perceptions of how ethical issues should be addressed and what is ethically correct behavior for an organization.

EXHIBIT 11.4
ACHE *Code of Ethics**

PREAMBLE

The purpose of the *Code of Ethics* of the American College of Healthcare Executives is to serve as a standard of conduct for members. It contains standards of ethical behavior for healthcare executives in their professional relationships. These relationships include colleagues, patients or others served; members of the healthcare executive's organization and other organizations; the community; and society as a whole.

The *Code of Ethics* also incorporates standards of ethical behavior governing individual behavior, particularly when that conduct directly relates to the role and identity of the healthcare executive.

The fundamental objectives of the healthcare management profession are to maintain or enhance the overall quality of life, dignity and well-being of every individual needing healthcare service and to create an equitable, accessible, effective and efficient healthcare system.

Healthcare executives have an obligation to act in ways that will merit the trust, confidence and respect of healthcare professionals and the general public. Therefore, healthcare executives should lead lives that embody an exemplary system of values and ethics.

In fulfilling their commitments and obligations to patients or others served, healthcare executives function as moral advocates and models. Since every management decision affects the health and well-being of both individuals and communities, healthcare executives must carefully evaluate the possible outcomes of their decisions. In organizations that deliver healthcare services, they must work to safeguard and foster the rights, interests and prerogatives of patients or others served.

The role of moral advocate requires that healthcare executives take actions necessary to promote such rights, interests and prerogatives.

Being a model means that decisions and actions will reflect personal integrity and ethical leadership that others will seek to emulate.

I. **THE HEALTHCARE EXECUTIVE'S RESPONSIBILITIES TO THE PROFESSION OF HEALTHCARE MANAGEMENT**

The healthcare executive shall:

A. Uphold the *Code of Ethics* and mission of the American College of Healthcare Executives;

B. Conduct professional activities with honesty, integrity, respect, fairness and good faith in a manner that will reflect well upon the profession;

C. Comply with all laws and regulations pertaining to healthcare management in the jurisdictions in which the healthcare executive is located or conducts professional activities;

(continued)

Exhibit 11.4
ACHE *Code of
Ethics* (continued)*

D. Maintain competence and proficiency in healthcare management by implementing a personal program of assessment and continuing professional education;

E. Avoid the improper exploitation of professional relationships for personal gain;

F. Disclose—and when appropriate, avoid—financial and other conflicts of interest;

G. Use this *Code* to further the interests of the profession and not for selfish reasons;

H. Respect professional confidences;

I. Enhance the dignity and image of the healthcare management profession through positive public information programs; and

J. Refrain from participating in any activity that demeans the credibility and dignity of the healthcare management profession.

II. **THE HEALTHCARE EXECUTIVE'S RESPONSIBILITIES TO PATIENTS OR OTHERS SERVED**
The healthcare executive shall, within the scope of his or her authority:

A. Work to ensure the existence of a process to evaluate the quality of care or service rendered;

B. Avoid practicing or facilitating discrimination and institute safeguards to prevent discriminatory organizational practices;

C. Work to ensure the existence of a process that will advise patients or others served of the rights, opportunities, responsibilities and risks regarding available healthcare services;

D. Work to ensure that there is a process in place to facilitate the resolution of conflicts that may arise when values of patients and their families differ from those of employees and physicians;

E. Demonstrate zero tolerance for any abuse of power that compromises patients or others served;

F. Work to provide a process that ensures the autonomy and self-determination of patients or others served;

G. Work to ensure the existence of procedures that will safeguard the confidentiality and privacy of patients or others served; and

H. Work to ensure the existence of an ongoing process and procedures to review, develop and consistently implement evidence-based clinical practices throughout the organization.

(continued)

Exhibit 11.4
ACHE *Code of*
*Ethics**
(continued)

III.   THE HEALTHCARE EXECUTIVE'S RESPONSIBILITIES TO THE ORGANIZATION
The healthcare executive shall, within the scope of his or her authority:

A.   Lead the organization in prioritizing patient care above other considerations;

B.   Provide healthcare services consistent with available resources, and when there are limited resources, work to ensure the existence of a resource allocation process that considers ethical ramifications;

C.   Conduct both competitive and cooperative activities in ways that improve community healthcare services;

D.   Lead the organization in the use and improvement of standards of management and sound business practices;

E.   Respect the customs, beliefs and practices of patients or others served, consistent with the organization's philosophy;

F.   Be truthful in all forms of professional and organizational communication, and avoid disseminating information that is false, misleading or deceptive;

G.   Report negative financial and other information promptly and accurately, and initiate appropriate action;

H.   Prevent fraud and abuse and aggressive accounting practices that may result in disputable financial reports;

I.   Create an organizational environment in which both clinical and management mistakes are minimized and, when they do occur, are disclosed and addressed effectively;

J.   Implement an organizational code of ethics and monitor compliance; and

K.   Provide ethics resources and mechanisms for staff to address organizational and clinical ethics issues.

IV.   THE HEALTHCARE EXECUTIVE'S RESPONSIBILITIES TO EMPLOYEES
Healthcare executives have ethical and professional obligations to the employees they manage that encompass but are not limited to:

A.   Creating a work environment that promotes ethical conduct;

B.   Providing a work environment that encourages a free expression of ethical concerns and provides mechanisms for discussing and addressing such concerns;

C.   Promoting a healthy work environment, which includes freedom from harassment, sexual and other, and coercion of any kind, especially to perform illegal or unethical acts;

D.   Promoting a culture of inclusivity that seeks to prevent discrimination on the basis of race, ethnicity, religion, gender, sexual orientation, age or disability;

E.   Providing a work environment that promotes the proper use of employees' knowledge and skills; and

F.   Providing a safe and healthy work environment.

(continued)

Exhibit 11.4
ACHE *Code of Ethics** (continued)

V.   THE HEALTHCARE EXECUTIVE'S RESPONSIBILITIES TO COMMUNITY AND SOCIETY

The healthcare executive shall:

A.   Work to identify and meet the healthcare needs of the community;

B.   Work to support access to healthcare services for all people;

C.   Encourage and participate in public dialogue on healthcare policy issues, and advocate solutions that will improve health status and promote quality healthcare;

D.   Apply short- and long-term assessments to management decisions affecting both community and society; and

E.   Provide prospective patients and others with adequate and accurate information, enabling them to make enlightened decisions regarding services.

VI.   THE HEALTHCARE EXECUTIVE'S RESPONSIBILITY TO REPORT VIOLATIONS OF THE CODE

A member of ACHE who has reasonable grounds to believe that another member has violated this *Code* has a duty to communicate such facts to the Ethics Committee.

Source: ACHE (2017).

*As amended by the Board of Governors on November 13, 2017.

Creating and Maintaining Ethics in a Healthcare Organization

The top leaders and managers of an HCO are responsible for creating and maintaining the ethics of the organization. However, they do not, and should not, make all the decisions about ethical issues that arise in the HCO. **Senior managers should create organization structures, processes, and cultures that enable managers, supervisors, employees, physicians, staff, and others throughout the organization to make ethics decisions in their areas of responsibility.** Senior managers take the lead in creating and maintaining ethics for the entire HCO; managers at lower levels take the lead in their own departments and work units. The president of a health research institute is responsible for ethical performance of the entire organization. Shannon, director of neuroscience research, is responsible for ethical performance in her division.

How can leaders create structures, processes, and cultures to strengthen ethical performance throughout their HCOs? Think back to earlier parts of this chapter and to prior chapters to fully appreciate the approaches listed in exhibit 11.5.

Here is an example of leading an HCO's employees to follow ethics guidelines: The CEO of a large hospital in South Carolina hired a young vice president. The CEO told the new vice president, "I'm going to give you a lot of responsibility and one piece of advice. Every time you get ready to make a decision, ask yourself how you would feel if your decision was reported on the front page of the morning newspaper." The vice president remembered and benefited from that advice—especially when making decisions with ethical implications.

EXHIBIT 11.5

Approaches to
Achieving Ethical
Performance in
HCOs

Approach	Principles, Tools, and Methods
Organizing the HCO	• Organize work, tasks, positions, groups, systems, and resources to support the HCO's ethics, and support people dealing with ethical questions.
	• Organize an ethics advisory committee or create an ethicist position to advise the HCO's employees, physicians, supervisors, and others who want help with ethical dilemmas or distress. The committee or ethicist should be available for all ethics situations (not just medical ones).
	• Write and promote ethics rules, policies, processes, procedures, and a code of conduct—all to guide employees in ethical situations. Ensure that these documents are based on input from all appropriate stakeholders (not just managers or selected stakeholders). Include processes for how to avoid ethical problems, how to make ethical decisions, and how to contact an ethics advisory committee for help.
	• Appoint a compliance officer or position. Monitor the HCO's ethical performance and compliance with its ethics. Hold employees and others accountable for compliance with ethical standards, principles, policies, and codes.
	• Organize hotlines and whistle-blower mechanisms and processes for employees to report possible violations of the HCO's ethics. When violations are reported or found through monitoring, investigate and take appropriate action to prevent reoccurrence.
	• Allocate sufficient resources to implement structures, processes, positions, policies, and an ethical climate. To the extent possible, allocate available resources in such a way that ethical problems, dilemmas, and distress are lessened.

(continued)

Staffing the HCO	• Write job descriptions to reflect or even explicitly state ethical principles. • Award merit pay, incentives, and other compensation in a way that encourages positive ethics. • In performance reviews, evaluate workers on how well they follow ethical standards. Evaluate managers on how well they and their employees follow ethical principles. • During orientation of new staff, emphasize ethical principles and explain how staff can get help when faced with ethical questions. • Train and educate staff about the HCO's ethical climate and principles. Ensure employees know the structures, processes, and resources available to handle ethical situations. • Require managers to do an ethics self-assessment annually to monitor their own ethics and identify possible improvements. • Ensure that employees feel safe when asking ethics questions or reporting ethics violations. • Provide supportive counseling to employees, such as for moral distress and grief related to ethics situations.	**EXHIBIT 11.5** Approaches to Achieving Ethical Performance in HCOs *(continued)*
Leading the HCO	• State clearly and often the HCO's ethics and ethical climate. • Be a role model for the HCO's ethics. Live the HCO's ethics. Personally support the desired ethics—even if doing so is politically difficult because important stakeholders disagree. • Lead the development of an appropriate ethical culture and climate. Create a culture in which asking ethical questions and discussing ethics problems becomes "the way we do things here." Avoid a culture that emphasizes teamwork so much that an employee who has ethical concerns remains silent to be "a team player." • When leading meetings, allow time for participants to ask questions and express concerns about the ethics of an issue or decision. • Motivate employees by using reinforcement, goal setting, Maslow's hierarchy of needs, and other approaches to drive ethical behavior. • Use a leader's power—highly ethical leaders may have referent charismatic power (in addition to other powers) when influencing others about ethics. • Regularly monitor the ethical performance of the HCO.	

CHECK IT OUT ONLINE

ACHE provides a lot of resources to its members, many of which are available on its website. The ACHE Ethics Self-Assessment tool is freely available at www.ache.org/about-ache/our-story/our-commitments/ethics/ethics-self-assessment. This survey poses statements to rate yourself on, such as "I fulfill the promises I make" and "I respect the practices and customs of a diverse patient population while maintaining the organization's mission." Healthcare managers can use the ACHE Ethics Self-Assessment to consider their own ethics related to healthcare leadership. Students can use it to learn more about ethics in HCOs. Check it out online and see what you discover.

Looking ahead to chapter 13 on decision making, managers can use decision-making principles, tools, and methods for ethical decisions. Leaders must create a fair process in which decision makers carefully consider the views and values of *all* stakeholders who might be affected by a decision (Nelson 2015). This process ensures that conflicting views and values are considered *before* the decision is made. This approach, known as *procedural justice*, uses fair procedures when making ethical decisions. It is useful when responding to the types of challenges, issues, and developments identified in chapter 1—health disparities, mergers, demographic trends, use of social media, patients' engagement in their health, physician employment, cost reduction, genetics in healthcare, and others. Chapter 13 explains more about how to make such decisions.

ONE MORE TIME

Culture in an organization is "the set of values, norms, guiding beliefs, and understandings that is shared by members of an organization and taught to new members as the correct way to think, feel, and behave" (Daft 2016, 386). It evolves from forces inside and outside the organization. Because an HCO's culture is mostly invisible, employees interpret it by observing and listening to what goes on in the HCO. Culture strongly affects staff behavior, goal achievement, stakeholder satisfaction, and the HCO's performance and survival. To successfully lead an organization, managers must deliberately shape and influence the organization's culture so that it becomes what they think is best for the organization given its environment, mission, goals, plans, and so forth. Culture change is not easy, but it can be done by managing the forces and factors that affect culture. By organizational socialization, employees learn their organization's culture, including what is and is not acceptable behavior. Managers and leaders should try to develop a strong, consistent culture throughout the entire HCO. Yet, they must also let departments, work units, and teams develop their own subcultures (within the main culture) that are best for these individual parts of the organization.

An organization's culture includes its ethics, which are moral principles of right and wrong. Four common ethical principles in healthcare are autonomy, beneficence, justice, and nonmaleficence. In HCOs, managerial ethics, medical ethics, professional ethics, and social responsibility ethics are all important. Ethics in HCOs come from personal ethics of staff (especially leaders), the organization itself, and external sources such as accreditation standards and laws. Leaders can use management tools and methods to shape ethics and culture in HCOs.

(T) FOR YOUR TOOLBOX

- Model of forces and factors that influence HCO culture
- Model for interpreting an HCO's culture
- ACHE *Code of Ethics*
- Approaches to achieving ethical performance in HCOs

FOR DISCUSSION

1. Discuss the factors that shape culture in HCOs. Why do individual HCOs have different cultures?

2. How can you interpret the culture of an organization? Discuss your interpretation of the culture of your college or university.

3. Describe examples of subcultures within an overall HCO culture. What are the pros and cons of having subcultures?

4. Discuss examples of medical ethics, professional ethics, and managerial ethics in HCOs.

5. What captured your interest in the ACHE *Code of Ethics*? How do you feel about the ethical responsibilities of the healthcare management profession?

6. What can managers do to achieve ethical performance in their HCOs?

CASE STUDY QUESTIONS

These questions refer to the Integrative Case Studies at the back of this book.

1. Disparities in Care at Southern Regional Health System case: Explain how the ethical principles of autonomy, beneficence, justice, and nonmaleficence are relevant in this case. Explain how the four types of ethics—medical ethics, professional ethics, managerial ethics, and social responsibility—are relevant in this case.

2. How Can an ACO Improve the Health of Its Population? case: Explain how the ethical principles of autonomy, beneficence, justice, and nonmaleficence are relevant in this case. Explain how the four types of ethics—medical ethics, professional ethics, managerial ethics, and social responsibility—are relevant in this case.

3. "I Can't Do It All!" case: How would you describe the organization culture of Healthdyne? Using exhibit 11.1, explain how Mr. Brice could use specific forces and factors to change the culture to what you think he would want.

4. Increasing the Focus on Patient Safety at First Medical Center case: Explain how Dr. Frame could use specific forces and factors to change the culture to what you think she would want.

 RIVERBEND ORTHOPEDICS MINI CASE STUDY

Riverbend Orthopedics is a busy group practice with expanded services for orthopedic care. It has seven physicians and a podiatrist, plus about 70 other employees. At its big, new clinic building, Riverbend provides extensive orthopedic care. Several technicians provide diagnostic medical imaging, from basic X-rays to magnetic resonance images. The physicians perform surgery in their own outpatient surgery center with Riverbend's own operating nurses and technicians. Therapy is provided by three physical therapists and one part-time contracted occupational therapist. In addition to staff providing actual patient care, the clinic has staff for financial management, medical records, human resources, information systems/technology, building maintenance, and other administrative matters. Occasional marketing work is done by an advertising company. Legal work is outsourced to a law firm. Riverbend is managed by a new president, Ms. Garcia. She and Riverbend have set a goal of achieving "Excellent" ratings for patient experience from at least 90 percent of Riverbend's patients this year.

(continued)

RIVERBEND ORTHOPEDICS MINI CASE STUDY *(continued)*

Riverbend's organization culture has evolved somewhat accidentally based on physicians emphasizing clinical care and Ms. Garcia emphasizing financial control. There has not been any conscious effort to shape the organization culture. She feels that might have to change.

MINI CASE STUDY QUESTIONS

1. To help Riverbend achieve its goal, identify at least five "values, norms, guiding beliefs, and understandings" that should be taught to and shared by Riverbend's staff.

2. Using this chapter, explain in detail how Ms. Garcia could shape and influence Riverbend's organization culture so that it helps lead physicians and employees to achieve the patient experience goal.

REFERENCES

American College of Healthcare Executives (ACHE). 2017. *ACHE Code of Ethics.* Amended November 13. www.ache.org/about-ache/our-story/our-commitments/ethics/ache-code-of-ethics.

Daft, R. L. 2016. *Organization Theory and Design,* 12th ed. Mason, OH: South-Western Cengage.

Dye, C. F. 2017. *Leadership in Healthcare,* 3rd ed. Chicago: Health Administration Press.

Griffin, R. W., J. M. Phillips, and S. M. Gully. 2017. *Organizational Behavior: Managing People and Organizations,* 12th ed. Boston: Cengage Learning.

Hamric, A. B., E. G. Epstein, and K. R. White. 2014. "Moral Distress and the Healthcare Organization." In *Managerial Ethics in Healthcare: A New Perspective,* edited by G. L. Filerman, A. E. Mills, and P. M. Schyve, 137–58. Chicago: Health Administration Press.

Haraden, C., and A. Frankel. 2004. "Shuttling Toward a Safety Culture: Healthcare Can Learn from Probe Panel's Findings on the Columbia Disaster." *Modern Healthcare* 34 (1): 21.

Jacob, S. 2013. "Baylor, Scott & White First Tackled Cultural Fit in Merger Due Diligence." *D CEO Healthcare*. Published October 30. http://healthcare.dmagazine.com/2013/10/30/baylor-scott-white-first-tackled-cultural-fit-in-merger-due-diligence.

Jarrett, M. P. 2017. "Patient Safety and Leadership: Do You Walk the Walk?" *Journal of Healthcare Management* 62 (2): 88–92.

Johnson, J. A., and C. C. Rossow (eds.). 2019. *Health Organizations: Theory, Behavior, and Development*, 2nd ed. Burlington, MA: Jones & Bartlett Learning.

Kash, B. A. 2016. "Interview with Jayne E. Pope, RN, FACHE, CEO of Hill Country Memorial Hospital." *Journal of Healthcare Management* 61 (5): 307–10.

Kaufman, K. 2017. "The New Role of Healthcare Integration." In *Futurescan 2017: Healthcare Trends and Implications 2017–2022*, edited by I. Morrison, 2–6. Chicago: Society for Healthcare Strategy & Market Development and Health Administration Press.

Nelson, W. A. 2015. "Making Ethical Decisions." *Healthcare Executive* 30 (4): 46–48.

Peters, T., and R. Waterman. 1982. *In Search of Excellence*. New York: Harper & Row.

Rorty, M. V. 2014. "Introduction to Ethics." In *Managerial Ethics in Healthcare: A New Perspective,* edited by G. L. Filerman, A. E. Mills, and P. M. Schyve, 1–18. Chicago: Health Administration Press.

Thomas, N. B. 2017. "Leading with Compassion." *Healthcare Executive* 32 (2): 80–81.

Van Dyke, M. 2017. "Building on Success to Conquer Patient Harm." *Healthcare Executive* 32 (2): 21–30.

Walston, S. L. 2017. *Organizational Behavior and Leadership in Healthcare: Leadership Perspectives and Management Applications*. Chicago: Health Administration Press.

CHAPTER 12

CONTROLLING AND IMPROVING PERFORMANCE

You can't manage what you don't measure.

Common management expression

LEARNING OBJECTIVES

Studying this chapter will help you to

➤ define and describe control;

➤ identify types of performance that managers must control;

➤ explain how managers control performance using a three-step approach;

➤ describe control tools and techniques, including data visualization; and

➤ understand how Six Sigma, Lean, and high reliability are used for performance improvement.

HERE'S WHAT HAPPENED

Managers measured the performance of Partners HealthCare and realized not all expectations were met. Some aspects of performance did not compare well to standards and target performance levels. At Faulkner Hospital (part of the Partners health system), 27 percent of discharged heart failure patients had to be readmitted within 30 days. That outcome was worse than the national rate. Managers saw a need to improve the quality of patient care for heart failure. They redesigned the patient care process for treating heart failure and then continued to measure outcomes. The redesign used telehealth to enable Partners' staff to monitor heart patients at home after discharge from the hospital. Also in the redesigned process, staff taught patients self-care for their heart problems so they could stay healthy. After changing the structure and process of care, managers continued to measure readmission rates. They also measured other aspects of performance, such as the percent of patients who learned more about heart failure, the percent who were able to gain control over their heart failure, and the percent who were confident they could independently manage their heart failure. Results showed a 51 percent decrease in heart failure readmissions, high patient satisfaction, and $8,155 net savings per patient because of reduced readmissions.

As seen in the preceding Here's What Happened, managers must control their organization's performance. Partners' managers realized some performance was "out of control" when they compared actual results to planned results. So they made changes to improve performance, continued to measure the results, and brought performance "in control."

How do managers control and improve performance? This chapter explains how. It begins by defining and describing the management control function. Controlling and improving performance is the fifth and final management function (as we learned in chapter 2), and it interacts with the other four functions. Four of the ten managerial roles identified by Henry Mintzberg (described in chapter 2) involve controlling: the roles of monitor, entrepreneur, disturbance handler, and resource allocator. Next, the chapter discusses types of performance that managers must control in healthcare organizations (HCOs). Managers can do this by using the three-step control method and control tools and techniques that are described. Sources of data and examples of data visualization are presented. The chapter finishes with explanations of Six Sigma, Lean, and high reliability approaches to performance improvement in HCOs. Exhibits show tools, graphs, and diagrams that managers use to visually understand and improve work processes and performance. This chapter will help you prepare for operations management work, which some students choose for careers.

What Is Control?

Recall from chapter 2 that managers control performance by comparing actual performance to preset standards and making corrective adjustments if needed to meet those standards (Dunn 2016). Thus, managers do three things to **control** performance:

1. Set performance standards.

2. Measure actual performance and compare it to the standards.

3. Improve performance if it does not meet the standards.

control
To monitor performance and take corrective action if performance does not meet expected standards.

What are some examples of control? A thermostat is a mechanical device that controls the performance of a heating and cooling system to achieve a preset, expected temperature. It measures one dimension of performance: temperature. Often, we are interested in several dimensions of performance, such as when we drive and control a car. The car measures its speed, fuel consumption, engine temperature, and other dimensions of performance. Drivers measure comfort and other dimensions. We compare the actual speed measurements to speed standards posted on signs, and we adjust the car's performance if necessary. We steer the car so that it performs according to the standards on Google Maps. All these actions enable us to control multiple dimensions of performance to accomplish our goals of getting to our destination safely, on time, and without a speeding ticket. The driving example involves both mechanical and human control systems.

Organizations are not machines. They are composed of people, which makes control more challenging. Fortunately, effective methods are available that managers can use to control their organizations. Although managers do not use a steering wheel, they do use management tools to steer their HCOs. What have you already learned from this book that you could use to steer performance in an HCO? Try to list at least five tools. We next examine dimensions of control in HCOs.

Control in Healthcare Organizations

HCOs have lagged behind other industries in controlling and improving their performance (McLaughlin and Olson 2017). However, forces in HCOs' external environments—especially those pertaining to healthcare financing, reimbursement, and payment—have led HCOs to do more to control performance. Recall that chapter 1 reported trends for payment based on value rather than volume of care. As a result, HCOs are adapting to pay-for-performance models based on standards of quality, patient experience, coordinated care, outcomes of care, cost of care, and other expectations.

What other aspects of performance do you think HCOs must control? Name an HCO, and then list a few dimensions of performance you think it should control. One way to think about this is by using the *stakeholder approach* (studied in chapter 1). For example, patients often expect convenient scheduling of appointments, short wait times when they arrive for appointments, and accurate diagnosis and treatment. Employees often expect fair compensation, reasonable workloads and schedules, and respect from their managers. What are the performance expectations and standards of vendors, accreditors, the state health department, and other stakeholders?

The *structure/process/outcome approach* is another way to think about types of performance HCOs must control. These three performance dimensions were developed by Avedis Donabedian (1966, 1988) primarily for medical care. They were later extended to other kinds of work. Managers should realize that structures and processes strongly affect outcomes. Thus, to improve outcomes, managers should improve structures and processes.

structure measures
Measures of resources, staff, equipment, competencies, inputs, facilities, and characteristics of the organization; how the organization is set up.

◆ **Structure measures:** These measures include available resources, staff, equipment, competencies, inputs, facilities, and characteristics of the HCO. They reflect how the organization is (or was) set up. The rehabilitation facility is accredited; the community health center included three health coaches, one nutritionist, and one behavioral health counselor; the medical group has an electronic health records system; and the public health department had two health inspectors.

process measures
Measures of the work that is done, how it is done, and the activities performed.

◆ **Process measures:** These measures include what work is done, how it is done, and which activities are involved. They reflect the HCO in action after someone presses the "on" button. The outpatient surgery center verifies insurance information for its patients, the hospital made 17 medication errors, and telehealth remotely monitors blood pressure readings of rural patients.

outcome measures
Measures of results and effects.

◆ **Outcome measures:** These measures include what happens (or happened) as a result of the structures and processes. They reflect the results and effects. The physician group achieved 5 percent growth in pediatric market share, 90 percent of cardiac rehabilitation patients are able to work, and 12 percent of the hospital's patients were readmitted within 30 days. Partners HealthCare examined several outcome measures in the opening Here's What Happened.

As we learned in chapter 1, stakeholders have begun actively holding HCOs accountable for better value (an outcome). If performance outcomes do not meet performance standards, what should managers do? According to Donabedian's research, managers should change structures, processes, or both.

To control the performance of an entire HCO, managers must control the structure, process, and outcome performance of individual parts of the HCO. These parts include departments (e.g., laboratory), work units (e.g., microbiology), shifts (e.g., second shift), and workers (e.g., lab techs). Managers must also control how the many parts work together (the coordination studied in chapter 5) because organizations are systems of interrelated parts. Today's management tip: **Quality problems are often caused by the system rather than by a person.** Quality expert W. Edwards Deming believed that only about 15 percent of quality problems were caused by faulty workers, whereas the other 85 percent were caused by faulty systems, processes, and management (Warren 2014). Managers in HCOs are therefore adjusting how they manage their organization and how they try to improve quality. For example, many HCOs are using scripts (structures) to carefully control staff interactions (processes) with patients, families, and others, in order to improve patient experience (outcomes). UCLA Health has scripted standardized tasks and behaviors that all employees must perform when interacting with patients (UCLA Health 2018):

With everyone on every encounter, we commit to:

- **Connect** with **Compassion** by addressing the patients as Mr./Ms. or by the name that they prefer.
- **Introduce** yourself with **Integrity** by stating your name and your role.
- **Communicate** with **Teamwork** what you are going to do, how long it is going to take, and how it will impact the patient.
- **Ask** with **Discovery** by anticipating the patient needs, questions, or concerns.
- **Respond** with **Respect** to patient questions or requests with immediacy.
- **Exit** with **Excellence** by ensuring all of the patient's needs are met.

A THREE-STEP CONTROL METHOD

Recall the three steps used to control performance mentioned earlier in this chapter. The next few sections explain the steps in depth with examples for HCOs. By following these steps, you will be better prepared to control performance:

1. Set performance standards.

2. Measure actual performance and compare it to the standards.

3. Improve performance if it does not meet the standards.

These steps should be viewed as a continual cycle.

STEP 1: SET PERFORMANCE STANDARDS

Managers often establish standards (also called targets). Perhaps you do the same in your life. In chapter 3 we learned that managers plan goals and decide what they want to accomplish during the next year, month, week, shift, and so forth. During implementation planning

TRY IT, APPLY IT

> Think of examples of controlling performance in your daily life. Do you control your use of time? Use of money? Academic performance? Performance in a sport or hobby? If so, describe how you control your performance. What other control methods could you use? Discuss your ideas with your classmates.

and project planning, they set standards and targets by which to compare and judge actual performance. Standards are expressed using metrics (numerical measurements) of things that can be measured. Here are examples of targets in healthcare:

◆ 8 percent reduction in cost per chemotherapy procedure this year

◆ 20 percent reduction in number of patient care disparities by October 1

◆ 3 percent gain in social media followers next month

◆ 6 hours of training for each patient navigator during August

key performance indicator
A metric linked to a target or standard of performance.

A **key performance indicator** (KPI) is a metric linked to a target (McLaughlin and Olson 2017). KPIs are directly linked to an organization's strategic goals (Walston 2017). A KPI generally shows how close (above or below) actual performance is to the target—and thus how close the organization is to achieving a target or goal. Viewing a KPI, a manager can quickly see how her department's performance compares to the target. Performance management apps and programs often show KPIs using colored visual gauges so managers quickly see, for example, that actual performance is at 78 percent of the target.

Imagine a dental practice in Austin whose patients complain about long waits after arriving for scheduled appointments. A goal is set for 80 percent of patients each month to wait less than 5 minutes after arrival. At the end of the first month, the KPI shows 84 percent of patients waited less than 5 minutes. The KPI gives the practice manager a quick way to assess whether the practice is achieving its goal.

Suppose Greg manages a community health education center in Omaha. He sets targets for which classes will be offered, when each new class will begin, and how many people will enroll in each class. Greg creates standards when he organizes jobs and work, such as a standard of 24 hours to respond to a customer's inquiry. He sets staffing targets, such as less than 10 percent employee turnover per year. Greg sets targets that are SMART: specific, measurable, achievable, realistic, and time related.

Managers set standards and targets based on external and internal factors. External factors include accreditation standards, licensure requirements, government regulations, and industry standards. The Joint Commission and the Malcolm Baldrige National Quality Award have criteria for quality in HCOs. Websites now publicly report data about HCOs' prices, quality, outcomes, and other measures. Professional associations such as the Society for Human Resource Management provide benchmarks, which are standards of performance based on best practices. All these external sources of data and information influence managers as they set their performance targets.

Managers also consider internal factors when setting expectations and targets. As noted earlier, an organization's mission, goals, strategic plans, and implementation plans will identify essential standards and targets. Managers should also think about available internal funds, leadership capabilities, and organization culture that influence goals and targets. Recall from chapter 3 that the strategic planning process requires an HCO to identify its strengths and weaknesses. Managers must consider these factors when making realistic targets (rather than wild guesses).

Stakeholders—both internal and external—influence managers as they set targets. Internally, if employees express frequent complaints about parking, managers may set targets of adding 50 parking spaces by March 1 and increasing employees' satisfaction with parking to 95 percent by March 15. Externally, when lenders set target dates for repayment of loans, a physician-recruiting company must accept those targets. **Managers should consider expectations of stakeholders when setting performance targets.**

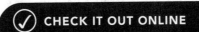

CHECK IT OUT ONLINE

As part of control, managers use publicly available online data to compare their HCOs' performance with that of similar HCOs. Managers of HCOs can use these data to find the "best" performance in their area and determine a reasonable target for next year. Hospital Compare (www.medicare.gov/hospitalcompare/) is a national source of HCO clinical care performance data. Many states also provide comparative performance data for hospitals, nursing homes, surgery centers, home care agencies, or physician practices. Florida Health Finder (www.floridahealthfinder.gov) and Illinois Hospital Report Card (www.healthcarereportcard.illinois.gov) are two examples. Check it out online and see what you discover.

After considering external and internal factors, managers set targets for the future. The targets are reflected in organization documents, such as strategic plans, budgets, staffing plans, job descriptions, policies, rules, inventory stock levels, and Gantt charts.

STEP 2: MEASURE ACTUAL PERFORMANCE AND COMPARE IT TO STANDARDS

The second step for control is to measure and compare actual performance to standard performance. Suppose Nina manages a chronic pain clinic in Las Vegas. She had set a target of serving 25 patients per day at her clinic. Now she must measure the actual number of clinic patients served per day and compare that number to 25 to determine if performance was better than, worse than, or equal to the target. As a manager, you will be accountable for measuring performance in your area of responsibility. You can't manage what you don't measure (as the chapter opening quote told us).

Where do all the data for measuring actual performance come from? If you take a job in an existing department or program, some measurement systems will probably be in place (although you might want to update them). If you are helping to start a new program or HCO, you will have to create systems to gather performance data.

Managers obtain data from inside their HCO. Some types of data capture may be centralized for the whole HCO, such as for patient billing. Other types of data capture might be decentralized to individual departments, such as clinical procedure completion times. Health and medical records, financial accounts, registration files, payroll records, and inventory reports have useful data. Department records usually have operational statistics for the department's workload, inputs, outputs, and activities to produce the outputs. Many data are automatically entered into extensive digital databases and data warehouses that managers can search. More data are available through surveys, such as patient satisfaction surveys and employee attitude surveys. These surveys might be quantitative, with check boxes and numerical ratings (e.g., a scale of 1 to 5). Or, they might be qualitative, allowing for comments and explanations beyond a single number. Qualitative data also come from organized focus groups, customer interviews, informal conversations, observations, town hall meetings, Snapchat messages, phone calls, and other feedback from stakeholders.

External data are also very useful. Managers can obtain these data from documents, digital reports, conversations, licensure agency proceedings, accreditation surveys, government databases, customers, supply chain partners, and other stakeholders and sources. Additional data may come from the many external databases found online (e.g., those mentioned earlier in the Check It Out Online box).

Managers should be thoughtful about which data they use for metrics and control. Many data are automatically captured by computers, barcode scanners, and other devices and then moved to cloud storage. Automatic capture and storage of massive amounts of data can create problems if too many metrics are reported for managers to sort through. Too many data may overwhelm end users because time, effort, and resources are required to process, report, and interpret data and metrics. Another concern is that data for some metrics might not be easily available because they are confidential or hard to collect. Problems arise when frontline workers must frequently stop and record data. They may feel that this task wastes their time and interferes with their "real" work. Accurate, valid, and reliable data are usually not free, so managers must ensure that the value of the data exceeds the cost of accurately collecting and processing it. The number of metrics used should be few enough that significant additional resources are not needed for data collection, processing, and reporting. No more than 20 metrics should be used in a large HCO or multifacility system, and fewer are needed in smaller organizations (Langabeer and Helton 2016). Measures should be useful, accurate, easily available, easily understood, and calculated the same way over time (Spath 2018).

Managers often use quantitative performance measures, such as counts, frequencies, percentages, ratios, averages, and other metrics. These data can be presented in charts, graphs, tables, maps, and other data visualizations that help managers see the main points. Examples are shown in exhibits 12.1 through 12.5. Some people say that every picture tells a story. Every chart, graph, and exhibit also tells a story. What story do you think is told by each of these exhibits?

Managers use a *line graph* (sometimes called a run chart) to show performance data trends, such as trends for customers' tweets (exhibit 12.1). Managers use a *bar graph* (sometimes called a bar chart) to show and compare performance data, such as performance

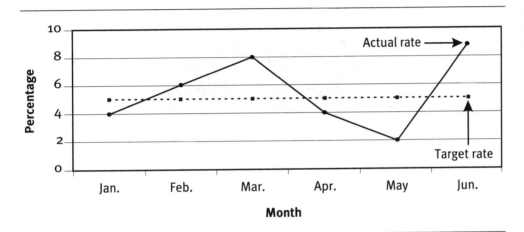

EXHIBIT 12.1
Line Graph or
Run Chart

Source: Spath (2018).

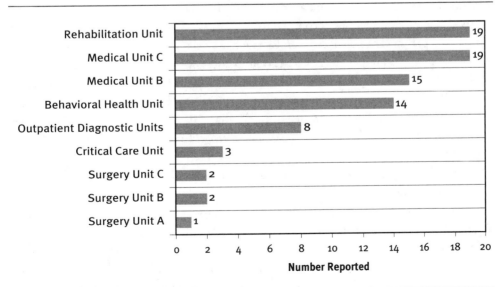

EXHIBIT 12.2
Bar Chart

Source: Spath (2018).

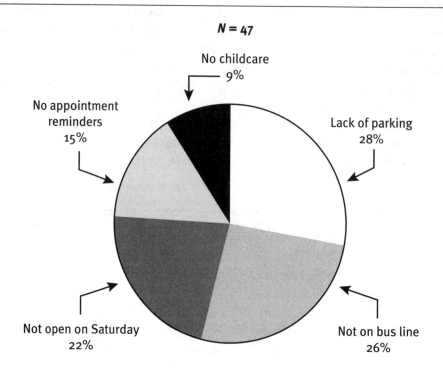

Source: Spath (2018).

data for multiple patient care units (exhibit 12.2). Managers use a *pie chart* to show how all performance data are divided into data categories—for example, how all patient complaints are divided into five categories of complaints (exhibit 12.3). Managers use a *control chart* to show actual performance data and trends—such as rejected claims—compared to performance standards. An upper control limit (UCL) and lower control limit (LCL), shown in exhibit 12.4 as thick gray lines, define the range within which performance is considered normal. Within this range, performance can vary and still be considered normal (Spath 2018). A center mean line shown in exhibit 12.4 as a dashed gray center line is another standard for comparison. Managers use a *tabular report* (sometimes called a table of data) to show performance data, such as patient satisfaction results, in a readable format (exhibit 12.5). Another example of a tabular report is shown in exhibit 5 of the Partners HealthCare case, which appears at the back of this book.

Many HCOs use scorecards and dashboards to report performance measures in a single report. These graphics generally report performance for a specific period, such as a day, a month, or a year. They may show any number of measures (e.g., the ones found throughout this chapter), depending on which measures managers decide to include. The graphics can be easily produced and revised to show different measures selected by the managers at

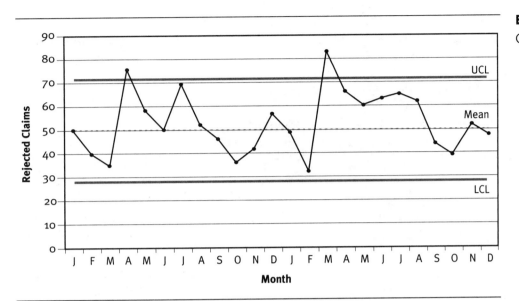

EXHIBIT 12.4
Control Chart

Source: Spath (2018).

EXHIBIT 12.5
Table of Data

Survey Questions	Mean Score N = 47
Overall, how would you evaluate:	
1. The quality of the mental health services you received	3.5
2. The helpfulness of the staff members	3.0
3. The courtesy shown you by the staff members	3.8
4. Staff's attention to privacy during treatment sessions	4.0
5. The professionalism of the staff members	3.9
6. The extent to which your mental health needs were addressed	3.6
7. The availability of appointments	3.5
8. The effectiveness of the medication and/or treatment you received	3.8
9. The degree to which staff members respected your confidentiality	4.1
10. Opportunities to participate in decisions about your treatment	3.9

Scale: 1 = Poor   2 = Fair   3 = Good   4 = Very Good   5 = Excellent

Source: Spath (2018).

balanced scorecard
Report with
performance measures
typically for finances,
customer service,
internal business
processes, and growth
and learning; other
kinds of measures may
also be used.

any level of an HCO. **Balanced scorecards** were first developed in the 1990s to present a balanced view of an organization, rather than only a financial view. The scorecards typically (but not always) include measures that strongly affect strategic goals in four categories:

1. Financial (e.g., revenue, return on investment)

2. Customer service (e.g., new customers, client satisfaction)

3. Internal business processes (e.g., inventory levels, production errors)

4. Potential for growth and learning (e.g., new services, employee retention)

Some HCOs use more scorecard categories to focus on additional dimensions of performance. Managers can add measures that are important and remove measures that have become less urgent. For example, at a new chiropractic business that is barely paying its bills, managers could include "cash on hand" and "billed revenue" in the dashboard or scorecard. After the business becomes more financially stable, they could remove those measures and replace them with newer measures, such as "number of clients" and "employee satisfaction scores."

STEP 3: IMPROVE PERFORMANCE IF IT DOES NOT MEET STANDARDS

If the second control step shows performance does not meet expectations, managers must use the third control step—improve performance. How? **Managers can apply the tools, methods, principles, theories, and techniques described in earlier chapters of this book to fix performance.**

Managers can first reconsider the goals, targets, and standards and decide if they are still realistic. Maybe a law changed or a new competitor emerged. Perhaps managers were far too optimistic in setting goals during the strategic planning process. For a variety of reasons, managers might realize that a target should be changed. (Of course, managers should not simply change the standard whenever performance does not meet the standard!)

If managers feel their standards should be maintained, then they must change the organization's structures, processes, or both to achieve satisfactory performance. What are some possibilities? Think back to previous chapters. Managers might have to adjust the job design, work design, organization design, decentralization, standardization, horizontal coordination, organization culture, motivation techniques, training, staffing ratios, work schedules, rules, work processes, performance appraisals, teams, project planning, or leadership styles. In the Here's What Happened at the beginning of this chapter, we saw that Partners HealthCare made some of these changes. Review the For Your Toolbox section at the end of each chapter and the defined terms throughout the chapters to think of other possibilities.

When you try to improve performance in an HCO, remember that it is a system of interrelated, interdependent parts. That means if one part is changed, other parts will be affected and might also have to change for the system (organization) to perform well. If technological parts of a system are changed, then human processes also have to change. For example, researchers studied HCOs' early attempts to use healthcare information technology (IT) systems (Kellermann and Jones 2013). Why did actual performance initially not achieve the performance standards of these IT systems? One common reason was that human work processes had not been changed to fit the new technology. For HCOs and their new technological systems to reach performance targets, work processes had to be redesigned, workers had to be trained in the new processes, and incentives had to be provided to motivate the workers to change.

Managers have plenty of possible adjustments that they *could* make. Which ones *should* they make? That depends on the situation. It is a problem to be analyzed and solved. Managers can use three tools to analyze performance problems: a cause-and-effect diagram, a process map, and root-cause analysis. A **cause-and-effect diagram** (also called a *fishbone diagram*) can be used to identify possible causes of performance problems. Exhibit 12.6 is an example of a cause-and-effect diagram. This tool can be used to dig down to factors that contribute to good performance or bad performance. The performance (effect) is stated in the "fish head" on the right side of the diagram. The fish skeleton (cause) is left of the fish head and leads to the head. In exhibit 12.6, the horizontal spine of the fish connects to

cause-and-effect diagram
A tool that visually identifies which factors might affect performance.

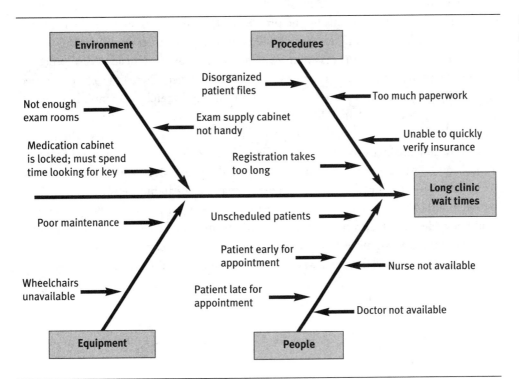

Exhibit 12.6
Cause-and-Effect (Fishbone) Diagram

Source: Spath (2018).

four diagonal fishbones that represent four types of factors that might cause the problem (effect) in the fish head.

The four main fishbones (categories of factors) are the

1. environment in which the work is performed,

2. equipment used to perform the work,

3. procedures done to perform the work, and

4. people who perform the work.

These four types of factors can be used to identify possible causes of performance problems. Managers can add other fishbones if necessary for additional categories of factors.

Clinic staff can brainstorm *possible* factors in each of these four categories that *might* cause the performance problem. In exhibit 12.6, "Disorganized patient files" is a factor in the Procedures category that might cause the problem of long clinic wait times. Staff could drill down to identify subfactors that might cause the disorganized files factor. Although not shown in the exhibit, "Lack of staff training" could be a subfactor that causes the "Disorganized patient files" factor, which in turn causes the problem of long clinic wait times. After the clinic staff has suggested possible factors and subfactors, they use data to figure out which ones actually are causing the problem. Data and information gathered in the second step of the control method can help them uncover the problem.

Another tool is the **process map,** which managers use to visualize work processes that create a product or service. A **process** is a set of tasks, activities, and steps performed sequentially to transform resource inputs into outputs and thereby accomplish a specific outcome (Langabeer and Helton 2016, 76). A process map (also called a *flowchart*) is shown in exhibit 12.7. This tool enables managers to identify, arrange, and analyze the flow of tasks, activities, and steps required to complete a process and create an output, such as a medical image. Managers can use this tool to initially plan a new work process or revise an existing process. Causes of process problems may be apparent. Steps that do not add any value to the process may be found. Perhaps resource inputs, tasks, activities, and steps should be added, deleted, combined, rearranged, or simplified to make the process easier, faster, less complicated, more accurate, less error prone, more convenient, more efficient, less costly, or better in some other way. This is sometimes called *process engineering*.

To understand how to create a process map, study the following steps (McLaughlin and Olson 2017, 140–41):

1. Assemble and train a team of people who are involved in the process that will be mapped.

process map
A tool that identifies and shows in sequence the flow of tasks, activities, and steps required to complete a process.

process
A set of tasks, activities, and steps performed sequentially to transform resource inputs into outputs and thereby accomplish a specific outcome.

2. Determine the boundaries (beginning and end) of the process and level of detail wanted.

3. Brainstorm and then arrange in sequence the tasks and steps in the process at the desired level of detail; this may be done with sticky notes on a table or wall.

4. Create a formal process map using appropriate symbols and digital drawing software.

5. Ask relevant people to review the chart; make changes as needed.

An interesting way to diagnose problems is to prepare a process map of how the work process was originally designed and then compare it to a process map of how the work is actually being performed. Managers may discover that workers are not following the proper process. Perhaps they are using shortcuts or work-arounds. These charts force managers to think through work processes and how to improve them.

Managers may also apply **root-cause analysis** (RCA) as a tool to identify and correct the underlying cause(s) of a performance problem. RCA is a structured problem-solving technique to find and fix the ultimate cause of a problem rather than the visible symptoms of the problem (McLaughlin and Olson 2017). It requires understanding what happened, why it happened, and how to prevent it from happening again. To do this, managers may repeatedly ask "Why?" until the root cause of a problem has finally been found. Here is an example (McLaughlin and Olson 2017, 145–46):

> **root-cause analysis**
> A structured problem-solving technique to find and fix the ultimate cause of a problem rather than the visible symptoms of the problem.

1. A patient received the wrong medication.

    ◆   Why?

2. The doctor prescribed the wrong medication.

    ◆   Why?

3. Relevant information was missing from the patient's chart.

    ◆   Why?

4. The patient's most recent lab test results were not entered into the chart.

    ◆   Why?

5. The lab technician sent the results, but they were in transit.

The *why* questioning could keep going. Brainstorming, observation, surveys of customers and employees, and cause-and-effect diagrams can also be used for RCA (Langabeer

Exhibit 12.7
Process Map

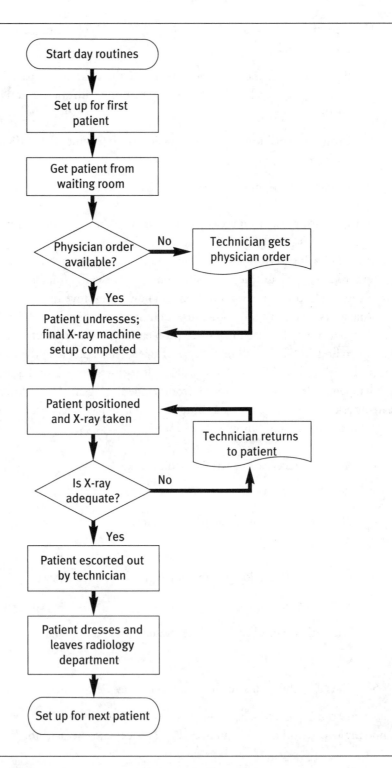

and Helton 2016). The main point: Dig deeply to find and fix the underlying cause of a problem.

QUALITY IMPROVEMENT PROGRAMS AND METHODOLOGIES

Thus far, this chapter has mostly focused on the three-step approach by which managers control performance in their organizations. This approach helps control quality and is often used in quality improvement (QI) programs. Organizations have used various forms of QI for decades. We now examine three QI programs that are used in HCOs. Six Sigma and Lean are both common; high reliability is becoming more common.

SIX SIGMA

The **Six Sigma** quality management program strives to eliminate defective products and services by eliminating variation in systems (McLaughlin and Olson 2017). Its performance standard is extremely high: no more than 3.4 defects, problems, or errors per 1,000,000 opportunities. This performance level is pursued by using the five-step DMAIC cycle for improvement projects: define, measure, analyze, improve, and control. The DMAIC cycle takes basic methods from Deming's Plan-Do-Check-Act cycle of improvement, expands them to five steps, and applies them with greater rigor to reduce variation and defects in business processes. The following list explains the five DMAIC steps used in Six Sigma (Dunn 2016; McLaughlin and Olson 2017):

> **Six Sigma**
> A performance improvement program that aims to reduce variation and defects in work processes and outputs to meet customers' quality requirements.

1. **D**efine in measurable terms the quality problem that is to be solved or the quality process that is to be improved. Identify what customers think are essential characteristics of quality and what their minimal performance standards are.

2. **M**easure the current performance of the process and how well it meets customers' requirements. Gather detailed data for inputs, processes, and outputs.

3. **A**nalyze the data for causes of defects and problems. Use root-cause analysis to find true causes.

4. **I**mprove defective processes discovered in the prior step. Select and implement improvements based on probability of successful implementation and resolution of the problems. Measure results until outcomes meet standards.

5. **C**ontrol and maintain the improved process with continued monitoring, training, incentives, and structures as needed.

Six Sigma was developed by Motorola in the 1980s and then refined and used with much success by General Electric. Today it is used in many companies and HCOs because of its proven effectiveness. Managers provide extensive training to employees who work in teams applying Six Sigma to specific projects and processes. Employees may have specific roles on teams, such as team leader, recorder, or facilitator. They may earn proficiency designations (e.g., yellow belt, green belt, black belt) for competency in Six Sigma tools and methods including data collection, statistics, and cause-and-effect diagrams. A Six Sigma team cycles through the five steps to continually improve processes, eliminate process variation, reduce defects in products and services, and increase fulfillment of customers' expectations (Langabeer and Helton 2016).

LEAN PRODUCTION

Lean production
Design of work processes to reduce waste, increase efficiency and speed, and thereby produce more value for customers.

Lean production focuses on what is valuable to customers and designs work processes to produce value for customers (McLaughlin and Olson 2017). This approach includes removing waste to increase efficiency, speed, and quality. After waste is eliminated, more of the production time and activity adds value to the customer's service and experience. Managers remove the following types of waste (which often occur in HCOs) because they do not add value for the customer (Langabeer and Helton 2016, 92; McLaughlin and Olson 2017, 258):

- *Wait time*—when someone is waiting for someone or something to become available

- *Transit time*—when patients, workers, or equipment move somewhere else

- *Idle time*—when work is not being done because of system downtime or a planned break

- *Transition time*—when resources are cleaned after one patient and prepared for the next patient

- *Overproduction*—producing more than is needed, such as too many meals

- *Overprocessing*—extra processing and steps to accomplish a task, such as extra "clicks" and screen changes on a computer or device

- *Defects*—production of parts or services that have to be redone or thrown away

- *Inventory*—supplies, materials, work-in-progress, and finished products that are stored for future use

- *Unnecessary motion*—motion that does not add value to the product or service

Lean tries to eliminate all waste by striving for continual improvement (known as *kaizen*). The kaizen approach requires a change from "If it isn't broken, don't fix it" to "If it isn't broken, it can still be improved" (McLaughlin and Olson 2017, 276). A Lean organization keeps searching for—and finding—ways to improve its work processes to better serve customers. Managers of all HCOs can try to do the same.

Lean closely examines processes and workflows (called *value streams*) that provide a service to a customer. Each step of each value stream process—such as patient registration, insurance certification, patient transportation, and patient treatment—is analyzed using **value stream mapping**. This is a visual diagram of all steps in a process used to transform inputs to outputs when creating a product or service for customers (McLaughlin and Olson 2017). Managers use this Lean tool to find and eliminate wasted steps, wasted time, wasted supplies, wasted labor, and other waste that does not add value to the customer. Exhibit 12.8 shows a value stream map for a birthing center. The Lean team that developed the map over several weeks will use it to find and remove non-value-adding work while keeping the work that does add value for customers. For example, healthcare processes often have much wait time (as most of us have experienced). The value stream map identifies wait times in the birthing center. The Lean team will redesign the process where possible to decrease long wait times.

> **value stream mapping**
> A visual diagram of all steps in a process used to transform inputs into outputs when creating a product or service for customers.

The value-added time in a patient's process (such as in exhibit 12.8) is sometimes less than 5 percent of the total time the patient spends to complete the process (McLaughlin and Olson 2017, 261)! Managers in Lean organizations improve this by redesigning and standardizing how work is done (recall scientific management in chapter 2). The Using Chapter 12 in the Real World sidebar provides an interesting example of redesigning work processes at a US Department of Veterans Affairs (VA) health center. As a manager of an HCO, you will have many opportunities to improve processes to improve the patient experience.

Lean is more than a set of tools and methods (Barnas 2018). To really work, Lean must be a systematic approach to management. The organization's vision, purpose, goals, and strategies must first provide a clear, guiding North Star for Lean change and improvement. Transformational leadership and humble leadership will help. The Lean management system and philosophy must be fully embraced. Then the HCO can actually start using Lean tools and methods.

HIGH RELIABILITY

The Agency for Healthcare Research and Quality (AHRQ) defines high-reliability organizations (HROs) as "organizations that operate in complex, high-hazard domains for extended periods without serious accidents or catastrophic failures" (AHRQ 2018). One example is a military aircraft carrier that has aircrafts taking off and landing once a minute amid continually changing and risky, uncertain conditions.

EXHIBIT 12.8
Value Stream Map

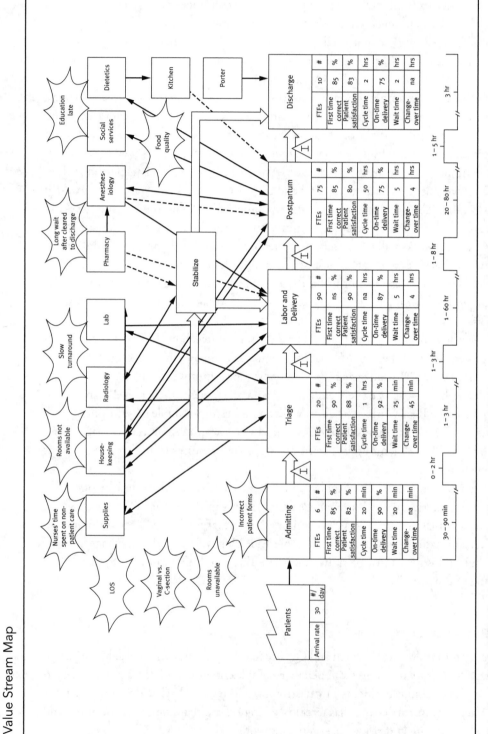

Note: Created with eVSM software from GumshoeKI, Inc., a Microsoft Visio add-on. FTE = full-time equivalent; LOS = length of stay; na = not applicable.

Source: McLaughlin and Olson (2017, 262).

🌐 **USING CHAPTER 12 IN THE REAL WORLD**

The Greenville VA Health Care Center in North Carolina used Lean to redesign work processes and produce more value for customers by removing waste and increasing efficiency, speed, and quality. Staff applied Lean in a population health program for veterans with hypertension. Before Lean, the steps to perform blood pressure (BP) checks varied. The variability resulted in inaccurate measurements, wasted time, and extra work because BP checks had to be redone. Lean principles standardized the steps to perform BP checks, thereby eliminating the variability, wasted time, and repeat work. Do it right the first time! A second problem before the Lean redesign was that some patients, after seeing a physician, then needed an appointment with a clinical pharmacist. This appointment often had to be scheduled on a later day, which caused extra travel, more wait time, and delayed care. After the Lean redesign, an interdisciplinary team (nurse, primary care provider, and clinical pharmacist) now provides patient-centered care with all required services in one appointment. This new process improves care and reduces wasted time. Lean redesign used cultural competence to redesign care so it fit military veterans' preferences for group appointments. A successful pilot project involving 20 patients is now being expanded to serve more than 400 patients per year (Forte 2018).

Becoming an HRO involves creating a mind-set. In an HRO, everyone is always on high alert to anticipate problems, detect them early (e.g., a strange smell), and respond quickly before a small problem becomes a big problem (e.g., a raging fire). This mind-set is a continual way of thinking and behaving while working, rather than a project that begins and ends. An HRO has five essential characteristics (AHRQ 2018; Federico 2018):

1. *Preoccupation with failure.* People in HROs think about potential failure, realizing that new threats can occur unexpectedly anytime, anywhere. They are highly attuned to small signs of danger. A lack of mistakes leads to intense concern about the imminent next one.

2. *Reluctance to simplify.* People in HROs do not simplify or shortcut their understanding of work processes and why things may (or did) fail. They go beyond shallow surface explanations and dig more deeply because work is

complex. RCA is applied. Reflective thinking and continuous learning are used.

3. *Sensitivity to operations.* People in HROs stay very aware of work conditions and any variance from what is expected. This situation awareness means people develop an understanding of their current work in relation to the bigger picture and what is going on around them. They are sensitive to how a process change can affect other processes.

4. *Deference to expertise.* People in HROs believe those who are closest to a work process know the most about it. In an emergency, a person of low status or less seniority may know the most about the situation. Deference is given to local expertise rather than hierarchical authority. Everyone is expected to share concerns with others, and the organization climate encourages speaking about potential safety problems.

5. *Commitment to resilience.* People in HROs practice assessing and responding to risky challenges. They develop skill in quickly identifying potential safety threats and responding before harm occurs. They feel empowered and safe to speak up about risks and problems.

The high-reliability approach to safety performance is not yet common in healthcare (Federico 2018). Some large hospitals and healthcare systems, such as Johns Hopkins Medicine in Maryland, have been implementing it to improve patient safety and avoid medical errors. Others are considering it. However, before trying to implement the five characteristics of high-reliability thinking, hospitals should first ensure leaders are committed to pursuing zero harm and creating a strong culture of safety and process improvement (AHRQ 2018). Ascension, a large healthcare system that operates in 24 states, committed in 2011 to become a high-reliability organization. In its evolution toward high reliability, Ascension has realized several key points (Hendrich and Haydar 2017):

◆ "Healthcare leaders at all levels must be adamant in creating a safe environment for care."

◆ "Complacency lurks around every corner" and must be overcome.

◆ "Capital and operating budgets challenge even the willing," yet funds and resources for safety must be made available.

◆ "Patients are persons: Disclosure is the right thing to do" when safety fails.

◆　"Safety is not an initiative" or a program; it is a transformation of the organization's culture that influences outcomes.

Today, "the U.S. healthcare system is realizing how critical the HRO model is . . . for healthcare institutions to prevent patient harm" (Buell 2018, 24). Future healthcare managers should learn more about this approach as they prepare for their careers.

CONTROLLING PEOPLE

Earlier in this chapter we learned that performance problems are usually caused by the system a person works in, rather than by the person. We have studied how to improve systems, structures, and processes to improve performance. Yet controlling and improving performance does involve people, so let's now think about controlling people. Which tools and methods can you think of from previous chapters to control human behavior? Leadership, supervision, job descriptions, motivation, performance appraisals, progressive discipline, training, power, authority, rewards, punishments, culture, values, and rules. Excellent—you thought of many useful tools!

Managers use these tools to appropriately control people to help control organization performance. We know people are not all alike, so what works for Miraya might not work for Tony. What works for baby boomers might not work well for Generation Z. Professional workers may expect more self-control and peer control than authoritarian control of their performance. In general, organizations have been changing to rely more on organization culture and values and less on bureaucratic rules and supervision to guide employees' performance (Daft 2016). When employees strongly embrace organization values, their performance is controlled more by those values and less by managerial authority and supervision.

Another important trend is the increased use of evidence, data, analytics, benchmarks, and monitoring systems to help people know their current performance—often in great detail and frequency. This was noted in chapter 8 in connection with performance appraisals. Even physicians who have historically relied on their own professional judgment are now using these tools and analytics to improve their performance.

Finally, for managers to successfully control their HCOs, they must control themselves and their own performance. This book has offered some ideas for improving one's performance. We will address this topic more fully in chapter 15 on professionalism. As a manager, you should continually strive to improve your own performance so that you can contribute more to your HCO, serve as a role model, and manage others effectively.

Managers at all levels of an HCO must control the performance of their work units, departments, and entire organization. They control performance by following a three-step process: (1) set performance standards, (2) measure actual performance and compare it to the standards, and (3) improve performance if it does not meet the standards. This approach is used to control many dimensions of performance, such as patient experience, costs, diversity, value, productivity, quality, satisfaction, health status, and dozens of others. Managers should pay attention to structure measures, process measures, and outcome measures of performance. Outcome measures have become more important, yet all measures matter because structures and processes create the outcomes. Internal and external information is used to set standards and targets that are SMART: specific, measurable, achievable, realistic, and time related.

Managers collect, analyze, and display data to compare actual performance to target performance. This requires effective data collection systems and data visualization methods. If performance does not reach targets, managers can use cause-and-effect diagrams, process maps, root-cause analysis, and other tools to analyze problems and develop solutions. Managers of HCOs use Six Sigma, Lean, and high-reliability approaches to control and improve performance in HCOs. They also apply the tools and techniques studied throughout this book.

(T) FOR YOUR TOOLBOX

- Three control steps

- Structure, process, and outcome measures

- Standards, targets, and key performance indicators

- Line graph (run chart)

- Bar graph (bar chart)

- Pie chart

- Control chart

- Tabular report (table of data)

- Cause-and-effect diagram

- Process map (flowchart)

- Root-cause analysis

- Six Sigma

- DMAIC cycle

- Lean production

- Value stream mapping

- High-reliability organization

FOR DISCUSSION

1.   What are some types of performance that a manager would have to control for a home health care agency? A health insurance company? A primary care clinic? An outpatient surgery facility? A mental health counseling center? A medical supply store?

2.   Describe the three-step approach that managers use for control. Which step do you think would be the most difficult? What could you do to make that step easier?

3.   Compare and contrast what a manager can show in a line graph, bar chart, pie chart, and control chart.

4.   Discuss the Six Sigma, Lean, and high-reliability approaches for performance improvement.

5.   How can a manager control employees so that their HCO achieves its performance targets?

CASE STUDY QUESTIONS

These questions refer to the Integrative Case Studies at the back of this book.

1.   Hospice Goes Hollywood case: What do you think are Hollywood Hospice's performance goals in this case? Which performance metrics would be useful for this HCO? Suggest performance targets for Hollywood Hospice. Describe the kinds of data managers should collect to analyze performance. Which charts or graphs from this chapter would you use to visually present performance data to the hospice's leaders?

2.   How Can an ACO Improve the Health of Its Population? case: What do you think are Vandalia Care's performance goals in this case? Which performance metrics would be useful for Vandalia? Suggest performance targets for the ACO. Describe the kinds of data the ACO should collect to analyze performance. Which charts or graphs from this chapter would you use to visually present performance data to the ACO's leaders?

3.   Increasing the Focus on Patient Safety at First Medical Center case: What do you think are FMC's performance goals in this case? Which performance metrics (departmental and centralized) do you think are needed? Suggest performance targets for the HCO. Describe the kinds of data the HCO should collect to analyze performance. Which charts or graphs from this chapter would you use to visually present performance data to FMC's leaders?

4.   Managing the Patient Experience case: Identify and describe performance improvement terms, concepts, tools, and methods from chapter 12 that are evident in this case.

RIVERBEND ORTHOPEDICS MINI CASE STUDY

Riverbend Orthopedics is a busy group practice with expanded services for orthopedic care. It has seven physicians and a podiatrist, plus about 70 other employees. At its big, new clinic building, Riverbend provides extensive orthopedic care. Several technicians provide diagnostic medical imaging, from basic X-rays to magnetic resonance images. The physicians perform surgery in their own outpatient surgery center with Riverbend's own operating nurses and technicians. Therapy is provided by three physical therapists and one part-time contracted occupational therapist. In addition to staff providing actual patient care, the clinic has staff for financial management, medical records, human resources, information systems/technology, building maintenance, and other administrative matters. Occasional marketing work is done by an advertising company. Legal work is outsourced to a law firm. Riverbend is managed by a new president, Ms. Garcia. She and Riverbend have set a goal of achieving "Excellent" ratings for patient experience from at least 90 percent of Riverbend's patients this year.

Assume that Riverbend has received "Excellent" ratings from only 58 percent of its physical therapy patients. Many of these patients complain specifically about how much time their physical therapy appointments take.

MINI CASE STUDY QUESTIONS

1. Draw a detailed process map of a physical therapy appointment at Riverbend that had more steps, delays, and backups than necessary. Then draw a revised process map showing a faster, more efficient process for the appointment.

2. Explain to Ms. Garcia how Lean management could help Riverbend achieve its goal with physical therapy patients.

REFERENCES

Agency for Healthcare Research and Quality (AHRQ). 2018. "High Reliability." Updated August. https://psnet.ahrq.gov/primers/primer/31.

Barnas, K. 2018. "Sustaining a Lean Transformation." *Healthcare Executive* 33 (1): 54–57.

Buell, J. M. 2018. "Sustaining a Safety Culture: Your Core Value." *Healthcare Executive* 33 (2): 20–27.

Daft, R. L. 2016. *Organization Theory and Design*, 12th ed. Mason, OH: South-Western Cengage.

Donabedian, A. 1988. "The Quality of Care: How Can It Be Assessed?" *Journal of the American Medical Association* 260 (12): 1743–48.

———. 1966. "Evaluating the Quality of Medical Care." *Milbank Memorial Fund Quarterly* 44 (2): 166–206.

Dunn, R. T. 2016. *Dunn and Haimann's Healthcare Management*, 10th ed. Chicago: Health Administration Press.

Federico, F. 2018. "Is Your Organization Highly Reliable?" *Healthcare Executive* 33 (1): 76–79.

Forte, J. 2018. Interview with the author, April 26.

Hendrich, A., and Z. Haydar. 2017. "Building a High-Reliability Organization: One System's Patient Safety Journey." *Journal of Healthcare Management* 62 (1): 13–17.

Kellermann, A. L., and S. S. Jones. 2013. "What It Will Take to Achieve the As-Yet-Unfulfilled Promises of Health Information Technology." *Health Affairs* 32 (1): 63–68.

Langabeer, J. R., and J. Helton. 2016. *Healthcare Operations Management*, 2nd ed. Burlington, MA: Jones & Bartlett Learning.

McLaughlin, D. B., and J. R. Olson. 2017. *Healthcare Operations Management*, 3rd ed. Chicago: Health Administration Press.

Spath, P. L. 2018. *Introduction to Healthcare Quality Management*, 3rd ed. Chicago: Health Administration Press.

UCLA Health. 2018. "CICARE." Accessed September 5. www.uclahealth.org/patient-experience/cicare.

Walston, S. L. 2017. *Organizational Behavior and Leadership in Healthcare: Leadership Perspectives and Management Applications*. Chicago: Health Administration Press.

Warren, K. 2014. "Quality Improvement: The Foundation, Processes, Tools, and Knowledge Transfer Techniques." In *The Healthcare Quality Book*, 3rd ed., edited by M. S. Joshi, E. R. Ransom, D. B. Nash, and S. B. Ransom, 83–107. Chicago: Health Administration Press.

CHAPTER 13

MAKING DECISIONS AND SOLVING PROBLEMS

A problem well stated is a problem half solved.

John Dewey, philosopher and pioneer of
educational reform

LEARNING OBJECTIVES

Studying this chapter will help you to

➤ define and describe decision making;

➤ explain who makes decisions;

➤ describe the rational decision-making approach and its limits;

➤ explain the satisficing, intuition, incremental, evidence-based, and garbage can
approaches to decision making;

➤ identify barriers to decision making;

➤ describe sources and uses of data for decision making; and

➤ know how to resolve conflict with decisions.

HERE'S WHAT HAPPENED

Partners HealthCare faced serious problems in the areas of quality of care and financial risk. At all levels of the organization, managers had to make decisions to solve these problems and resolve conflicts. They had to diagnose problems, consider alternative ways to solve them, and decide which solutions to try. Yet, before they performed these steps, managers first had to decide who should make the decisions and which decision-making approaches to use. Should they use a rational approach, a political approach, an evidence-based approach, an intuitive approach, or some other approach? After making one decision, managers often had to make other decisions. For example, managers decided to use telehealth to solve the readmission problem — and that led managers to decide when, where, and how to implement the telehealth technology. They had to decide on new positions, responsibility and authority for positions, whom to hire, work schedules, patient care policies, and other matters. Conflict was inevitable, and when some nurses and primary care physicians resisted, the Connected Cardiac Care program managers resolved those conflicts. To do so, they first had to decide which approach to use — accommodating, compromising, collaborating, or something else.

Managers at Partners HealthCare continually made decisions, solved problems, and resolved conflicts to achieve the organization's goals and mission. These activities are a big part of what managers do at every level of a healthcare organization (HCO). Although decisions at higher levels have bigger consequences than decisions at lower levels, managers at all levels make decisions to solve problems and resolve conflicts. Imagine the decisions HCOs are making now in response to the exciting trends and developments described in chapter 1!

Managers make decisions to perform all five main management functions—planning, organizing, staffing, leading, and controlling. Several of Mintzberg's management roles (discussed in chapter 2) involve making decisions and solving problems: monitor, disturbance handler, resource allocator, and negotiator. Decision making affects management activities described in other chapters. Conversely, management activities discussed in other chapters affect how decisions are made. For instance, recall that organizing work (chapters 4 through 6) includes centralization and decentralization of authority to make decisions, which affects how decisions are made throughout an organization. Think about how different approaches for leading and influencing (chapters 9 through 11) affect how managers make decisions, solve problems, and resolve conflict.

How do managers make decisions? Well, how do *you* make decisions? Flip a coin? Throw a dart? Compare pros and cons of several options? Just do what worked before? Follow instincts? Go with the first idea that comes to mind? All of the above? None of the above?

This chapter explains how managers at all levels of an HCO can make decisions to solve problems and resolve conflicts. First, it describes decision making and identifies the types of decisions managers make. Then it explains several approaches that managers use to make decisions. The main approach, which is based on rational thinking and analysis, is not always feasible or realistic. Thus, managers may use other methods, which are explained. Barriers to effective decision making and uses of data and big data in decision making are also discussed. The final section of the chapter explores how to resolve conflict, which involves making decisions.

DECISION MAKING AND DECISIONS

Some authors say decision making is "choosing from among alternatives to determine a course of action" (Liebler and McConnell 2004, 141). These writers do not directly include implementation in their definition, yet their decision-making process does include evaluating implemented decisions. Another writer defines organizational decision making as "the process of identifying and solving problems" (Daft 2016, 468), which seems to imply that a solution is implemented. Other writers agree that decision making is choosing from among alternatives, and the steps in their decision-making approach include implementation (Griffin, Phillips, and Gully 2017). Based on these perspectives, in this book **decision making** is defined as the process of choosing from among alternatives to determine and implement a course of action. Drawing attention to implementation forces managers to make decisions that are realistic and can be implemented.

Managers have to make two types of decisions and solve two types of problems (Daft 2016). **Programmed decisions** are well defined, routine, easily diagnosed, and easily solved with existing decision rules, formulas, algorithms, and procedures. Programmed decisions can be made with high confidence that the chosen alternative will succeed and solve the problem. For example, when should I see a dentist? How many boxes of gloves should we have available each day at each clinic? How many custodians will be needed to clean the clinics next month?

Alternatively, **nonprogrammed decisions** are new, unusual, and hard to define, diagnose, and understand. They present fuzzy alternatives with uncertain cause and effect relationships. Creative thinking and difficult judgments are likely to be needed. For example, when the United States enacted the Affordable Care Act, HCO managers throughout the country wondered, How will this healthcare reform law affect us? What should we do? They struggled to define the decisions to be made, to describe alternative courses of action, and to anticipate how alternatives might play out and with which consequences. The new healthcare law was extremely comprehensive, with many new reforms, and it was not clear how those reforms would affect HCOs and their stakeholders. Recall from chapter 3 that nonprogrammed problems and decisions often arise during strategic planning.

decision making
The process of choosing from among alternatives to determine and implement a course of action.

programmed decisions
Decisions that are well defined, routine, easily diagnosed, and easily solved with existing decision rules, formulas, algorithms, and procedures.

nonprogrammed decisions
Decisions that are new, unusual, hard to define, and hard to diagnose; they present fuzzy alternatives with uncertain cause and effect relationships and without existing decision rules to follow.

Do you suppose managers use the same decision-making methods for programmed and nonprogrammed decisions? Think about this question as you study the decision methods in this chapter.

WHO MAKES DECISIONS?

Individuals throughout an organization make decisions, and so do groups, committees, teams, and HCOs. Experienced senior managers make decisions, and so do inexperienced managers in their first week on the job.

We can categorize decisions as *individual* and *organizational*. Individual decisions are made by a single person—such as you, a webpage designer, a grant writer, or a diversity coordinator. Organizational decisions are made by groups of people in an organization—such as a website design task force, the department of clinical research, or a group of managers that is developing more diversity and inclusion. Group decisions have become more common as a way to bring many kinds of expertise and viewpoints into the decision process. Another benefit is that more stakeholders are involved in the decision, which creates more support for it. However, as we saw in chapter 6, involving more people in decision making means more time and cost.

Who actually *makes* the decision is not always the same as who *provides input* for the decision. Some people provide advice, consultation, helpful analysis, brainstorming, or other assistance but do not then make the decision. A manager who is dealing with a problem must determine who will make the decision to solve the problem. Recall from chapter 6 that groups use different methods to make decisions. At one extreme, a manager might use an autocratic approach and make the decision alone. At the other extreme, a manager might use a delegated approach and let a subordinate or group decide without

---

(→) TRY IT, APPLY IT

As a manager, your involvement in making a specific decision can range on a continuum from complete to almost none—that is, from autocratic to delegated. Try to think of situations in which you made an autocratic decision, delegated a decision, and used an approach that was somewhere in between autocratic and delegated. Discuss your examples with classmates. This practice will help you understand that managers must determine how much to involve other employees and stakeholders in organizational decisions.

the manager. In between the autocratic and delegated approaches, a manager might share decision making with subordinates to get their participation. For example, the manager might obtain input from group members and then make the decision alone. Group members might vote democratically to decide what to do. A manager might build consensus among a group of people for an idea that everyone generally agrees with. A manager who is dealing with a problem that requires a decision must first decide

◆ who will provide input, analysis, brainstorming, and consultation; and

◆ who will make the decision and how (e.g., majority vote, consensus).

METHODS FOR MAKING NONPROGRAMMED DECISIONS

Managers make decisions in different ways. Programmed decisions are the easy ones and can be made by following an appropriate decision rule. For example, in deciding when to schedule a dental appointment, many of us follow a common decision rule: See a dentist every six months. However, two cautions apply to this type of decision (Griffin, Phillips, and Gully 2017). First, managers must ensure that the problem or situation really is routine and that a programmed decision would be appropriate. Second, managers must apply an appropriate decision rule.

The rest of this section will explain methods for making nonprogrammed decisions. These are the harder ones, such as deciding where to live after graduation. We begin with the rational approach, which will probably seem familiar to many people. It is common yet idealistic. We will learn why this approach is hard to follow completely, and then we will consider other approaches.

RATIONAL APPROACH

As the name suggests, **rational decision making** is based on logical reasoning and deliberate analysis to arrive at the best decision. You have probably used this method (at least partially) to make a decision, such as which college to attend. Individuals, groups, committees, and teams use this method in organizations.

The rational approach is shown below in eight steps (Daft 2016, 471–73). Some variations of the approach combine steps (e.g., Dunn 2016; Griffin, Phillips, and Gully 2017). The first four steps *identify the problem* and the decision that must be made. Identifying the problem is important, as the quote at the beginning of this chapter indicates. The last four steps *solve the problem* by making and implementing a decision. Each of the eight steps builds on what was done in the previous steps. Decision makers are supposed to follow the steps in sequence, from 1 to 8. However, they sometimes back up to redo

rational decision making
The process of making a decision based on logical reasoning and deliberate analysis.

earlier steps. See exhibit 13.1 for applications of the rational approach to a student's decision and an HCO's decision.

1. *Monitor the decision environment.* Review external and internal information, check results, and detect performance problems.

2. *Define the decision problem.* Describe a detected performance problem by gathering more information about it, such as who, what, where, and when.

3. *Specify the decision objectives.* State what is to be accomplished by the decision, and identify the desired outcomes. Talk with people who are involved. Seek varied perspectives.

4. *Diagnose the problem.* Analyze the information gathered to determine why the problem happened, and explore causes of the problem. Dig deeply below the problem's superficial symptoms.

5. *Develop alternative solutions.* State what could be done to solve the problem. What are the options? Think creatively and brainstorm possibilities. Consult relevant online sources, such as professional associations and other HCOs.

6. *Evaluate the alternatives.* Judge how well each alternative solution would achieve the decision objectives and outcomes. Consider pros and cons, likely consequences, and stakeholders' views.

7. *Choose the best alternative.* Select the best alternative to achieve the decision objectives.

8. *Implement the chosen alternative.* Put the chosen alternative into effect—make it happen.

Chapter 11 discussed ethics and suggested that HCOs should have a process for deciding how to resolve ethical problems. Managers and ethics committees often follow a process similar to this rational model. They define the problem, diagnose it, develop alternative solutions, consider the pros and cons of those solutions, pick the solution they think is right, and implement it. Participants in this process give extra attention to ethics by considering the following (Nelson 2015):

◆ The values and preferences of all stakeholders who would be affected by the decision

◆ The ethical consequences of alternatives

◆ Which ethical principles (e.g., beneficence) support each possible solution

◆ Whether any solution violates an ethical principle (e.g., justice)

Rational Decision-Making Steps	Student Example: Renting an Apartment	HCO Example: Lab Productivity
1. Monitor the decision environment	Apartment listings show rents are starting to rise.	Internal reports show the number of lab tests performed per lab tech declined 4 percent this year and is now 7 percent below industry standards.
2. Define the decision problem	On September 1, rent for my current one-bedroom apartment will rise to $1,000 per month, which is more than I can afford.	Tests per tech are 3 percent above standards on the first shift and 8 percent below standards on the second shift; automated tests per tech equal standards; manual tests per tech are 11 percent below standards.
3. Specify the decision objectives	I want to spend no more than $900 per month on rent in the next academic year and live somewhere that offers the same safety, comfort, and convenient location as my current apartment.	Lab tests per tech should equal the industry standards for our kind of lab tests and equipment.
4. Diagnose the problem	Landlords have to cover their rising costs; my current apartment will be upgraded with new appliances and my rent will rise.	The second-shift chief tech job is vacant; the second-shift workload declined 9 percent since last May 1.
5. Develop alternative solutions	Negotiate a $900 rate with my landlord; move to a cheaper one-bedroom apartment; join a friend in a two-bedroom apartment for $700 per month per person.	Promote a second-shift tech into the chief tech job to supervise staff; create a productivity incentive system for the second shift; advertise the lab to bring more work to the second shift.
6. Evaluate the alternatives	Consider cost, location, safety, and comfort.	Consider costs, feasibility, effects on the entire lab, and the likelihood of increasing the second shift's tests per tech.
7. Choose the best alternative	Move in with my friend for $700 per month.	Promote a second-shift tech into the chief tech job to supervise staff.
8. Implement the chosen alternative	Let my current lease expire, sign a new lease, move my stuff, and notify my family and friends.	Promote the tech, provide supervisory training and mentoring, and monitor results.

EXHIBIT 13.1

Examples of the Rational Decision-Making Process

Note: Based on the eight-step process of Daft (2016, 471–73).

Rational decision making generally makes sense, and managers often use it. Yet sometimes managers do not rely on it. Why? **Human ability to be rational is limited** (Daft 2016; Griffin, Phillips, and Gully 2017). The human brain can process a limited amount of information, consider a limited number of factors, and evaluate a limited set of alternatives. Even the brains of world-champion chess grand masters eventually become "full" and cannot consider one more alternative move. Further, human brains are not robotic; they are affected by personality, emotions, biases, personal values, experiences, situations, and pressures. These may cause decision makers to be (or at least seem to be) irrational instead of rational. Also, some problems are just too complex to accurately describe and diagnose. Finally, in today's world, there just may not be enough time for decision makers to gather all the information, much less analyze it. The result is **bounded rationality.** There are boundaries (limits) to how rational a person can be and how rational decision making can be. Then what happens? Because of bounded rationality, managers often make decisions using other approaches. These are explained next.

bounded rationality
Limits to human
rational decision
making.

SATISFICING APPROACH

Herbert Simon developed the satisficing approach to decisions (Daft 2016; Walston 2017). This method assumes that people are not capable of making the best decision among all possible alternatives. **Because of bounded rationality, people cannot (and do not) make the choice that will maximize outcomes and results.** Instead, they conduct a limited search for alternatives and choose an early solution that will achieve their minimum acceptable results. They **satisfice**—that is, they decide on a satisfactory alternative that will suffice. A manager might "kind of" follow the rational model but hurries along, takes shortcuts, and settles on a solution that is good enough. This approach is easier and faster, requires fewer resources, and involves less conflict than the ideal pursuit of the best solution. Managers realize that better alternatives probably exist, yet they also realize that not all problems need the best solution—they just need an acceptable solution. Perhaps you have used this approach to decide which shirt to buy or to choose which apartment to rent. Individuals and organizations often satisfice when making decisions (Daft 2016; Walston 2017).

satisfice
To decide on a
satisfactory (rather
than the best) solution
that will suffice.

Some organizational decisions are made by groups and coalitions rather than by just one person. Groups are also likely to satisfice. There are even more barriers to the rational approach for an organizational decision than for an individual decision. With more people involved, there are more personal biases, hopes, fears, favors to repay, and so forth. It becomes challenging for all group members to analyze all possible solutions and agree on a best solution. Some groups cannot even agree on what *best* means! Group members typically want to finish the decision-making meeting to get back to their other work that is piling up. So they agree on the first simple solution that everyone can live with. It probably is not the best solution, but it meets their minimum requirements. To enable the process, a group member might informally confer with a few other members before a meeting and compromise toward a satisficing solution.

INTUITION APPROACH

Instead of using rational analysis, individuals sometimes make a decision by using **intuition**. With this approach, a manager bases the decision on experience, hunches, feelings, or unconscious processes rather than on conscious logical thinking and reasoning (Daft 2016; Griffin, Phillips, and Gully 2017). Good intuition is the result of years of experience and enormous amounts of information stored in the subconscious, so it is not arbitrary. Managers find this approach useful when time is short, problems are complex, precedents do not exist, and facts are scarce. Even when rational decision making can be used, managers may supplement it with intuition. For example, an HCO manager in Billings might use the rational approach and tentatively decide to hire Allen as the new community outreach specialist. However, before she tells the human resources director her decision, she wants to "sleep on it" and let her unconscious intuition determine if Allen is a good choice. In the morning, her intuition will let her know if she is comfortable with that decision.

> **intuition**
> The process of knowing, believing, or deciding based on experience, hunches, or unconscious processes rather than on logical conscious thinking and reasoning.

The origins of intuition are not fully understood, although experience seems to help it develop. People may not be able to fully explain their intuition or justify intuitive decisions. Yet, they can sometimes use intuition with good results for decision making. Intuition can be developed, and managers can practice intuitive thinking by paying more attention to their inner mind and feelings about choices. Managers can learn to use the intuitive approach to complement the rational approach and help overcome bounded rationality. This process takes years of experience, and new managers should be cautious about relying solely on intuition.

✓ CHECK IT OUT ONLINE

Intuition for decision making can be improved—for example, by paying more attention to one's inner mind, inner voice, and feelings about choices. A clear, quiet mind helps intuition, so turn off the technology, stop texting, and meditate for a while to become more aware of your inner thoughts and feelings. Jot down notes while letting your mind wander. Visit an online bookseller and read customers' reviews of books or DVDs on intuition. Find one that fits your style. Check it out online and see what you discover.

INCREMENTAL APPROACH

Sometimes an HCO might begin a rational decision-making process but then proceed through the steps with pauses, backups, interruptions, redos, and only gradual progress. Decision making can be incremental, with a series of small decisions that eventually create a big decision. Carlos might say, "If we try to figure out the whole solution and decide everything at once, by the time we do, the situation will have changed, and we'll have to figure it out again." Instead, he and his team take two steps forward and one back (and maybe a step sideways) to further diagnose the problem or revise an earlier small decision. **Incremental decision making** does not follow an orderly, linear sequence of steps.

    In 2010, the Affordable Care Act was enacted with a five-year implementation plan. Many HCOs began incrementally deciding how to adapt to the new law. Managers knew they would have to gradually figure out what to do as parts of the law were implemented, courts ruled on legal challenges to the law, and the government's implementation plans were modified. Deciding what to do required incremental decision making. Managers do the same with other complex decisions; these may take a year or longer. They think, "Let's get started, and we'll keep figuring it out as we go." This approach is common for nonprogrammed decisions that must be newly created. It works best in HCOs that value learning, experimentation, change, and innovation (which are discussed in chapter 14). Some HCOs encourage this trial-and-error approach as a way to learn, especially for complex problems that are too big to solve all at once.

EVIDENCE-BASED APPROACH

Managers sometimes use **evidence-based management** for decision making to overcome people's struggles to be fully rational. This approach is similar to rational decision making and more intensely applies that method. Managers use it to avoid bounded rationality, blinders, biases, groupthink, flawed assumptions, and closed-mindedness (Hellriegel and Slocum 2011).

    "Evidence-based practice is about making decisions through the conscientious, explicit and judicious use of the best available evidence from multiple sources by

1. Asking: translating a practical issue or problem into an answerable question

2. Acquiring: systematically searching for and retrieving the evidence

3. Appraising: critically judging the trustworthiness and relevance of the evidence

4. Aggregating: weighing and pulling together the evidence

5. Applying: incorporating the evidence in the decision-making process

6. Assessing: evaluating the outcome of the decision taken

to increase the likelihood of a favorable outcome" (Barends and Briner 2014).

    The evidence-based approach begins with a careful statement of the problem to be solved. As new evidence is examined and logically applied to the problem, managers might

---

incremental decision making
The process by which a big, complex decision is gradually made from a series of small decisions during a lengthy time period that may involve backing up to further diagnose problems, rethink ideas, and revise prior choices.

evidence-based management
An approach to making decisions through the conscientious, explicit, and judicious use of the best available evidence from multiple sources.

further refine the problem. This intelligent approach searches for relevant information from multiple sources (Barends and Briner 2014; Briner, Denyer, and Rousseau 2009):

◆ External scientific research evidence

◆ Internal evidence from the local setting, context, or organization

◆ Experiences, expertise, and professional judgments of practicing managers

◆ Preferences, values, and views of relevant stakeholders

In this approach, managers systematically acquire and use the best evidence available. They pay careful attention to which evidence and information is relevant and how accurate, valid, and reliable it is. They give greater weight to some evidence than to other evidence. This approach moves the rational process closer to the idealized version. Managers apply discipline and ask each other tough questions to avoid quick fixes, faddish answers, and educated guesses (Hellriegel and Slocum 2011). However, because of its systematic thoroughness, the evidence-based approach requires more resources, time, and staff. Evidence-based management decision making has been used for healthy transitions programs, integrated chronic disease management, perioperative services, nursing productivity, and a hospital evacuation because of a hurricane (Kovner and D'Aunno 2016).

Garbage Can Approach

Garbage can decision making is even less sequential and step-by-step than the incremental approach. It was conceived by Michael Cohen, James March, and Johan Olsen to understand decision making in very organic, messy organizations characterized by uncertainty, change, and disorder (Daft 2016). Garbage can decision making occurs in freewheeling, chaotic organizations in which streams of people, problems, solutions, and decision opportunities are coming, going, and changing (Daft 2016, 490). Rather than explain how a particular decision is made, this approach explains how a pattern of decisions is made in an organization.

Imagine an organization's monthly meeting in a conference room, which presents an opportunity for making decisions. Some people who are present were not at the prior meeting. Some arrive late or leave early and are therefore not present for all discussions and decisions. Others take calls on their cell phones during the meeting and are not paying attention. Ideas are thrown into the discussion, perhaps as solutions in search of a problem. Information is limited and obscure. Decision makers do not understand the causes of problems or know if they will be solved by proposed solutions. If they do *x*, it might cause *y*, but then again it might cause *z*, or it might not cause anything. Managers decide to try something; if it doesn't work, they can try something else later.

garbage can decision making
Seemingly random organizational decision making resulting from evolving streams of problems, solutions, participants, and decision-making opportunities.

The garbage can approach to decision making might seem surprising. When used in an organization, it may leave some people wondering, "What were they thinking?" Yet some freewheeling, nonbureaucratic organizations do use this method as an alternative to the rational process (Daft 2016). Managers should realize that this type of decision making might occur in their HCO if its meetings are too loose, unstructured, and chaotic. Some suggest that HCO medical staffs and universities use this approach (Walston 2017):

BARRIERS TO EFFECTIVE DECISION MAKING

Managers should strive to avoid or overcome the following common barriers to decision making (Daft 2016; Dye 2017; McConnell 2018; Walston 2017):

- ◆ Unwillingness to confront problems (or the *real* problems); avoidance, delay, procrastination

- ◆ Inability to admit a previous decision was wrong and is not working

- ◆ Defining a problem in such a way that it is solved too easily and quickly

- ◆ Not diagnosing a problem well enough to really solve it

- ◆ Hurrying and not devoting enough time to decision making

- ◆ Having a closed organization culture or closed leadership style

- ◆ Being risk averse or afraid to try a new idea; exercising too much caution; being stuck in a rut

- ◆ Wishful thinking, unrealistic optimism, hubris, and overestimating the ability to handle problems

- ◆ Accepting only favorable information, avoiding unfavorable information, and rejecting useful information because of its source

- ◆ Biases, personal agendas, and conflicts of interest

- ◆ Organization politics and political behavior

- ◆ Not involving the right people in the decision

- ◆ Using an inappropriate approach to decision making

- ◆ Groupthink, conformity, playing it safe, copycat thinking, and copycat decisions

To avoid the all-too-common last barrier, consider this classic advice from longtime management consultant and writer Peter Drucker (1967, 148): "The first rule in decision-making is that one does not make a decision unless there is disagreement." Deborah J. Bowen, FACHE, CAE, the president and CEO of the American College of Healthcare Executives, adds that "leaders should cultivate the art of productive disagreement" (Bowen 2016, 8).

DATA FOR DECISION MAKING

For effective decision making, managers need data—sometimes lots of data—with which to analyze problems and evaluate alternative solutions. Where do the data come from? How do managers use it? Organizations often use both quantitative and qualitative sources of data and methods rather than rely on only one approach (Daft 2016; McLaughlin and Olson 2017):

Quantitative Data and Methods

◆ Written and digital files, reports, and records; databases; scorecards; and other sources inside an HCO have useful quantitative data, as do external reports, websites, and databases.

◆ Computer programs and apps with probability models, operations management methods, linear programming models, decision trees, mathematical formulas, scheduling systems, statistical programs, and comparison matrices use quantitative data to make decisions to solve problems. These and other management science techniques can easily process dozens and even hundreds of quantitative variables to reach decisions—far more than humans can process. However, such techniques are less useful for capturing people's qualitative feelings, judgments, and experiences.

Qualitative Data and Methods

◆ Discussions, interviews, focus groups, and conversations with people inside and outside the HCO provide useful qualitative data and information.

◆ Delphi technique, nominal group technique, brainstorming, intuition, devil's advocate approach, expert opinion, and pro/con discussions use qualitative data to make decisions to solve problems.

In larger HCOs, specialized internal staff conduct data gathering and analysis to help the actual decision makers. Larger HCOs have been hiring many data analysts, decision scientists, and researchers to do this work. Smaller HCOs with less need and fewer funds may contract with external consultants for help with data. Computer software and apps have become more user friendly, enabling managers to more easily analyze data.

Data analytics is done to obtain insights that enable smarter decisions and better outcomes (McLaughlin and Olson 2017, 205). HCOs use three types of analytics:

1. *Descriptive analytics* condenses large amounts of data into a few meaningful pieces of information. Examples include performance statistics for quality, finances, utilization, compliance, labor use, and other key performance indicators.

2. *Predictive analytics* forecasts probabilities of future events and outcomes. Examples include predicting which prior patients might unnecessarily use the (costly) emergency department and how much a 5 percent increase in salary would affect employee retention.

3. *Prescriptive analytics* recommends solutions to problems and questions. Examples include optimal staffing of a rehabilitation facility, minimizing risk of patient injury, and maximizing use of expensive medical equipment.

The growth of analytics and big data has resulted from massive—sometimes unimaginably massive—amounts of available data and the development of technology to use it. Every two years, the volume of healthcare data doubles (Ebadollahi 2017). Google scientists were able to analyze and predict in the United States, almost in real time, the spread of winter flu by studying the frequency of certain flu-related search terms in its billions of daily searches (Daft 2016). Analysts run computer models with hundreds of variables to better understand how social determinants of health (e.g., food and housing) affect use of costly emergency departments. In the future, decision support systems will be more commonly used with expanded data sets to better solve problems and improve performance. Artificial intelligence will also be used for clinical and managerial decisions as a way to overcome the bias that humans have in their decision making (Radick 2017). The Using Chapter 13 in the Real World sidebar describes how a real HCO uses analytics for population health.

An organization must strive to have its information available at the right time in the right place in the right form for the right people. Doing this requires effective **knowledge management**—a system for finding, organizing, and making available an organization's knowledge, including its experience, understanding, expertise, methods, judgment, lessons learned, and know-how (Daft 2016; Hellriegel and Slocum 2011). It includes both codified knowledge in written documents and tacit knowledge in people's heads. Tacit knowledge is insight, know-how, intuition, experience, judgment, and expertise. Compared to codified knowledge, it is harder to find, gather, organize, store, and make available to others in the organization. Yet, tacit knowledge comprises much of an organization's unique, valuable knowledge. Managers use information technology (IT) to manage codified knowledge relatively easily. Managing tacit knowledge is more challenging, and it depends on person-to-person interactions, professional networks, and face-to-face connections.

Suppose managers of an HCO in New Brunswick want to enable staff to share tacit knowledge. They can facilitate these relationships so that employees can easily find

knowledge management
A system for finding, organizing, and making available an organization's knowledge, including its experience, understanding, expertise, methods, judgment, lessons learned, and know-how.

USING CHAPTER 13 IN THE REAL WORLD

To improve population health in the Seattle area, Providence St. Joseph Health uses big data and analytics to identify and solve problems. This health system has a population health data coordinating council, a senior director of population health informatics, and other groups and positions that help gather and use data to identify and solve health problems in local communities. They are expanding the collection and use of data for social determinants of health (not ordinarily included in medical records) and integrating it with clinical data. This enables the health system to make better decisions about where and how to invest its resources to best improve population health. For example, big data and predictive analytics enable proactive decisions and problem solving to reduce the population's costly visits to the emergency department (Buell 2018).

and interact with people who have the right tacit knowledge. Face-to-face meetings, team huddles, and discussions are useful. Work spaces can be designed to encourage and enable conversations. Managers can also invest in telecommunication systems, Skype, FaceTime, social media, and other technology to enable conversations for sharing tacit knowledge. To more widely share knowledge, tacit knowledge can be codified in documents, captured in Instagram videos, blogged, tweeted, and posted online and in social media. The knowledge can be e-codified to share within the company or beyond.

TRENDS IN DECISION MAKING

The external environment of most HCOs has become more complex and less certain. As a result, HCOs' decisions have also become more complex and less certain. HCOs face more nonprogrammed decisions that do not fit their playbooks. Compared to decisions made in the past, today's decisions usually involve more factors, more alternatives, more information, and more stakeholders' interests. Thus, some HCOs and decision makers use deliberate evidence-based decision making, involve more people, and make more group (rather than individual) decisions.

On the other hand, the environment is changing rapidly, so HCOs feel they must make decisions rapidly. Pressure to make complex decisions quickly has led some managers to use more satisficing, intuition, and incremental decision making. HCOs are now more willing to allow trial and error, followed by learning. They make an incremental decision, try it, learn from it, adjust, and try again. (Does this method remind you of the define, measure, analyze, improve, and control cycle in chapter 12?) Some HCOs have begun actively encouraging a trial-and-error approach.

Finally, the workforce and decision makers in most HCOs have become more culturally diverse. Decision makers should take the time to understand relevant views, concerns, and ideas of different cultures that are involved in a decision or that will be affected by the decision. Doing so takes more time and patience amid pressure to make fast decisions.

These trends are general and do not apply to every situation and organization.

RESOLVING CONFLICT

Conflict and decision making have a reciprocal relationship—they affect each other. A moderate amount of conflict can improve decision making by opening up closed thinking, expanding understanding, developing creative ideas, and avoiding groupthink. Good decision making depends on first examining all conflicting ideas, views, and alternatives. The flip side is that conflict can be resolved by good decision making.

Some conflict (but not too much) is both normal and useful in HCOs. When there is too little conflict, managers might stimulate it to gain the benefits of conflict (Walston 2017). But if there is too much conflict that is not managed well, it can be harmful and ruin an organization. The Joint Commission, which accredits HCOs, states that conflict is common and can produce positive change. However, if leaders do not manage conflict, healthcare quality and safety may be threatened. Thus, a conflict management process is required for accreditation (Joint Commission 2015, 106).

CAUSES OF CONFLICT

Conflict is normal in HCOs because of causes that are normal in HCOs. It occurs among individuals and groups. The following causes of conflict occur naturally, so managers should expect them in their HCOs (Daft 2016; Dye 2017; McConnell 2018; Walston 2017). Some of the examples provided here are healthcare related:

◆ *Goal incompatibility.* Goals include decreasing costs but increasing weekend staff; goals include innovation along with consistency.

◆ *Differences in perceptions, values, beliefs, cognition, emotions, cultures, and views.* Physicians and managers think differently; staff members are diverse in terms of gender, age, culture, and other characteristics, so they have different views.

◆ *Task interdependence and required cooperation.* A nurse hands the surgeon a scalpel; the restaurant server waits for the cook to finish a pizza.

◆ *Competition for scarce resources.* There is not enough time, information, power, money, space, prestige, staff, equipment, or other resources to meet everyone's needs and wants; three employees requested a laptop, but only one is available.

◆ *Unclear or overlapping expectations.* People are unsure what to do or when to do it (often because of unclear communication); the policy says to "perform equipment maintenance daily," but the first shift staff leaves the maintenance for the second shift and vice versa.

These causes of conflict might be worsened by other factors, including time pressure, poor communication, past history, unreasonable rules, personalities, or someone just having a bad day. Take a few minutes to think of examples you have heard about or experienced.

CONFLICT RESOLUTION MODEL

Kenneth W. Thomas and Ralph H. Kilmann (1974, 2018) developed a model to resolve conflict that has been used for more than 40 years. Managers, human resource professionals, negotiators, mediators, executive coaches, and others use it in many organizations today, including in HCOs (Dye 2017; McConnell 2018).

The model consists of five styles for resolving conflict—collaborating, competing, compromising, accommodating, and avoiding (see exhibit 13.2). Which approach should a manager use to resolve conflict? The answer depends on *how assertive* and *how cooperative* she chooses to be, which depends on her temperament and the situation (Thomas and Kilmann 2018). In other words, the approach depends on *concern for oneself* and *concern for others*. Depending on whether assertiveness is high, medium, or low and cooperativeness is high, medium, or low, a person uses one of these five styles to resolve conflict (also shown in exhibit 13.2). Each approach is sometimes appropriate and sometimes not so appropriate, as shown in exhibit 13.3. (The styles might remind you of the leadership styles discussed in chapter 9.)

A manager decides which style to use after evaluating the situation. In other words, the best approach is contingent. (Sound familiar?) When you are a manager or supervisor, you can use the guidelines in exhibit 13.3 to evaluate conflict and then choose the style that seems right for the situation. Studies have found that in general (but not always), managers who collaborate are more successful, are more often found in high-performing organizations, and are viewed more positively by others than managers who do not collaborate (Hellriegel and Slocum 2011). In contrast, managers who use the competing or avoiding styles are more likely to be viewed negatively. The compromising style is generally viewed positively by others. Views of the accommodating style are mixed and do not permit clear conclusions.

Exhibit 13.2

Five Styles for
Resolving Conflict

Collaborating	Competing	Compromising	Accommodating	Avoiding
Exchanging information, examining differences, and being creative to reach a win–win solution to fully satisfy everyone (*high assertive and high cooperative*)	Using your power to force acceptance of your position while ignoring the concerns of the other person (*high assertive and low cooperative*)	Everyone giving and taking to reach a mutually acceptable, partly satisfying, and convenient solution (*medium assertive and medium cooperative*)	Neglecting your own concerns to satisfy the concerns of the other person; yielding to someone else; self-sacrificing (*low assertive and high cooperative*)	Not trying to satisfy anyone's concerns; withdrawing from the conflict by postponing or ignoring it (*low assertive and low cooperative*)

Source: Data from Thomas and Kilmann (2018).

Additional Suggestions for Managing Conflict

New managers should learn to use the conflict resolution model developed by Thomas and Kilmann. It is an excellent tool for managers, supervisors, and others in HCOs. What else can managers do to successfully manage conflict?

Earlier we learned that The Joint Commission requires that HCOs have a conflict resolution process for accreditation. Managers can follow such a process. Dye (2017, 255) offers the following steps:

1. Declare that a conflict exists, so that everyone formally realizes it and uses proper processes to resolve it.

2. Give reasons why the conflict exists and ensure the conflict is not based on personal hostility or malice.

3. Enlist a neutral person to clarify issues in the conflict and seek input from all concerned participants.

4. Consider only one conflict at a time; do not let participants bring up others until the first conflict has been resolved.

5. Require everyone involved in the conflict to participate and not hide.

6. Maintain a fair discussion, with opportunities for participants to assert and defend themselves.

7. Clearly state the outcome of the conflict and the agreement that ends it; declare the conflict has ended.

Collaborating	Competing	Compromising	Accommodating	Avoiding
The outcome matters to everyone.	The outcome is extremely important to you.	There is no time now for collaboration.	The outcome does not matter to you, but it matters to someone else.	The outcome does not matter to you.
You want a win–win situation.	The outcome is needed for compliance with essential rules or laws.	The conflict involves incompatible goals.	You realize your position is wrong.	The conflict is beyond your control or cannot be solved.
There is time to carefully consider everyone's views.	The conflict must be quickly settled, such as in an emergency.	A quick but temporary resolution of a complex conflict is needed.	You are unlikely to get your way, so you pick your battles.	The conflict is not your responsibility.
You want everyone committed to the solution.	The conflict is with someone who takes advantage of cooperation.	A democratic approach is required.	It's important to get along with others; peace matters.	The conflict may resolve itself.
Problem-solving expertise is available.	The conflict involves an unpopular yet necessary matter.		Yielding now can help you get something else you want later.	
			You want others to try their ideas.	

EXHIBIT 13.3
When to Use Each Conflict Resolution Style

Sources: Data from Hellriegel and Slocum (2011); Ledlow (2009); Polzer, Neale, and Illes (2006); Thomas and Kilmann (2018).

Managers can of course use many other tools, methods, theories, and concepts from this book. Think back to what you learned in previous chapters about management, leading, motivating, using power, and so forth. The next two chapters explain additional useful concepts, including emotional intelligence and effective communication—both of which are essential for managing conflict.

A final suggestion is to seek expert help when necessary to resolve difficult conflicts that are harming your HCO. The expert could be someone in the HCO, such as a professional counselor who has experience in conflict resolution. Or, it could be an outside consultant, mediator, or arbitrator. An arbitrator allows disputants to present their views and input and then makes a decision (similar to a court judge) to resolve the conflict. A mediator leads conflicting parties through discussions, question-and-answer sessions, negotiations, and processes that guide the parties to decide themselves how to work out the problem. Sometimes a neutral, objective outsider can be effective in resolving difficult conflicts.

ONE MORE TIME

Managers in an HCO make decisions to solve problems and resolve conflicts to achieve the HCO's goals and mission. Making decisions is a big part of what managers do at every level of an HCO to perform all five main management functions—planning, organizing, staffing, leading, and controlling. Decision making is the process of choosing from among alternatives to determine and implement a course of action. Some decisions are programmed (i.e., routine, common) and can be decided with common decision rules, formulas, and procedures based on past experience.

Other decisions are nonprogrammed (i.e., nonroutine, uncommon) and are therefore harder to make. The external environment has become more complex and uncertain, so HCOs' decisions have also become more complex, uncertain, and nonprogrammed. Managers sometimes make these decisions alone but more often involve other people. They may take the rational approach, which uses deliberate analysis, explicit reasoning, and choosing from among alternatives to make the best decision. This approach makes sense, yet managers may find it hard to follow completely because of bounded rationality. Thus, they might partly follow the rational method and then use satisficing, intuitive, incremental, evidence-based, or garbage can approaches. Quantitative and qualitative data, big data, analytics, and knowledge management are essential for effective decision making.

Conflict is natural in HCOs because of conflicting goals, scarce resources, interdependent work, unclear expectations, and differences among people, groups, and departments. To resolve conflict, a manager may collaborate with, compete with, compromise with, accommodate, or avoid the other person(s). The proper approach depends on how assertive and how cooperative someone chooses to be, or how much concern for oneself and concern for others a person has. Although the collaborative style seems to work best in many situations, a manager should develop the ability to use each of the five conflict resolution styles when appropriate.

(T) FOR YOUR TOOLBOX

- Programmed and nonprogrammed decisions
- Rational decision making
- Satisficing decision making
- Intuition decision making
- Incremental decision making
- Evidence-based decision making
- Garbage can decision making
- Conflict resolution model

FOR DISCUSSION

1. Is satisficing really appropriate for managers, or is it just being lazy?

2. How do you feel about using intuition rather than rational thinking to make decisions?

3. Which barriers to effective decision making have you observed or experienced in a club, team, or group? What could have been done to overcome those barriers?

4. Several students talked about where they want to work after graduation. One student wants to work in an HCO that does not have conflict because working there will be less stressful. What do you think of that idea?

5. Discuss the pros and cons of the five conflict resolution styles. Which style(s) do you favor? How could you become better prepared to use all the styles?

CASE STUDY QUESTIONS

These questions refer to the Integrative Case Studies at the back of this book.

1. Disparities in Care at Southern Regional Health System case: What are some of the decisions that Mr. Hank and his HCO must make? Using terms, concepts, and decision-making approaches discussed in this chapter, explain how he and his HCO could make each of these decisions.

2. Hospice Goes Hollywood case: Referring to exhibits 13.2 and 13.3, which of the five conflict resolution styles do you think Ms. Thurmond should use to resolve the conflict? Justify your answer.

3. How Can an ACO Improve the Health of Its Population? case: What decisions does Ms. Dillow have to make? Using terms, concepts, and decision-making approaches discussed in this chapter, explain how she could make the decisions.

4. The Rocky Road to Patient Satisfaction at Leonard-Griggs case: Referring to exhibits 13.2 and 13.3, which of the five conflict resolution styles do you think Ms. Ratcliff should use to resolve the conflict? Justify your answer.

 RIVERBEND ORTHOPEDICS MINI CASE STUDY

Riverbend Orthopedics is a busy group practice with expanded services for orthopedic care. It has seven physicians and a podiatrist, plus about 70 other employees. At its big, new clinic building, Riverbend provides extensive orthopedic care. Several technicians provide diagnostic medical imaging, from basic X-rays to magnetic resonance images. The physicians perform surgery in their own outpatient surgery center with Riverbend's own operating nurses and technicians. Therapy is provided by three physical therapists and one part-time contracted occupational therapist. In addition to staff providing actual patient care, the clinic has staff for financial management, medical records, human resources, information systems/technology, building maintenance, and other administrative matters. Occasional marketing work is done by an advertising company. Legal work is outsourced to a law firm. Riverbend is managed by a new president, Ms. Garcia. She and Riverbend have set a goal of achieving "Excellent" ratings for patient experience from at least 90 percent of Riverbend's patients this year.

Ms. Garcia has often tried to use a rational and somewhat individual decision-making approach at Riverbend. This has caused some problems, and she wants to try other approaches. Assume that Riverbend currently has Excellent ratings from only 65 percent of its patients.

MINI CASE STUDY QUESTIONS

1. Discuss how Ms. Garcia and her management team could use tools from this chapter to make decisions and solve problems to reach the 90 percent goal.

2. Although the physicians all approved the 90 percent goal, Ms. Garcia feels that conflict might arise between her and Dr. Barr regarding *how* to achieve the goal. Which causes of conflict (described in this chapter) might create that conflict? Which conflict resolution style should Ms. Garcia use?

REFERENCES

Barends, E., and R. Briner. 2014. "Evidence-Based Practice—Insights from Key Domains: Management." Seminar at University of Edinburgh Business School, Scotland, May 2.

Bowen, D. J. 2016. "Cultivating Leadership Acumen Amidst Change." *Healthcare Executive* 31 (5): 8.

Briner, R. B., D. Denyer, and D. M. Rousseau. 2009. "Evidence-Based Management: Concept Cleanup Time?" *Academy of Management Perspectives* 23 (4): 19–32.

Buell, J. M. 2018. "The Health Continuum: Leveraging IT to Optimize Care." *Healthcare Executive* 33 (1): 10–19.

Daft, R. L. 2016. *Organization Theory & Design*, 12th ed. Mason, OH: South-Western Cengage.

Drucker, P. F. 1967. *The Effective Executive*. New York: Harper & Row.

Dunn, R. 2016. *Dunn and Haimann's Healthcare Management*, 10th ed. Chicago: Health Administration Press.

Dye, C. F. 2017. *Leadership in Healthcare*, 3rd ed. Chicago: Health Administration Press.

Ebadollahi, S. 2017. "The Power of Advanced Technologies to Transform Hospitals and Health Systems." In *Futurescan 2017: Healthcare Trends and Implications 2017–2022*, edited by I. Morrison, 17–21. Chicago: Society for Healthcare Strategy & Market Development and Health Administration Press.

Griffin, R. W., J. M. Phillips, and S. M. Gully. 2017. *Organizational Behavior: Managing People and Organizations*, 12th ed. Boston: Cengage Learning.

Hellriegel, D., and J. W. Slocum. 2011. *Organizational Behavior*, 13th ed. Mason, OH: South-Western Cengage Learning.

Joint Commission. 2015. *Hospital Accreditation Standards*. Oak Brook Terrace, IL: Joint Commission.

Kovner, A. R., and T. D'Aunno. 2016. *Evidence-Based Management in Healthcare: Principles, Cases, and Perspectives*, 2nd ed. Chicago: Health Administration Press.

Ledlow, G. R. 2009. "Conflict and Interpersonal Relationships." In *Health Organizations: Theory, Behavior, and Development*, edited by J. A. Johnson, 149–65. Sudbury, MA: Jones & Bartlett.

Liebler, J. G., and C. R. McConnell. 2004. *Management Principles for Health Professionals*, 4th ed. Sudbury, MA: Jones & Bartlett.

McConnell, C. R. 2018. *Umiker's Management Skills for the New Health Care Supervisor*, 7th ed. Burlington, MA: Jones & Bartlett Learning.

McLaughlin, D. B., and J. R. Olson. 2017. *Healthcare Operations Management*, 3rd ed. Chicago: Health Administration Press.

Nelson, W. A. 2015. "Making Ethical Decisions." *Healthcare Executive* 30 (4): 46–48.

Polzer, J. T., M. A. Neale, and J. L. Illes. 2006. "Conflict Management and Negotiation." In *Health Care Management: Organization Design and Behavior*, 5th ed., edited by S. M. Shortell and A. D. Kaluzny, 148–70. Clifton Park, NY: Thomson Delmar Learning.

Radick, L. E. 2017. "Artificial Intelligence in Healthcare: The Current, Compelling Wave of Interest." *Healthcare Executive* 32 (5): 20–28.

Thomas, K. W., and R. H. Kilmann. 2018. "An Overview of the Thomas-Kilmann Conflict Mode Instrument (TKI)." Kilmann Diagnostics. Accessed September 5. www.kilmanndiagnostics .com/overview-thomas-kilmann-conflict-mode-instrument-tki.

———. 1974. *Thomas-Kilmann Conflict-Mode Instrument*. Tuxedo, NY: Xicom Inc.

Walston, S. L. 2017. *Organizational Behavior and Leadership in Healthcare: Leadership Perspectives and Management Applications*. Chicago: Health Administration Press.

CHAPTER 14

MANAGING CHANGE

People's readiness for change depends on creating a felt need for change.

Thomas G. Cummings and Christopher G. Worley,
management scholars and authors

Studying this chapter will help you to

➤ describe change in healthcare organizations,

➤ explain a three-step approach to implementing small-scale change,

➤ explain an eight-step approach to implementing large-scale change,

➤ understand why people resist change and how managers can overcome resistance,

➤ explain how to use concepts and methods from prior chapters to implement change, and

➤ describe how organization learning and organization development can facilitate change.

HERE'S WHAT HAPPENED

The Partners HealthCare system was engaged in extensive change to adapt to its changing external environment, satisfy its stakeholders, and fulfill its mission. Partners changed some of its strategic goals, patient care delivery models, management systems, organization structure, clinical processes, communication policies, work technologies, staff positions, and performance measurements. Some changes were radical, such as a major redesign of patient care delivery, while others were incremental, with only minor adjustments to procedures. To successfully make these changes, managers used change management methods. For instance, senior managers demonstrated support for the changes by committing funds and resources to them. Employee "champions" were identified who understood the changes and could rally others to accept and support them. Managers provided specialized staff to implement new technologies and processes. The managers gave employees enough time to adapt to the changes in their work. New patient care systems were pilot tested with more than a hundred patients before expanding to more than a thousand. Managers evaluated many aspects of the changes and reported positive outcomes to overcome staff resistance. Although the changes affected many employees, managers successfully implemented the changes so that Partners could improve population health in its community.

As we learned in the opening Here's What Happened, healthcare organizations (HCOs) often change. In fact, they continually change. Some employees think that living with change is a survival skill for working in HCOs. While that might be true, merely surviving change is not enough for managers. **Because of their roles and responsibilities, all managers must lead and manage change for their HCO, not just change themselves.** By doing so, managers make important contributions to their HCOs. The ability to manage change is essential for managers' job success and career growth. This chapter will help you develop this skill.

 Managers deal with change when they perform the five management functions: plan-ning, organizing, staffing, leading, and controlling. We first learned about these functions in chapter 2. Planning, by nature, causes change as new goals and strategies are developed for the future. Organizing work, tasks, jobs, teams, and departments involves changing authority, responsibility, and supervisory relationships to fit new developments such as artificial intelligence. Staffing involves change as new tasks are added to jobs, people retire and are replaced, and compensation changes. Leading and motivating also require change because HCO workforces comprise four to five generations of employees with different motivators. Controlling is changing to embrace big data and analytics that continually compare precise performance measures with targets. Two of Mintzberg's ten managerial roles (discussed in chapter 2) clearly involve change: entrepreneur and disturbance handler. Although change management is not a distinct management function, it is part of performing the five basic management functions and the roles of managers.

Think about the changes mentioned in the opening Here's What Happened, changes described throughout this book, changes reported in the local news, and changes in your daily life. Many of these involve health, healthcare, and HCOs. When changes in HCOs succeed, they can help people lead healthier lives. Managers who help plan and implement the changes feel positive emotions afterward—satisfaction, accomplishment, joy, and sometimes relief. Yet, "despite the huge investment that companies have made in tools, training, and thousands of books . . . most studies still show a 60%–70% failure rate for organizational change projects—a statistic that has stayed constant from the 1970's to the present" (Ashkenas 2013). As bad as that failure rate is, it may be worsening as change becomes more complex, uncertain, and difficult.

This chapter will help you succeed with change. It begins by examining change in HCOs. We next learn a three-step process to implement small changes. Then we study an eight-step approach to implement large-scale organization change. Next, the chapter explains why people resist change and how managers can overcome resistance. The chapter then explores how managers use concepts, methods, and tools from prior chapters to implement change in HCOs. The final section presents organization learning and organization development to further enable successful change in HCOs. The chapter provides important tools to manage change, which managers use at all levels of an HCO.

CHANGE IN HEALTHCARE ORGANIZATIONS

Can you think of some changes in HCOs? Why do you suppose those changes occurred? Recall from chapters 1 and 3 that changes in the external environment often drive changes in HCOs. Chapter 1 lists trends and developments in the environment—such as workforce demographics, payment based on value, mobile health technology, and retail medicine—that are forcing change in HCOs. A medical practice in Minneapolis might move to a different facility, tighten the supply chain system, or implement telehealth. While much change in HCOs results from external factors, sometimes it is driven by internal factors. The volunteer services coordinator retires. The heating system keeps malfunctioning. Cheryl discovers a daily pattern of narcotics missing from the pharmacy. Some of these factors are predictable, and some are surprises.

Another reason for so much change is that one change leads to other changes. Most HCOs are complex and have many interacting parts. When the storeroom changes its schedule for delivering supplies to the clinics, the clinics then change their procedures for using and ordering supplies. A business that sells customer service training modules to HCOs sees complaints on social media about its high prices. In response, Kelly, the sales manager, decentralizes authority so that sales staff can adjust prices for customers. This sales department change causes Roberto in the accounting department to change corporate control mechanisms that monitor sales, prices, and revenues. Change in one department causes changes in other departments.

In HCOs, managers face two types of change. Radical change is big and revolutionary. Incremental change is smaller and evolutionary (Daft 2016). During the 1990s, change shifted (changed) toward radical change as consultants told managers to get rid of their old business models and create entirely new ones. Consultants said the external environment had changed so much and so fast that minor adjustments to the existing way would not be enough. Instead, major changes were required. But a few years later, leaders realized the downsides of radical, wholesale change (Abrahamson 2000). What do you think had happened? Rapid, extensive change had left too little time for organizations and people to recover and restabilize. There was too much turmoil and instability for everyone to function normally. Employees were fearful and overstressed. Managers were so busy with change that they did not perform other necessary work. Leaders realized that too much change implemented too quickly ruined an organization's core competencies without successfully developing new competencies. Managers learned to carefully manage the amount and pace of change.

✓ CHECK IT OUT ONLINE

How comfortable are you with change? Tests can help people judge their readiness for change and how well they accept change. Managers can use these tests when leading change in HCOs because readiness is needed for successful change. Some online tests take only a few minutes to complete. For example, try the Change-Readiness Assessment at www.ecfvp.org/files/uploads/2_-change_readiness_assessment_0426111.pdf (from a website for a leadership class taught by T. J. Jenney at Purdue University). Check it out online and see what you discover.

MANAGING ORGANIZATION CHANGE

Literature and research on managing organization change offer useful lessons and models. Taken together, these models emphasize the importance of not only a shared, big-picture vision but also a carefully developed implementation plan with flexibility to adapt (Kash et al. 2014). We next examine two models for change that are often used in organizations—including HCOs.

SMALL-SCALE CHANGE

unfreeze
Create dissatisfaction with the current way and motivate people to want change.

refreeze
Lock in the new way and make it the correct way of doing something.

Kurt Lewin developed a systematic three-step process for change in the mid-twentieth century that is still popular and effective today. He viewed change as a movement from an old way to a new way of doing something. The three steps are (1) **unfreeze**, (2) move, and (3) **refreeze** (see exhibit 14.1). They are explained in this section based on the work of Cummings and Worley (2015) and Griffin, Phillips, and Gully (2017). An example at an HCO's business office for fundraising was created to illustrate the three steps.

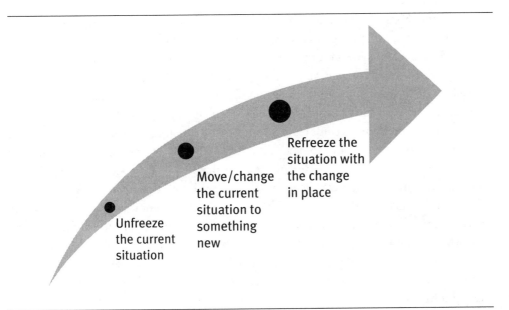

Exhibit 14.1
The Three-Step
Change Process

Source: Data from Cummings and Worley (2015); Griffin, Phillips, and Gully (2017).

Step 1: Unfreeze the way something is done.

◆ Clear out old ideas to make room for new ideas.

◆ Explain why change is needed; weaken the forces that maintain the status quo.

◆ Describe clearly what will change, what will not change, and how jobs will be affected.

◆ Motivate people to want to change; make them feel dissatisfied with the current way.

◆ Alter how people think about the situation; help people see how the future could be better.

◆ Lead people to feel change is possible and can succeed.

◆ Begin to overcome resistance.

If this first step is done well, people will be committed to make the change succeed. Better yet, they will persist if difficulty arises.

Throughout healthcare, many nonprofit health associations, charities, foundations, and interest groups raise funds to help people with their health. You have probably heard of some, such as the American Cancer Society, American Lung Association, and Children's

Hunger Fund. Some are national, with state and local offices. Others are regional or local. To obtain donations, the organizations must work well with clients, donors, and other stakeholders. Let's imagine a business office at such an HCO near Alexandria.

The business office manager, Mr. Remson, held a staff meeting. He reviewed social media feedback (used to monitor performance as part of the control process) that indicated some people who called the business office were unhappy about staff performance. More specifically, the social media comments revealed that the staff members were not helpful or polite when taking phone calls from clients and families. One caller even followed up with a letter complaining about the staff. Mr. Remson shared the feedback and letter with the nine business office employees. He explained that an impolite, uncaring way of handling phone calls (as perceived by the callers) harmed the reputation of the business office and the entire HCO. Mr. Remson added that a bad image would lead to fewer clients, fewer donations, and perhaps job losses. He suggested that employees try the "mother" test: "Ask yourself, 'Is this how I would want someone to talk to my mother?'" Mr. Remson next read telephone guidelines from a business etiquette website. He asked for feedback, opinions, and input from each employee, and discussion followed. One employee noted that HCOs are supposed to provide an excellent customer experience in every interaction. Mr. Remson agreed and told the staff they should do that. Then he expressed confidence in them.

Step 2: Move to the new way of doing it.

- ◆ Move to the new methods, processes, techniques, structures, culture, behaviors, policies, procedures, training, tools, work settings, and people.

- ◆ Reorganize work, jobs, and tasks and the way they are performed.

- ◆ Use the new way.

- ◆ Exert energy and effort to overcome inertia (i.e., the existing way).

- ◆ Set control mechanisms to measure new performance.

This step applies management principles learned earlier in this book to change the way work is performed. For example, work standardization is applied.

At the business office, each employee was given a list of telephone etiquette standards to follow (e.g., answer a call by the third ring, introduce yourself, control the tone of your voice). Job descriptions were changed to specifically state that telephone etiquette was an important part of the job. Employees took turns calling each other pretending to be a client, and staff practiced the new standard way of handling phone calls. During practice calls, employees sometimes backed up for a redo as they learned the new way. There were a few funny moments. Mr. Remson continued to emphasize that excellent customer service is a core value and that the new telephone guidelines show the correct way to handle phone calls to ensure excellent service. He added that calls would be electronically monitored for quality control purposes.

Step 3: Refreeze the way it is done.

- ◆ Reward and reinforce the new way.

- ◆ Prevent employees who favor the old way from punishing (e.g., rejecting, scorning) employees who use the new way.

- ◆ Make the change the new normal and part of the daily routine.

- ◆ Stabilize the new way with repetition to strongly establish it.

- ◆ Link the new way to the rest of the organization (e.g., the organization culture, reward systems).

If this third step is not done well, people may drift back to the old way, especially if the new way becomes too hard.

Back at the business office, Mr. Remson continually emphasized the new telephone standards and commended staff when he heard them following the guidelines. He individually asked employees about their experiences with and feelings about the changes. These conversations enabled him to identify a "change champion," who then helped promote the new way with the office staff. After the first week, the change was going well. The staff celebrated their progress with a cake, and one employee felt safe joking with Mr. Remson about a call she handled. Resistance gradually faded, and employees accepted the new way. It then became automatic.

All three steps must be done well for the change to take root and succeed. At the front end, inadequate unfreezing and lack of readiness to change are frequent causes of failure. If you are managing change, invest the time needed to prepare people and unfreeze. At the back end, sometimes too little effort is made to refreeze after change has begun. If you are managing change, invest the time needed to refreeze. That will help the change "stick."

EIGHT-STEP APPROACH TO LARGE-SCALE CHANGE

In the 1990s, John P. Kotter developed a useful eight-step approach to create and sustain large-scale change in organizations. The steps are described in this section based on Cummings and Worley (2015) and Dunn (2016). This approach builds on the three steps for small-scale change. Steps 1 through 4 unfreeze the old way, steps 5 and 6 move to a new way, and steps 7 and 8 refreeze the situation with the new way in place. After studying these steps, you will realize that managers must *provide plenty of time* and not try to rush a large change. For example, the first step may take weeks to allow people time to hear about a proposed change, think about it, talk with others about it, think more about it, ask questions about it, and gradually understand how it could affect them individually and collectively.

Managers can use principles and methods from previous chapters of this book when they perform these eight steps. For example, the chapters on leadership and organizing teams have useful ideas. Think about how you could use the concepts, tools, and methods you have already learned to execute these eight steps.

Step 1: Establish urgency.

◆ Show a real need that cannot wait any longer; explain why the change is essential.

◆ Describe a real or potential crisis.

◆ Create dissatisfaction with the way things are now.

◆ Describe a great opportunity or vision that must be pursued.

◆ Realize that merely identifying a problem does not create urgency.

Step 2: Create a guiding coalition.

◆ Line up influential supporters at all levels of the organization.

◆ Enlist the support of people whose input and commitment are needed to make change happen.

◆ Create a project team to implement the change.

Step 3: Develop a change vision.

◆ Create a clear, simple, and easily understood statement of what the future will be.

◆ Tell how the future can be better than the current situation.

◆ Provide a sense of direction that motivates people.

◆ Ensure the vision statement makes sense to people at all levels of the organization.

Step 4: Communicate the change vision.

◆ Enable the guiding coalition to clearly communicate the change and its benefits.

◆ Communicate the change repeatedly in multiple ways, both formally and informally.

◆ Ask people what they know about the proposed change.

◆ Seek feedback and input from others about the change.

◆ Constantly repeat and reinforce the change vision message.

Step 5: Empower broad-based action.

◆ Give others permission to try the change.

◆ Revise policies, procedures, rules, and structures to enable the change.

◆ Provide training, practice, and support for the change.

◆ Let people take risks and learn from mistakes when trying the change.

◆ Support and reward the early adopters of the change.

◆ Continually work to overcome resistance.

Step 6: Create short-term wins.

◆ Arrange some quick, easy successes with the change.

◆ Publicize and celebrate the early wins and their benefits.

Step 7: Consolidate gains.

◆ Reward success to keep the change momentum going.

◆ Build on early successes to expand the change.

◆ Train more people to use the change.

◆ Show how success with the change benefits workers and other stakeholders.

◆ Redesign organization structure and processes to "lock in" early successes with the change.

Step 8: Anchor new approaches in the culture.

◆ Make the change part of what is valued and considered correct in the organization.

◆ Reward and reinforce the change to make it "the way we do things here."

◆ Hire and promote people who support the change.

◆ Ingrain the change in the culture to make it permanent.

Note that the second step—creating a guiding coalition—includes creating a project team to implement the change. So let's briefly return to project management, which we studied in chapter 3. Recall that project managers work to ensure assigned projects are completed within established constraints of time, budget, risk, scope, quality, and available resources (Project Management Institute 2017; Schwalbe and Furlong 2013). This work helps an HCO implement change. To ensure projects are completed, a project manager forms a project team based on the specific requirements of the project. This requires careful thought and choices (explained in chapter 6 on teams). The project manager and team then use management tools and project management tools to implement the project (change). When managers implement a project—such as a population health project, a clinical integration project, or a mobile health project—they should think of their project also as a *change project* and use appropriate change methods.

The Here's What Happened at the beginning of this chapter described Partners HealthCare managing change. The entire Partners HealthCare case study is in an appendix at the end of this book. Read the full case for more detail about what Partners did to successfully implement large-scale change.

RESISTANCE TO CHANGE

Forces outside and inside an HCO push *for* change. Yet, simultaneously, other forces push back *against* change. The resistance comes from an essential part of every HCO: people who work there! Not everyone resists change, but there will be some who resist, push back, and perhaps try to block the change. "Employees often go through the stages of anticipation, denial, anger, bargaining, depression, and, finally, acceptance" (McConnell 2018, 401). Some will ignore the change, some will cynically scorn it, some will quietly worry about it, some will accept it, and some will resist it. Let's consider a public health department in New York City. For a single proposed change, such as a different work schedule, employees may range from highly supportive to highly resistant. The manager communicates the same information to all employees. But employees have unique personalities, past experiences, biases, current life stressors, and other factors that might lead them to resist.

Employees at all levels, including managers, may resist change. This is why the two models for implementing change (small-scale and large-scale) include actions to overcome resistance. When managers plan and lead change, they should expect resistance, noncompliance, and perhaps outright defiance. In the Here's What Happened at the beginning of this chapter, some staff resisted change at Partners HealthCare. Resistance is a natural part of the change management process. Be ready for it. This topic is explored further by studying people, organizations, and the nature of healthcare.

WHY PEOPLE RESIST CHANGE

Pop quiz: Name the five human needs in Maslow's hierarchy of needs. (This is an open-book quiz, so feel free to check chapter 10.) After recalling these five needs, imagine a change that might interfere with your fulfilling one of these needs. You are not exactly sure about the proposed change, yet you worry it might interfere with fulfilling one of these basic human needs. Do you feel like resisting the change? Thinking about Maslow's needs gives us a framework for understanding reasons people resist change (see exhibit 14.2). **People often resist changes at work because they fear the changes might reduce satisfaction of their needs.** They fear a possible loss of something they value. Even though people do not know for certain that they will experience loss, they worry that they *might* lose something. Uncertainty and the unknown create fears and worry, which cause resistance.

Another reason people resist change is that they do not understand how it might benefit them. Exhibit 14.2 could be redone to show that a change might *increase* fulfillment of Maslow's needs. A change might lead to *more* job pay, security, friendships, esteem, and growth. Sometimes people do not perceive the possible benefits of change, which leaves them worried about loss instead.

Why else do people in organizations resist change? They may not see the reason for the change and may not understand why it is needed. They may ask, "Why do we have to go through all this change?" or "What's the purpose?"

Next, let's assume employees understand the purpose of a change and feel that overall it will benefit them. Yet, they still might resist. Why? Because they think the change is unrealistic or even impossible. There is not enough time, expertise, or resources, or there are too many obstacles and restraints to accomplish the change.

EXHIBIT 14.2
Changes at Work and Effects on Maslow's Needs

Changes at Work	Effect on Needs
Job might become too routine and less fulfilling; job might not use my abilities; job might provide less chance for growth and professional development	Less self-fulfillment; less self-actualization
Job might become lower status and less important; job might be less respected by others; job might lose power and resources; job change is bad for my professional image	Less esteem; less respect from others
Job might not let me work with my favorite coworkers; job might break up my work group; job might not conform to peer group norms, so peers reject me	Less affiliation, friendship, love, and belonging
Job might become unsafe; job and resources might become less secure; new boss creates insecurity; less control of my work schedule; fear of failure in new job	Less security; less safety
Job (and paycheck) might be eliminated; work hours (and pay) might be reduced	Less certainty about meeting basic needs (e.g., food, shelter)

Finally, some people resist change to spite or get revenge on a manager or organization. Workers who feel mistreated and have a grudge can resist or even sabotage change out of revenge. These workers may feel their actions are justified and resist change openly or secretly.

ORGANIZATION CHARACTERISTICS THAT MAY IMPEDE CHANGE

Like people, organizations have personalities, past experiences, biases, current life stressors, and other factors that may impede change (Griffin, Phillips, and Gully 2017). Recall from chapter 4 that organizations range from very mechanistic to very organic. Do you recall which type has rigid, specialized tasks and strict hierarchy, control, rules, and authority? Right—the mechanistic type. Organizations that are too mechanistic may have **structural inertia** that deters change. In contrast, organizations with an organic structure have flexible, shared tasks and loose hierarchy, control, rules, and authority. An organic structure supports new ways and change.

structural inertia
Resistance to change created by organization structures and systems.

Organizations often create structures and systems to control work and create stability (Griffin, Phillips, and Gully 2017). These include job descriptions, policies, procedures, training, rewards, punishments, performance appraisals, and other mechanisms designed to control performance. They create structural inertia—resistance to change due to structures and systems. That is good for stability and predictability, but it inhibits change. Extra effort and energy is required to overcome structural inertia to work in a new way. Rather than make the extra effort, people may resist the new way. They keep doing things the usual way. They might even say, "I like doing it the usual way because I can be on autopilot."

Other organization characteristics can also impede change. Recall from chapter 11 what comprises organization culture: values, norms, guiding beliefs, and understanding shared by members as the correct way to think, feel, and behave. Some organizations have a culture in which employees believe they are not allowed to question their managers, dare not make mistakes, and should respect tradition. Although that type of culture has some advantages, it also has the disadvantage of blocking change. Other cultures value innovation, asking questions, learning by trial and error, and trying new and creative ideas. That type of culture supports change.

Several other characteristics of organizations can deter change (Griffin, Phillips, and Gully 2017; Longenecker and Longenecker 2014). Organizations that have limited resources and tight budgets are less able to try new ideas and spend money on change that might fail. Some organizations lack the leadership, teamwork, and cooperation needed for change. Organizations in stable environments feel less pressure to change than do organizations in frequently changing environments. Finally, some organizations have commitments such as contracts with labor unions, supply chain partners, banks, physicians, and others. Some have legal commitments with accountable care organizations, joint ventures, strategic alliances, innovation partnerships, and other interorganization structures. These organization commitments—some of which may last for years—may restrict how an organization is allowed to change. (On the other hand, some commitments may require certain changes.)

HEALTHCARE CHARACTERISTICS THAT MAY IMPEDE CHANGE

We next consider several characteristics of healthcare that can impede change in HCOs. In general, the pace of successful change in healthcare and HCOs has been slow. We learned in chapter 12 that HCOs have lagged behind other industries in controlling and improving their performance (McLaughlin and Olson 2017). The healthcare characteristics listed in exhibit 14.3 help to explain why. These statements are general and do not apply to every worker and HCO. For example, when managers use transformational leadership and teams, their HCOs are less affected by these factors. Still, managers in HCOs should be mindful of these healthcare characteristics when they attempt to manage change.

HOW PEOPLE RESIST CHANGE

People may resist change aggressively or passively, directly or indirectly, openly or secretly (McConnell 2018). At one extreme, workers may openly, aggressively resist change. Nurses have marched in the streets with protest signs about proposed changes. An individual worker may refuse to comply with a change, such as when an employee feels the change is unsafe. Direct, aggressive resistance is easy to detect, so it is less common. Workers are more likely to resist indirectly. They usually want to be viewed as team players rather than troublemakers, so they may resist a change without directly refusing to comply. Instead, they take more sick time, arrive late, "forget" to do something, violate minor rules, or cooperate less. Their resistance may be seen in sloppy work, less work, and barely acceptable work. Workers may also resist a change in their current job by moving to a different job in the same organization or a different one.

Characteristic of Healthcare	How It Impedes Change
Healthcare involves risk to patients amid uncertainty and with big consequences.	Staff is averse to experimentation needed for successful change.
Staff interactions are often based on professional hierarchy, identities, and status.	Staff does not naturally collaborate, which is needed for organization changes.
Identity and self-image of many workers are strongly linked to one's profession and only weakly to one's organization.	Staff interest in organization change may be weak.
Relationships between healthcare staff and managers are based on transactions, self-interests, and conflicting goals.	Healthcare staff and managers may struggle to pursue shared organization change.

EXHIBIT 14.3
Healthcare Characteristics That Impede Change

Source: Data from Nembhard et al. (2009).

People exhibit different degrees of sincerity in their resistance. Some people may speak up to stop a change that they sincerely believe (rightly or wrongly) will harm people or the HCO. Recall from chapter 8 that employees have a right to protection from harm, and they have some rights (within boundaries) to express their views about work. On the other hand, as mentioned, some people resist change as a form of revenge. Their opposition to change is not sincere.

In the long run, employees are usually better off accepting a reasonable change in their job or organization. Continued resistance can make a worker obsolete and unable to function in the new work world. Employees, especially managers who lead others, should accept that change is inevitable and will soon be coming to a workplace near them. Lower-level managers and supervisors who adjust to change—and help their staff adjust to change—are respected by high-level executives and are more likely to advance in their careers.

People in HCOs resist change for many reasons. Some of these reasons are illustrated in the adjacent Using Chapter 14 in the Real World, which is about change in primary care medical practices. Think about this the next time you visit a primary care office.

FORCE FIELD ANALYSIS

force field analysis
Graphical technique that shows and evaluates the strength of various forces that are *for* and *against* a change.

Besides developing the three-step process for change explained earlier in this chapter, Kurt Lewin created **force field analysis.** This graphical technique shows and evaluates the strength of various forces that are *for* and *against* a change (McLaughlin and Olson 2017). Managers use the tool to judge if a proposed change can be implemented and to plan how to implement a change that has been approved. Managers can assess and then lessen resistance to the change.

For any change, there are forces that will drive (enable) the change and other forces that will restrain (block) the change. What forces can you think of? Which ones were described earlier in this chapter? Common forces may include resource availability, history and tradition, laws, powerful stakeholders, organization structures, organization values, social expectations, entrenched interests, costs, and people's attitudes, needs, and values. Each of these forces might be for or against a particular change. The forces will vary in their strength. A force field analysis of a specific change lists each *driving force*—and its strength—that would enable the change. The analysis does the same for each *restraining force* that would block the change. An example of this analysis is shown in exhibit 14.4. The change would create a new way for nursing staff from one shift to hand over patients to incoming staff on the next shift.

A manager can add up the strength of forces for and against a change. In exhibit 14.4, the restraining forces total 21 and are stronger than the driving forces, which total 19. Thus, currently the change is likely to fail. The manager can see that he must strengthen

USING CHAPTER 14 IN THE REAL WORLD

A large, multidisciplinary health system implemented change in its primary care clinics to increase efficiency, reduce costs, improve customer experience, and better utilize primary care physicians (Gray, Harrison, and Hung 2016). Medical assistants (MAs), whose training includes an associate degree or less, had been performing various lower-level clerical, administrative, and clinical tasks. The change redesigned patient care processes and shifted more tasks to MAs and away from physicians. An MA was assigned to each physician to act as a "flow manager." The MA would manage the flow of that physician's patients through their appointments and the clinics. In this role, each MA guided her physician during the day, monitored and handled some of the physician's e-mail, determined the schedule, and handled other tasks previously done by the physician. MAs had to be more proactive and directive to instruct their physician what to do.

Some MAs and physicians resisted this change for several reasons. One major reason was that their two jobs differed greatly in prestige, power, education, and work traits. Some physicians were reluctant to yield so much control to an MA. Some said they did not see any benefit from it. Some felt unsafe and insecure in letting go of certain tasks. Some were not used to being directed. Perceived status was affected. One physician implied the change was not realistic, saying the clinic was asking too much of MAs. Meanwhile, some MAs felt awkward about having their work scrutinized by physicians and about directing physicians. Some felt their working relationships had become more difficult. MAs had to learn and use new skills that made some MAs uncomfortable. Some MAs viewed the change as just extra work piled on them. However, other MAs "found the change rewarding and satisfying" (Gray, Harrison, and Hung 2016, 188). Some MAs and physicians adjusted to the change fine and benefited from it. Others did not.

driving forces, reduce restraining forces, or both. How can he do that? He might redesign the change. For example, he could revise the way confidential information is shared during shift change handovers to ensure no disclosure occurs. That would weaken or remove a strong restraining force and make the change more likely to succeed. The manager could also use the three-step change model to unfreeze the ritualism and tradition that restrain the proposed new way of doing end-of-shift handovers. That would further increase the likelihood of successful change. Many other ideas for overcoming restraining forces and resistance—based on prior chapters—are described next.

EXHIBIT 14.4
Force Field
Analysis

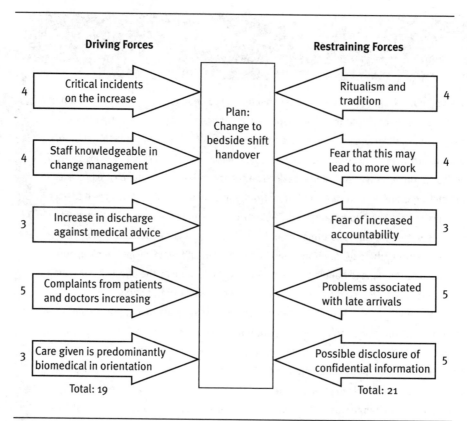

Source: McLaughlin and Olson (2017, 163).

OVERCOMING RESISTANCE TO CHANGE

Although managers must try to minimize resistance to change, they do not have to eliminate it. Managers should keep this in mind especially when undertaking large-scale change that will affect many people throughout an HCO. Dealing with possible or actual resistance might be frustrating to eager managers who want to implement the change. Yet, if managers don't do enough at the beginning to minimize resistance, it will block change and frustrate them later.

So what should managers do? Here are suggestions from this book and other sources (Daft 2016; Dunn 2016; Griffin, Phillips, and Gully 2017; Longenecker and Longenecker 2014; McConnell 2018). These ideas add depth and detail to the two change models studied earlier. Ideas are grouped into four broad, interrelated categories:

1. Involve relevant people in planning, deciding, and implementing the change.

2. Explain the change multiple times and in varied ways to employees and other stakeholders.

3.   Apply leadership principles and methods.

4.   Realize that people change at different times and speeds.

These ideas work best when managers have trusting relationships with others and have the organization structure, culture, and resources to enable change. If these factors are missing, managers will struggle to overcome resistance because people will not believe them or not feel safe trying new ideas. The organization and employees first should be ready for change.

Involve relevant people in planning, deciding, and implementing the change. This activity begins in the planning stage of management when decisions are being made for plans and how to implement them. Managers should involve the right people in making plans and decisions so that they "buy in" to the decision and will support it. For example, when planning an implementation schedule (see chapter 3), a manager should think about who will be affected by the change and who is needed to help it succeed. If the compliance staff must all move to a new location, involve them in planning the move. Their involvement will strengthen their commitment to the change and help create a realistic plan and schedule. The timing for involving people will vary depending on the change, the people, the timing, and other factors. A manager needs good judgment (which can be developed through experience) to determine when to involve which people. If in doubt, involving people sooner is usually better than doing so later.

Explain the change multiple times and in varied ways to employees and other stakeholders. This recommendation is related to the first one. As implementation proceeds, a manager must explain the change to a wider group of people who need to know about it. The timing for this explanation will vary depending on how particular people will be involved. It will also depend on the extent to which they were involved in the decision to make a change or to implement it.

As patiently and openly as possible, explain the who, what, why, where, when, and how of the change. Emphasize the purpose of the change and make a compelling case for it. Suggest how it might affect specific groups of people, such as second-shift workers, former cancer patients, and visitors younger than age 18. Try to reduce uncertainty by addressing pros and cons. Be prepared for questions and answer them sincerely. Empathy and honesty will help; superficial buzzwords and vague promises will not. Depending on the nature of the change, anticipate and do not overreact to criticism, frustration, denial, and anger from others. Allow people to express feelings, and then sincerely acknowledge and respond to their feelings. Tap in to the social media grapevine and informal networks to discover and correct inaccurate gossip and rumors. These steps can reduce resistance.

Provide sufficient time for people to get information, think about it, and follow up later with questions. People who resist are unlikely to change overnight, so allow them time to gradually accept the change. Repetition and multiple methods of communication may be required depending on the change, the number of people involved, and other factors. Chapter 15 on professionalism and communication offers more advice on this topic.

Managers should be willing to "change the change" when necessary to resolve people's valid concerns. For example, a medical office decided to change to open-access scheduling, which was expected to improve patients' access to appointments. The staff began implementing the change, but turmoil arose. The leader assessed the situation and had to decide whether to push ahead or back off. He decided to back off the change rather than force it. Open-access scheduling was still a good idea, but he acknowledged the staff did not understand it well enough to implement it. So he and the staff stepped back, revised the change plan and schedule, learned more about open scheduling, and tried again. Then they achieved the desired change (Reinertsen 2014).

Apply leadership principles and methods. Think back to earlier chapters on leadership, conflict resolution, motivation, power, and culture. Use knowledge and tools from those chapters to implement change and overcome resistance. For example, establish clear, compelling goals. Identify and clarify tasks, roles, responsibilities, and accountabilities for the change. Apply conflict resolution methods appropriately. Strive for win–win collaboration and be flexible when possible. Compromise and negotiation can help overcome resistance.

Don't be quick to use managerial authority to force change. Although that approach might sometimes be necessary (e.g., to comply with a court decision), it will likely irritate employees and cause indirect resistance, such as rule infractions and absence from work. Softer forms of power, such as persuasion and appeal to the greater good, may suffice to influence resisters. Apply principles of motivation. For example, a change might create opportunity for job growth or job autonomy that could motivate some workers. Be a role model for change and help create a culture of change that values experimenting, trying new ideas, learning from mistakes, and taking reasonable risks. In this culture, workers will feel more secure about trying a change, not succeeding at first, and practicing until they get it right.

Realize that people change at different times and speeds. A manager should judge people's readiness for a proposed change. (Change readiness can be assessed using a survey such as the one mentioned in this chapter's Check It Out Online.) Think about which groups in general and which key individuals in particular must help the change succeed. When judging the readiness of workers on a scale of 1 to 10, some will be 1, some 10, and most will be in between. Some people thrive on change and become bored without it; they might be ready for change before the managers are. Others wait to follow the crowd; they will be ready after a majority has tried the change and has told coworkers it is not too bad. Some people delay and avoid change for reasons given earlier. Manage the pace of change, but do not try to move everyone at the same pace. Support people as they proceed through the change process. Enlist early adopters of change as change champions to lead others.

→ TRY IT, APPLY IT

Think about a big change you've seen in an organization. It might be an organization where you did an internship, held a part-time job, or now go to college. Use what you have learned in this chapter to analyze how the change was managed. What was the change and its purpose? Who led and managed the change? Do you recall if any steps from the three-step change model were used? Were any steps from the eight-step change model applied? What was done to deal with resistance? Discuss your ideas with classmates.

When you are a manager, realize that overcoming resistance to change is not the same as creating commitment to change. For example, Alice does not resist changing to a new method of setting individual goals—but that does not mean she really supports it. Alice might not exert herself much to accomplish the change and might not help sell it to others. If the change falters, she won't do much to strengthen it. **Remember that lack of resistance is not commitment.** "I don't have a problem with it" does not mean "I am committed to making it succeed."

ORGANIZATION LEARNING AND ORGANIZATION DEVELOPMENT

To help their HCOs continually and successfully change, managers can use two approaches that focus on the organization as a whole rather than on a particular person, project, or change.

"**Organization learning** (OL) enhances an organization's capability to acquire and develop new knowledge" (Cummings and Worley 2015, 582). It goes beyond individual learning by individual employees. Instead, OL enables the entire organization to discover, produce, store, and reuse knowledge to benefit the organization. In rapidly changing external environments, OL is essential and can be a valuable competitive advantage.

Managers may design their organization's structures and processes to enable OL. For example, teams are better for OL than vertical hierarchies are. Employee empowerment and participation in decision processes enables OL. For OL to flourish, the culture must value learning, discovery, openness, teamwork, and sharing. People are not blamed for failure; instead, the culture encourages them to learn from failure. An organization's performance appraisal and reward systems promote OL and help the organization learn.

organization learning
A process that enhances an organization's capability to acquire and develop new knowledge.

Knowledge management (see chapter 13) further enables OL. Employees gather knowledge and share it throughout the organization via wikis, blogs, networks (electronic and personal), searchable databases, conversations, and other ways of sharing both tacit and documented knowledge (Griffin, Phillips, and Gully 2017). Furthermore, managers encourage employees to review and reflect on experiences, projects, successes, and failures. People who were involved in a project confer quickly, openly, and honestly to discuss what was supposed to happen, what did happen, why there were differences, and what they learned (Griffin, Phillips, and Gully 2017, 581). In addition to learning, reflection develops trust among participants. Managers can design other structures and processes to support OL to improve their HCO's ability to change.

Organization development (OD) also helps HCOs to continually and successfully change. As defined in chapter 2, OD is "a process that applies . . . behavioral science knowledge and practices to help organizations build their capability to change and to achieve greater effectiveness" (Cummings and Worley 2015, 1). This approach establishes an organization's social systems and culture that facilitate changing human behavior in the organization. Going beyond training, OD uses team building, interdepartmental activities, employee participation, conflict resolution, organization redesign, process redesign, culture change, group dynamics, respect, trust, autonomy, fairness, and employee empowerment (Cummings and Worley 2015; Daft 2016; Johnson and Rossow 2019). When these are blended together in an organization, change becomes more possible.

ONE MORE TIME

Managers at all levels of an HCO must successfully manage change. Change is constant, so this ability is important for managers' job success and career growth. Although change management is not a distinct management function, it is used when performing the five basic management functions: planning, organizing, staffing, leading, and controlling. Managers make changes in an HCO because of external factors, internal factors, and previous changes in the HCO. Some changes are radical and others are incremental; both types are needed.

Small-scale change can be implemented using Lewin's three steps: unfreeze, move, and refreeze. Large-scale change can be managed with Kotter's eight-step approach, which builds on the three steps for small-scale change; managers should establish urgency, create a guiding coalition, develop a change vision, communicate the change vision, empower broad-based action, create short-term wins, consolidate gains, and anchor new approaches in the organization culture. They can also apply project management techniques to keep change within budget and on schedule.

People often resist change. Common reasons include fear of not being able to fulfill wants and needs, fear of losing something valuable, not understanding the reasons for change, not understanding the benefits of change, feeling change is not possible, and inertia. Resistance may be evident or hidden. Managers use force field analysis to judge the forces for and against change and to reduce resistance to a proposed change. To reduce resistance, managers should involve people who will be affected by the change in planning and implementing that change, explain the change multiple times in multiple ways to stakeholders, apply leadership principles and methods, and realize that people change at different times and speeds. Organization learning and organization development can help HCOs become more capable of accomplishing change.

 FOR YOUR TOOLBOX

- Lewin's three-step approach to change
- Kotter's eight-step approach to large-scale change

- Force field analysis
- Organization learning
- Organization development

FOR DISCUSSION

1. Consider in detail Lewin's three-step process for change. Which of the three steps do you think would be hardest? How could you develop your ability to apply this change process?

2. Describe with specific examples how at least five management theories, principles, methods, or tools studied in other chapters could be used in Kotter's eight-step process for large-scale organization change.

3. Think about a change that you resisted at your college or workplace. Why did you resist the change? Why do people in general resist change?

4. How can managers overcome resistance to change?

CASE STUDY QUESTIONS

These questions refer to the Integrative Case Studies at the back of this book.

1. Disparities in Care at Southern Regional Health System case: At the end of the case study, what change does Mr. Hank want to make? Using information in the case study, plus any inferences you want to make, conduct a force field analysis for his desired change. Explain how Mr. Hank could apply Kotter's eight-step process to achieve his change.

2. Hospice Goes Hollywood case: Using information from this chapter, explain why you think the hospice's clinical staff resist the change proposed by Ms. Thurmond. Describe how she could use Lewin's three-step process to implement her change.

3. "I Can't Do It All!" case: What change does Mr. Brice want to make? Describe how Mr. Brice could use Lewin's three-step process to implement his change.

4. Increasing the Focus on Patient Safety at First Medical Center case: What change does Dr. Frame want to implement? Using information in the case study, plus any inferences you want to make, conduct a force field analysis for the proposed change.

5. The Rocky Road to Patient Satisfaction at Leonard-Griggs case: Using information from this chapter, explain why you think the office staff resist the change for implementing patient surveys. Describe how Ms. Ratcliff could use Lewin's three-step process to implement her change.

RIVERBEND ORTHOPEDICS MINI CASE STUDY

Riverbend Orthopedics is a busy group practice with expanded services for orthopedic care. It has seven physicians and a podiatrist, plus about 70 other employees. At its big, new clinic building, Riverbend provides extensive orthopedic care. Several technicians provide diagnostic medical imaging, from basic X-rays to magnetic resonance images. The physicians perform surgery in their own outpatient surgery center with Riverbend's own operating nurses and technicians. Therapy is provided by three physical therapists and one part-time contracted occupational therapist. In addition to staff providing actual patient care, the clinic has staff for financial management, medical records, human resources, information systems/technology, building maintenance, and other administrative matters. Occasional marketing work is done by an advertising company. Legal work is outsourced to a law firm. Riverbend is managed by a new president, Ms. Garcia. She and Riverbend have set a goal of achieving "Excellent" ratings for patient experience from at least 90 percent of Riverbend's patients this year.

To achieve the goal, Ms. Garcia wonders if employees should be using standardized scripts for interactions with patients. (For an example, review Using Chapter 4 in the Real World.) This would be a change; some employees would consider it a big change.

MINI CASE STUDY QUESTIONS

1. To help Ms. Garcia think about the proposed change for scripted interactions with patients, prepare a force field analysis for the change. You may make reasonable assumptions and inferences.

2. Using information from this chapter, prepare a list of steps for Ms. Garcia to take to implement the change to standardized scripts.

References

Abrahamson, E. 2000. "Change Without Pain." *Harvard Business Review* 78 (4): 75–79.

Ashkenas, R. 2013. "Change Management Needs to Change." *Harvard Business Review*. Published April 16. https://hbr.org/2013/04/change-management-needs-to-cha.

Cummings, T. G., and C. G. Worley. 2015. *Organization Development and Change*. Stamford, CT: Cengage Learning.

Daft, R. L. 2016. *Organization Theory & Design*, 12th ed. Mason, OH: South-Western Cengage.

Dunn, R. 2016. *Dunn and Haimann's Healthcare Management*, 10th ed. Chicago: Health Administration Press.

Gray, C. P., M. I. Harrison, and D. Hung. 2016. "Medical Assistants as Flow Managers in Primary Care: Challenges and Recommendations." *Journal of Healthcare Management* 61 (3): 181–91.

Griffin, R. W., J. M. Phillips, and S. M. Gully. 2017. *Organizational Behavior: Managing People and Organizations*, 12th ed. Boston: Cengage Learning.

Johnson, J. A., and C. C. Rossow. 2019. *Health Organizations: Theory, Behavior, and Development*, 2nd ed. Burlington, MA: Jones & Bartlett Learning.

Kash, B. A., A. Spaulding, C. E. Johnson, and L. Gamm. 2014. "Success Factors for Strategic Change Initiatives: A Qualitative Study of Healthcare Administrators' Perspectives." *Journal of Healthcare Management* 59 (1): 65–81.

Longenecker, C. O., and P. D. Longenecker. 2014. "Why Hospital Improvement Efforts Fail: A View from the Front Line." *Journal of Healthcare Management* 59 (2): 146–57.

McConnell, C. R. 2018. *Umiker's Management Skills for the New Health Care Supervisor*, 7th ed. Burlington, MA: Jones & Bartlett Learning.

McLaughlin, D. B., and J. R. Olson. 2017. *Healthcare Operations Management*, 3rd ed. Chicago: Health Administration Press.

Nembhard, I. M., J. A. Alexander, T. J. Hoff, and R. Ramanujam. 2009. "Why Does the Quality of Health Care Continue to Lag? Insights from Management Research." *Academy of Management Perspectives* 23 (1): 24–42.

Project Management Institute. 2017. *A Guide to the Project Management Body of Knowledge (PMBOK Guide)*, 6th ed. Newtown Square, PA: Project Management Institute.

Reinertsen, J. 2014. "Leadership for Quality." In *The Healthcare Quality Book*, 3rd ed., edited by M. S. Joshi, E. R. Ransom, D. B. Nash, and S. B. Ransom, 355–74. Chicago: Health Administration Press.

Schwalbe, K., and D. Furlong. 2013. *Healthcare Project Management*. Minneapolis, MN: Schwalbe Publishing.

CHAPTER 15

PROFESSIONALISM AND COMMUNICATION

Emotional intelligence is now a critical employability skill at any level.

Cynthia Kivland, leadership development
counselor, coach, consultant, and author

LEARNING OBJECTIVES

Studying this chapter will help you to

➤ understand what professionalism means for managers,

➤ explain emotional intelligence for professionalism and management,

➤ explain cultural competence for professionalism and management,

➤ explain communication for professionalism and management,

➤ identify types of communication in healthcare organizations, and

➤ describe how to apply a communication model to avoid communication problems.

HERE'S WHAT HAPPENED

Throughout all levels of Partners HealthCare, managers worked to achieve Partners' mission, vision, values, goals, and strategy. Their work required professionalism, emotional intelligence, cultural competence, and communication. Professionalism—living up to ethical and professional standards—enabled managers to work with others to serve their community and profession. Emotional intelligence enabled managers to understand emotions in themselves and others and use that understanding to manage their behavior and personal relationships. Cultural competency helped managers understand and interact with people who were culturally different from themselves: patients, employees, volunteers, donors, community leaders, and other stakeholders. Partners' managers communicated often. They communicated with people inside and outside the organization, and with individuals and groups. They spoke in quick hallway conversations and in carefully planned speeches. They wrote formal documents and hurried text messages. They decided which information to share with which people using chosen words in chosen media. Intentionally (and sometimes unintentionally), their behavior and appearance communicated messages about themselves. Professionalism, emotional intelligence, cultural competence, and communication enabled managers to accomplish goals, serve others, and help people live healthier lives.

As seen in the opening Here's What Happened, professionalism, emotional intelligence, cultural competence, and communication were essential for managers at Partners HealthCare. We have followed their work and activity in fifteen chapters. In each Here's What Happened episode, managers had to use these four competencies. In any healthcare organization (HCO), managers at all levels—including new, entry-level managers—need these competencies to excel in their jobs. You know that managers perform five management functions (plan, organize, staff, lead, and control) and ten management roles (figurehead, leader, liaison, monitor, disseminator, spokesperson, entrepreneur, disturbance handler, resource allocator, and negotiator). Pause and think about how much these management functions and roles require professionalism, emotional intelligence, cultural competence, and communication!

This chapter, the final one, focuses on these four additional competencies that managers use while performing management functions and roles. It first teaches professionalism—what it means, why it is important, and how it is done. Next, we study emotional intelligence, followed by cultural competence. Then the chapter moves to communication. It defines communication and describes several important types of communication in HCOs. Next, it presents a model of the communication process to explain how to communicate effectively—and avoid a "communication breakdown." The chapter ends with tips for improving communication. By the end of this chapter, your healthcare management toolbox will be filled with tools for you to use in your career.

PROFESSIONALISM

Professionalism is the "ability to align personal and organizational conduct with ethical and professional standards that include a responsibility to the patient and community, a service orientation, and a commitment to lifelong learning and improvement." It includes "personal and professional accountability," "professional development and lifelong learning," and "contributions to the community and profession" (ACHE 2018, 2). Professionalism means that HCO managers "conduct professional activities with honesty, integrity, respect, fairness and good faith in a manner that will reflect well upon the profession" (ACHE 2017). Character, conduct, and quality are basic components of professionalism (Benson and Hummer 2014).

> **professionalism**
> The ability to align personal and organizational conduct with ethical and professional standards.

To better understand this concept, let's return to the American College of Healthcare Executives (ACHE) *Code of Ethics* discussed previously in chapter 11 (ACHE 2017). The preamble and the section directly pertaining to the healthcare management profession follow. Please read the sections slowly, pause occasionally, and think about what the content means for professionalism in healthcare management.

PREAMBLE

The purpose of the *Code of Ethics* of the American College of Healthcare Executives is to serve as a standard of conduct for members. It contains standards of ethical behavior for healthcare executives in their professional relationships. These relationships include colleagues, patients or others served; members of the healthcare executive's organization and other organizations; the community; and society as a whole.

The *Code of Ethics* also incorporates standards of ethical behavior governing individual behavior, particularly when that conduct directly relates to the role and identity of the healthcare executive.

The fundamental objectives of the healthcare management profession are to maintain or enhance the overall quality of life, dignity and well-being of every individual needing healthcare service and to create an equitable, accessible, effective and efficient healthcare system.

Healthcare executives have an obligation to act in ways that will merit the trust, confidence and respect of healthcare professionals and the general public. Therefore, healthcare executives should lead lives that embody an exemplary system of values and ethics.

In fulfilling their commitments and obligations to patients or others served, healthcare executives function as moral advocates and models. Since every management decision affects the health and well-being of both individuals and communities, healthcare executives must carefully evaluate the possible outcomes of their decisions. In organizations that deliver healthcare services, they must work to safeguard and foster the rights, interests and prerogatives of patients or others served.

The role of moral advocate requires that healthcare executives take actions necessary to promote such rights, interests and prerogatives.

Being a model means that decisions and actions will reflect personal integrity and ethical leadership that others will seek to emulate.

I. THE HEALTHCARE EXECUTIVE'S RESPONSIBILITIES TO THE PROFESSION OF HEALTHCARE MANAGEMENT

The healthcare executive shall:

A. Uphold the *Code of Ethics* and mission of the American College of Healthcare Executives;

B. Conduct professional activities with honesty, integrity, respect, fairness and good faith in a manner that will reflect well upon the profession;

C. Comply with all laws and regulations pertaining to healthcare management in the jurisdictions in which the healthcare executive is located or conducts professional activities;

D. Maintain competence and proficiency in healthcare management by implementing a personal program of assessment and continuing professional education;

E. Avoid the improper exploitation of professional relationships for personal gain;

F. Disclose—and when appropriate, avoid—financial and other conflicts of interest;

G. Use this *Code* to further the interests of the profession and not for selfish reasons;

H. Respect professional confidences;

I. Enhance the dignity and image of the healthcare management profession through positive public information programs; and

J. Refrain from participating in any activity that demeans the credibility and dignity of the healthcare management profession.

What caught your attention when you read the *Code of Ethics* excerpt? Did you notice how it indicates proper *character* and *conduct* for HCO managers when they interact with other people? It also guides a manager's behavior when working alone. Professionalism means HCO managers behave in ways that earn trust, confidence, and respect. Managers are honest, fair, competent, and respectful of others. They serve others and their community. In their work, they follow professional standards and governmental laws, act in good faith, and are accountable for what they do. Professional managers continually develop by evaluating themselves, improving themselves, and learning throughout their careers. They realize how their actions, behaviors, and decisions affect the health, well-being, and lives of patients, employees, and many other people.

You might think professionalism requires a lot of work. You're right—it does require a lot. Yet, on a day-to-day basis, as professionalism becomes habit, it becomes easier to achieve. Think of professionalism as doing a lot of the "little things" that you might already do. For example, common courtesy, dependability, and helping people are part of professional relationships. Maybe you often do these things; if so, you are on your way to becoming a professional manager. If you do these things only occasionally, well, that's something to build on as you prepare for your career. Of course, nobody is perfect, including someone chosen as "Manager of the Year"! Even senior managers with many years of experience are still improving their professionalism.

Realize that employees pay attention to what managers do—and don't do. Consciously and unconsciously, workers watch and judge managers. They might not call it "professionalism," but workers judge managers' character and conduct. This type of judgment is another reason that successful managers develop their professionalism. This chapter and others (e.g., chapter 11, which discusses ethical behavior) will help you develop your professionalism. Be sure to keep developing throughout your career.

EMOTIONAL INTELLIGENCE

We learned that professionalism includes a manager's character and conduct, including relationships with other people. This leads us to emotional intelligence (EI).

Emotional intelligence is the "ability to recognize and understand emotions in yourself and others, and your ability to use this awareness to manage your behavior and relationships" (Kivland 2014, 72). Deborah J. Bowen, FACHE, CAE, the president and CEO of ACHE, believes that EI is essential for strong relationships, guiding staff, implementing change, and a better work–life balance (Bowen 2016). Although there is some disagreement as to how much EI is separate from personality, it appears that EI is separate from other measures of ability and personality and that EI does relate to job performance (Griffin, Phillips, and Gully 2017, 110). Some experts believe that EI helps explain why leaders with average IQ often outperform those with the highest IQ. "Emotional intelligence

emotional intelligence
Ability to recognize and understand emotions in yourself and others, and then to use this awareness to manage your behavior and relationships.

is now a critical employability skill at any level and a key differentiator for recruiting and promoting leaders" (Kivland 2018, 68).

EI involves self-awareness, self-regulation, self-motivation, social awareness, and social skills. Self-regulation and self-motivation may be combined into self-management, so that EI consists of four core skills (Cummings and Worley 2015; Freshman and Rubino 2002; Goleman 1998, 2015; Kivland 2014, 2018):

1. *Self-awareness* is the ability to perceive your emotions accurately and be aware of them as they happen.

2. *Self-management* is the ability to use emotional awareness for self-control and to positively direct your behavior.

3. *Social awareness* is the ability and empathy to understand people's emotions and how people react to you.

4. *Relationship management* is the ability to use social skills to relate to and communicate with others to influence them.

Managers should develop and use these four EI skills. They also should realize that they are not the only people in an HCO who have EI. Everyone has it to some extent. Employees use their EI to judge managers' emotions, behaviors, and relationships. Imagine an adult day care center in Columbia where employees observe their supervisor and then share their EI perceptions with each other. Workers consciously study and unconsciously sense their manager's emotions. They might ask peers, "What kind of mood is he in today?" Then they figure out the best way to relate to their manager—or in some cases avoid him! Managers with good EI will create a positive vibe that attracts employees and strengthens them. But managers with poor EI will create a negative vibe that drives away workers and weakens them. Have you experienced these EI types in a job setting, group activity, team project, social situation, or business meeting?

Sensitivity to emotions (of oneself and others) and relationship skills are essential competencies for healthcare settings. For example, think about how Partners HealthCare managers had to rely on EI to interact with stakeholders while planning and implementing telehealth services in the Boston area. Think too of how much healthcare depends on interpersonal relationships, teams, and collaboration. That kind of interaction is not possible without good EI. For example, one manager who was not promoted to the chief operating officer position she was seeking received feedback that "others perceived her as all about results over relationships and unable to read social cues that signaled stress or lack of team buy-in" (Kivland 2018, 68). Recalling the leadership styles discussed in chapter 9, this manager seems to have had a high production orientation but low people orientation.

As is true of other behaviors and skills, a manager can improve EI with effort and practice (Dye 2017; Kivland 2018):

◆ A good first step is to pay attention to your emotions throughout the day—become more aware. Take notes or keep a journal for a week.

◆ Identify your emotional triggers and keep track of what causes negative feelings. Causes might be stress, conflict, personal criticism, difficult people, or bad news.

◆ Note if your behavior and mood change when a trigger occurs. Some people become aggressive, hostile, impatient, frustrated, anxious, or withdrawn in response to triggers.

◆ Actively seek (rather than passively await) honest feedback from others about your emotions and interpersonal relationships. Be open to feedback from stakeholders.

◆ Despite your busy job, be available, approachable, caring, and welcoming toward others. Attend important events organized by other people to show respect and better understand them.

◆ Actively listen (rather than merely hear). Absorb and reflect on what someone both thinks and feels. Avoid judgment.

◆ Accept both good news and bad news, both praise and criticism.

◆ Be willing to admit your mistakes and apologize.

◆ As you become more self-aware, adjust your workday, behavior, and interpersonal styles.

◆ When dealing with strong emotions, pause, take a deep breath, and take control of your actions.

◆ Adjust your schedule to include more free time for unexpected events. Then you will have more time and energy to be available, calm, pleasant, friendly, and patient with others.

◆ Use positive emotions when interacting with someone to create a positive (rather than negative or neutral) shared experience.

◆ Be vulnerable. Admit to not knowing everything, being uncertain, and needing help. Then trust others to help.

◆ Select and consult EI books, videos, and other resources.

◆ Work with a mentor, trainer, or coach. (For tips on finding a coach, see www.coachnet.org/coaching/.)

Recall from chapter 2 our definition of management: the process of getting things done through and with people. Because people (including managers) are strongly affected by emotions, managers must understand both their own emotions and those of others to get things done through and with people. Chapter 1 identified many different types of healthcare management jobs and HCOs. You will be better able to perform in all of those jobs and HCOs if you develop your EI. Plus, you will feel more satisfied and fulfilled!

CULTURAL COMPETENCE

cultural competence
The ability to interact effectively with people of different cultures.

For a high degree of professionalism, a manager must also have **cultural competence**. This involves consistently respecting and responding to the beliefs, practices, cultures, and languages of diverse populations. "Cultural competence is the ability to interact effectively with people of different cultures" (Substance Abuse and Mental Health Services Administration 2016). People are diverse in many aspects of culture and identity, such as race, ethnicity, faith and religion, gender, sexual orientation, disability, personality, social status, age, geographic origin, and other characteristics (Molinari and Shanderson 2014). Diversity leads to differences in languages, communication styles, behaviors, beliefs, values, lifestyles, appearances, work habits, and other aspects of life and work. Thus, people differ in their sense of time, etiquette, feelings about authority, professional behaviors, and seemingly minor things such as what to do when given a business card.

Understanding these differences and interacting well with diverse people can strengthen a business. It can improve moral legitimacy, legal compliance, creativity, expertise, decision making, and competitive advantage (Griffin, Phillips, and Gully 2017). HCOs can improve their patient experience and customer satisfaction by understanding patients' cultural preferences. For example, employees at a Veterans Administration healthcare center for military veterans respect and respond to military culture, values, behavior, and preferences. Employees realize that veterans with hypertension want to support each other as comrades. The center schedules veterans in group appointments so they can fight the hypertension battle together (Forte 2018).

Have you taken a college course to learn about cultural diversity, inclusion, and cultural competency? Many colleges offer and some require such a course, which can help you prepare for a career in healthcare management (and for living in today's society). "Living with and managing diversity has become a central theme in the twenty-first century" (Dunn 2016, 540).

As you may have realized, cultural competence overlaps and is intertwined with professionalism and EI. Although the competencies are different, they enable and support each other. For example, professionalism, the ability to align your personal and organizational conduct with ethical and professional standards, will help you be culturally competent. So too will your self-awareness, self-management, social awareness, and relationship management, which are part of EI. Cultural competence also requires—and reciprocally affects—your communication (studied later in this chapter).

What else can a manager use or do to become more culturally competent? Cie Armstead, director of diversity and inclusion at ACHE, offers several excellent ideas (Armstead 2016):

- Become more aware of your own culture and your effect on others.

- Learn about different types of people by using reliable, unbiased sources.

- Intentionally improve your cultural awareness and learn about other cultures.

- Be open to a wide range of experiences with different people and cultures; participate in events in which you will be in the minority.

- Try to understand and adjust yourself to the cultural needs of diverse people.

- Support and promote diversity and inclusion.

Chapters 1 and 7 explained that the future will bring more diversity to the US population and thus to the mix of patients, employees, and stakeholders in HCOs. So in addition to being culturally competent themselves, managers must create a culturally competent organization with inclusion for diverse populations. An HCO's buildings, equipment, staff, policies, structures, processes, and services should respect and respond to the beliefs, practices, cultures, and languages of diverse populations and cultures. Managers can use many tools, methods, techniques, and principles from this book to create a culturally competent organization. For example:

- During the strategic planning process, add diversity, inclusion, and cultural competency to the organization's mission, vision, values, and goals.

- Use project planning to plan and implement projects to achieve diversity, inclusion, and cultural competency.

- Assign cultural competency responsibilities and tasks to specific jobs and departments, and then hold those jobs and departments accountable.

- Use staffing methods to ensure the HCO has the right staff, training, incentives, and appraisals to support cultural diversity and competency.

- Use leadership and motivation methods to create an organization culture that values diversity and inclusion.

- Use control methods to set standards, monitor performance, and adjust the HCO's structures and processes so that the organization becomes more culturally competent.

- Because decisions and change will be necessary, use appropriate tools and methods for making decisions and implementing change.

The Check It Out Online sidebar in chapter 7 describes an excellent online resource for HCOs striving to become more diverse, inclusive, and culturally competent.

One last suggestion might surprise you. The Golden Rule—treating others as you wish to be treated—might not always be the best approach. For cultural competence, consider using the Platinum Rule: "Treat others as *they* wish to be treated" (Dolan 2013, 34).

The Check It Out Online sidebar in this chapter describes standards for culturally and linguistically appropriate services in healthcare. Such services connect cultural competence with communication, which is studied next.

COMMUNICATION

We now shift to communication, a word that has many definitions. Together, the following two definitions identify the *process* and expected *outcome* of communication:

◆ Communication is "transmitting a message from a sender to a receiver, through a channel and with the interference of noise" (DeVito 1986, 61).

◆ Communication is "the development of mutual understanding" (Liebler and McConnell 2004, 496).

The first definition identifies elements of the communication process—transmitting, message, sender, receiver, channel, and noise. The second definition reflects the desired outcome of communication—achieving mutual understanding. Based on these ideas, this book defines **communication** as transmitting a message to someone else to develop shared understanding. Communication involves a sender, message, message transmission via a channel, intended receiver, and noise that interferes with transmission. The rest of this chapter gives you tools and techniques to communicate well when managing HCOs.

communication
Transmitting a message to someone else to develop shared understanding.

TYPES OF COMMUNICATION

There are several kinds of communication in HCOs. They vary in how much managers can control them. Some communication is *one-to-one*—a maintenance supervisor talks with a carpenter, for example. Other communication is *one-to-group*—a maintenance supervisor talks with all the maintenance workers on first shift. Some communication is *group-to-group*—the first-shift maintenance workers talk with the second-shift maintenance workers. The more people who are involved, the harder it is for someone to control the communication.

Communication is sometimes *intentional* and sometimes *unintentional*. We often communicate intentionally, even thinking ahead about what to say or write. We communicate unintentionally when our actions, behavior, body language, and facial expressions accidentally communicate unconscious feelings and attitudes. **Managers control and shape intentional communication but not unintentional communication.** This difference in control matters because unintentional communication affects how employees interpret managers' intentional communication. If the two are not consistent, the sender and receiver may not reach a shared understanding.

Managers use *formal* communication—the official communication of the HCO's structure of managers, authority, policies, rules, and documents. HCOs also have *informal* communication—the unofficial communication among coworkers, peers, friends, carpoolers, relatives, and others that occurs outside the official organization structure. Informal communication might contradict formal communication and is usually not controlled by managers. This type of communication is more spontaneous and changes more quickly than formal communication.

Recall from chapter 4 that an informal organization has its own unofficial communication known as the *grapevine*. Is there a student grapevine at your college or university? Although managers cannot control the grapevine and informal communication in their HCOs, they should not ignore it. By paying attention to it, managers can better understand how employees feel about the HCO, their jobs, a planned change, and many other aspects of the HCO. For example, managers at one medical center regularly checked in with the grapevine to judge how staff felt about going live with a new computer system. Formal messages from employees indicated mild support, but informal messages reflected anxiety. So managers gave employees more training and practice in the new system before it went live. An HCO's grapevine is likely to be extensive, but it is not always accurate. It will carry official news, unofficial news, exaggerated news, gossip, and stories (fiction and nonfiction). The grapevine used to be mostly oral; now, digital grapevines and social media spread messages much more widely and rapidly.

 CHECK IT OUT ONLINE

The National Standards for Culturally and Linguistically Appropriate Services (CLAS) in health were created to improve healthcare quality and equity for diverse populations. By following CLAS guidelines, HCOs can respect and respond to diverse cultural health beliefs and practices, preferred languages, health literacy, and other communication needs. These standards are available at https://minorityhealth.hhs.gov/omh/browse.aspx?lvl=2&lvlid=53. Four of the 15 CLAS guidelines pertain to communication and language assistance (US Department of Health and Human Services Office of Minority Health 2018):

- Offer language assistance to individuals who have limited English proficiency and/or other communication needs, at no cost to them, to facilitate timely access to all healthcare and services.
- Inform all individuals of the availability of language assistance services clearly and in their preferred language, verbally and in writing.
- Ensure the competence of individuals providing language assistance, recognizing that the use of untrained individuals and/or minors as interpreters should be avoided.
- Provide easy-to-understand print and multimedia materials and signage in the languages commonly used by the populations in the service area.

Check it out online and see what you discover.

Direction	Explanation	Example
Downward	Communication to someone at a lower level in one's own vertical chain of command or hierarchy	A nursing supervisor tells a subordinate nurse about the work schedule.
Upward	Communication to someone at a higher level in one's own vertical chain of command or hierarchy	A housekeeper tells her supervisor about broken equipment.
Horizontal	Communication to someone at the same level of an organization and outside of one's own vertical chain of command or hierarchy	The marketing director explains advertising costs to the finance director.
Diagonal	Communication to someone at a higher or lower level of an organization and outside of one's own vertical chain of command or hierarchy	A computer tech explains a new online security procedure to the warehouse supervisor.

DIRECTIONS OF COMMUNICATION

Communication flows in all directions in an organization, as presented in exhibit 15.1. Vertical communication has always been common because it follows the vertical hierarchy and chain of command. Trends reflect increasing horizontal and diagonal communication. You may want to turn back to chapter 5 to refresh your memory about different organization structures and consider how communication might flow up, down, sideways, or diagonally.

Managers use **downward communication** with their subordinates to give directions, make assignments, offer feedback, control performance, motivate, and so on. It connects levels of the organization down the hierarchy. To communicate this way, managers use on-the-job spoken instruction, electronic communication tools, memos, social media, policy statements, morning huddles, job descriptions, phone calls, hallway conversations, written procedures, control reports, performance appraisals, and many other methods.

Subordinates use **upward communication** with their managers to provide feedback, describe progress, report problems, give input and advice, answer questions, and so on. It connects levels of the organization up the hierarchy. Upward communication methods

downward communication
Communication to someone at a lower level in one's own vertical chain of command or hierarchy.

upward communication
Communication to someone at a higher level in one's own vertical chain of command or hierarchy.

include written memos, e-mail, voicemail, wikis, intranets, face-to-face conversations, formal meetings, social media, phone calls, electronic communication systems, reports, worksite chats, and others. Earlier leadership chapters in this book, and the EI section in this chapter, made it clear that managers must create effective relationships and communication channels with subordinates so that they are willing to communicate upward and share (rather than hide) important information. A worker should realize his manager depends on him to provide essential information candidly, concisely, quickly, and accurately.

Employees, including managers, must communicate upward to keep their boss informed. This communication includes informing one's supervisor about bad news, which may be hard to do. Some people use vague words to communicate negative news and only hint at a problem. For example, they may say, "We're a little behind" instead of directly stating that the HCO is two months behind on a six-month project! That vague communication does not help. Managers respect employees who are professional enough to keep them properly informed (about both good and bad news).

Employees and managers use **horizontal communication** to communicate with their counterparts at the same level of the HCO. This type of communication is between people who are not in a supervisor–subordinate relationship (recall the discussion of mutual adjustment from chapter 5). Also called *lateral* or *sideways* communication, horizontal communication helps coordinate work between departments and across an organization. It breaks down silos that develop when communication is mostly vertical. Horizontal communication is essential for interprofessional patient care, project teams, and other collaboration. Electronic collaboration tools, worksite conversations, texts, e-mail messages, project meetings, intranets, social media, portals, and phone calls are some ways people communicate horizontally.

Employees and managers also use **diagonal communication**. This type of communication has become more common as organizations become more organic and adopt a culture of "we are all on the same team." It is enabled by fast, widespread electronic methods such as wikis, discussion boards, intranets, team tools, and social media. Traditional face-to-face conversations and phone calls are also used. Diagonal communication is useful for sharing information, input, and expertise throughout an organization. However, in organizations that strongly respect the vertical chain of command, people should be careful when using diagonal communication.

Changes in the external environment are leading HCOs to be more open with communication rather than locked into vertical patterns. For example, managers at a hospital in Lincoln may use groups, task forces, and project teams of employees drawn from multiple departments throughout the HCO. These groups and teams can bring together employees who are in diagonal relationships with each other in the organization chart. Open communication aligns with the trend of organizations being more natural, horizontal, adaptive, and collaborative. They share information digitally throughout the organization on mobile devices and via electronic media.

horizontal communication Communication to someone at the same level of an organization and outside of one's own vertical chain of command or hierarchy.

diagonal communication Communication to someone at a higher or lower level of an organization and outside of one's own vertical chain of command or hierarchy.

COMMUNICATION PROCESS

The purpose of communication is to create shared understanding. However, sometimes communication creates *mis*understanding. You have probably experienced communication breakdowns that resulted from ineffective communication. They confuse people, waste valuable resources, and cause harm in HCOs. To be effective in their jobs, managers must understand how communication occurs and how to create effective communication. The communication model in exhibit 15.2 can help you do that.

The model in exhibit 15.2 shows two people. The person on the left (sender) has an idea and wants the person on the right (receiver) to understand and share that idea. **Communication must transmit the idea from the sender's mind to the receiver's mind.** Here are the essential elements of communication:

- *Idea*—thought, opinion, concept, or feeling in the sender's mind

- *Sender*—person who has an idea to communicate with someone else

- *Message*—the sender's idea encoded (expressed) in words, icons, visuals, body language, behaviors, actions, or other ways

EXHIBIT 15.2
Communication
Model

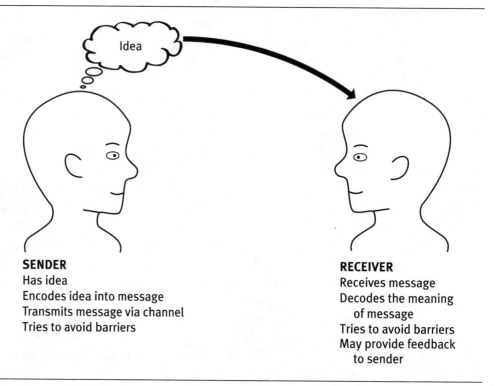

SENDER
Has idea
Encodes idea into message
Transmits message via channel
Tries to avoid barriers

RECEIVER
Receives message
Decodes the meaning
of message
Tries to avoid barriers
May provide feedback
to sender

◆ *Channel*—method or medium (e.g., phone call, text message, wiki, published report, Snapchat post, conversation, Skype call, handwritten sign, tweet) used to transmit the message from sender to receiver

◆ *Receiver*—person or people to whom the message is communicated

◆ *Barriers*—biases, distractions, and other obstacles that impede communication; also called *noise*

The following example shows how elements of the model work together to communicate. This simple example would happen very quickly with hardly any thought. Other communications (e.g., an important speech) would take much longer and involve much careful thought.

1. Sara Sender has an idea (where and when to go for lunch) in her mind that she wants to communicate to Ryan Receiver so that he has the same idea in his mind. Then they will share understanding of Sara's idea.

2. Sara considers how to encode her idea into a message and how to transmit the message using a communication channel. She considers possible barriers (environmental and personal) that could interfere with her encoding and sending the message or interfere with Ryan receiving and decoding her message.

3. Sara chooses text messaging as the channel to transmit her message to Ryan.

4. Sara encodes her idea (College Cafe @ 12:30 for lunch) into words and symbols. Then she adds a smiling emoji ☺ to reflect how she feels. Sara again considers possible barriers (noise) between herself and Ryan when choosing words and symbols to encode her idea.

5. Sara sends the encoded message to Ryan using the text message channel.

6. Ryan receives the text message.

7. Ryan decodes (interprets) the content and feeling of the message. He figures out what the message means to him.

8. Ryan clearly understands the idea that came from Sara. They have shared understanding.

Suppose Ryan wants Sara to know that he received her message and agrees with her. To accomplish this, he sends feedback to her. The feedback begins a new communication. Ryan now becomes the sender, and Sara becomes the receiver. Ryan follows steps 1–8 to send a text message ("Sure ok") to Sara. She receives and decodes Ryan's feedback message. Sara is happy to know they have shared understanding of where and when to go for lunch.

Communication may happen with or without feedback from the receiver to the sender. In this example, the receiver (Ryan) provided feedback to the sender (Sara) regarding her message to him. **Feedback from the receiver to the sender helps ensure shared understanding in communication.** It might even help avoid serious mistakes. Imagine a nurse in Tuscaloosa who, during a busy day, is listening on the phone (with background noise) to a physician (who is in a hurry) state a medication order that sounds like *4 mL* . . . or maybe it was *40 mL*. The nurse distinctly restates the order back to the physician to give feedback of how she understands the order. They confirm that they share the same idea: *4 mL*. Yet sometimes receivers do not provide feedback. Do you reply to every text you get? Do people give feedback after seeing a commercial on TV?

To plan a communication, which does the sender decide first—the encoded message or the channel by which to send the message? Think about how you have communicated. Often, the channel (e.g., text message, PowerPoint slides) is decided first, and then the actual message is created and encoded. Alternatively, a manager might encode a message first, such as composing a message in Microsoft Word and revising it to have the right tone and content. Then, the manager decides how to transmit the message—Facebook post now for employees, and later the monthly blog for the general public. The chosen communication channel (method) affects how the sender encodes the idea. The reverse is also true: How a message is encoded affects which channel to use. The sender must decide both while trying to avoid barriers that could block or distort communication. All of this is portrayed in exhibit 15.3.

Encoding Messages

verbal encoding
Using written or spoken words to represent ideas.

Messages may be encoded verbally or nonverbally. **Verbal encoding** uses words (written or spoken) to encode and represent ideas. This encoding depends on language, including variations based on dialects, slang, acronyms, grammar, and linguistics.

"When I use a word, it means just what I choose it to mean," said Humpty Dumpty. That makes it easy for Humpty, but not so easy for everyone else. Encoding ideas with

EXHIBIT 15.3
Encoding, Channels, and Barriers in Communication

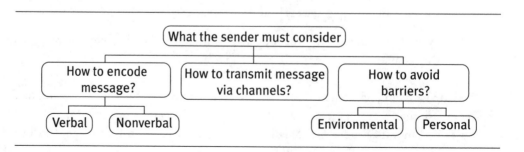

words can be tricky because words may mean different things to different people. A mother tells her son to "be home before dark" without realizing he will interpret *dark* differently than she does. Language is often imprecise (e.g., "I'll be there *soon*"), and words too often have multiple meanings that cause communication breakdowns. When encoding ideas into a message, managers should think about how the receiver might decode or interpret the words. Decoding will depend on various factors, which are discussed later in this chapter.

Problems arise in HCOs when a sender encodes a message with healthcare slang (e.g., "We bagged her") or acronyms (e.g., MI) that not everyone understands. Unknown slang and acronyms are so common in healthcare that webpages exist to help people decode healthcare messages (e.g., https://health.howstuffworks.com/medicine/healthcare/decoding-28-medical-slang-terms.htm). Although the receiver of a message can look up unknown slang and acronyms, some receivers just guess the meaning or skip that part of a message. Oops, we just lost shared understanding!

Nonverbal encoding is done without words. Nonverbal encoding includes diagrams, charts, icons, pictures, attire, objects, body language, gestures, touch, behavior, purposeful silence, actions, and lack of action (Drafke 2009; Dunn 2016; Griffin, Phillips, and Gully 2017). Words may be inadequate to sufficiently encode an idea, as reflected in the saying "A picture is worth a thousand words." PowerPoint presentations combine words with symbols to strengthen understanding. Managers encode nonverbally when words may be misinterpreted or to reinforce a verbal message. Nonverbal messages (e.g., tone of voice and behavior) should match verbal messages. If they disagree, then receivers perceive "mixed messages." Nonverbal messages are generally more powerful and more readily believed than verbal messages are. When these messages conflict, receivers believe the nonverbal message (Griffin, Phillips, and Gully 2017). As we've been told, actions speak louder than words. Thus, managers should manage the nonverbal messages they send—intentionally and unintentionally—by their tone of voice, posture, facial expressions, and other means.

> **nonverbal encoding**
> Representing ideas without using words, such as with icons, diagrams, attire, objects, body language, touch, behavior, and actions.

Recall from earlier in this chapter that a professional manager behaves in ways that earn trust, confidence, and respect. Professionalism includes how you present yourself—how you communicate nonverbal messages about yourself—to others. Have you ever seen someone who looked excited and someone else who looked tired? Nonverbal messages in gestures, facial expressions, handshakes, eye contact, and other body language communicate (sometimes unintentionally) feelings and attitudes. When manager Serika smiles, stands up straight, and moves quickly, other employees think she is happy and excited about her work. If she frowns, slouches, and trudges along, others think she is unhappy and tired of her work. **Employees observe and follow what managers do, so managers should consider how they present themselves and are perceived by others.**

You get only one chance to make a first impression, and it happens quickly. One communications expert claims that "people decide ten things about you within ten seconds of meeting you" based on your appearance and behavior (Bjorseth 2007, 52). Visit your college career center for advice on making a good first impression. Perhaps staff can record a video of you in a pretend meeting and review the video to offer coaching feedback. Some colleges offer an "Etiquette and Dining 101" course to help students develop self-presentation skills before going to job interviews.

Communication Channels

channels
Methods and media that transmit a message from sender to receiver.

How do managers transmit messages? They use **channels** of communication. Channels are the methods and media that carry an encoded message from sender to receiver. Each channel affects how a message is sent and how it is received. Also, how you encode a message affects how you transmit the message, and vice versa, so think about them together when deciding how to communicate. The earlier section on direction of communication included many channels that managers use, such as texts, wikis, teleconferences, posters, tweets, and hallway conversations.

Channels differ in information richness, which is how much information a channel conveys to create understanding (Griffin, Phillips, and Gully 2017). The richer channels (media) have more

◆ feedback and interaction between sender and receivers,

◆ transmission of multiple verbal and nonverbal cues (e.g., physical appearance, voice, pictures),

◆ language variety to express ideas in multiple ways, and

◆ personal focus and emotions.

Exhibit 15.4 shows communication channels in descending order of information richness. **Channels that convey both verbal and nonverbal information are rich in information and thus generally create understanding more quickly and accurately than less rich channels.** However, all channels have pros and cons, which are explained next based on work by Dunn (2016) and Griffin, Phillips, and Gully (2017).

Channels such as speeches, face-to-face discussions, video conferences, and a shouted "Yo, dude!" all transmit messages through *spoken words*. These channels convey a speaker's tone of voice, pauses, pronunciation, facial expressions, and other characteristics of speaking. As a result, they transmit information about feelings and emotion. These types of channels also enable immediate feedback, questions and answers, and clarification. However, even messages delivered through spoken channels are not always understood. Consider casual, spontaneous conversation. Very little time is spent encoding, transmitting, or decoding those messages, which sometimes reduces the understanding between speaker and receiver. Alternatively, some channels for spoken communication take more time to prepare and

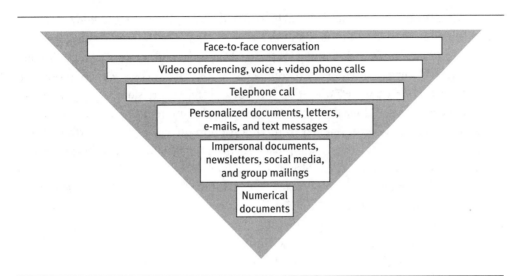

EXHIBIT 15.4
Information
Richness of Some
Communication
Channels (in
Descending Order)

transmit messages—such as formal speeches and video conferences—which improves understanding.

Other channels—such as formal reports, texts, groupware, PowerPoint slides, and handwritten notes taped to a wall—transmit messages through *written words*, perhaps with icons, pictures, exhibits, and other visuals. Advantages of written communication include a record of the communication and consistency so that everyone receives the same message. Written media are often viewed as more formal and official than oral media, and online writing is considered less formal than writing on letterhead with proper grammar and spelling. Written channels may require more time to carefully encode and decode messages, which can improve shared understanding. Thus, technical specifications that must be precise and accurate are conveyed in written documents that have been carefully encoded and proofread. Channels with written messages traditionally permitted slower feedback than channels with spoken information did. Now texting, online chat, and collaboration software enable quick written feedback. However, they tend to emphasize brevity and transmit less content, which can reduce understanding. Written channels are less rich than spoken channels because they do not convey as much emotional information. To partly overcome this problem, some senders use emojis such as ☺ and ☹ or different font effects (e.g., boldface), styles (e.g., all capital letters), and punctuation (e.g., multiple exclamation points) to convey feelings.

Which channels should a manager use in an HCO? It depends. As is true for many other aspects of managing, no single approach is always best. Managers can consider each communication situation and judge which channel would be best. Which channel would fit with the HCO's culture? Which would work best for people who will receive and decode the message? Which channel would avoid barriers and a communication breakdown? Which channel would create shared understanding?

Face-to-face conversation is best for personal, sensitive, and complex communication, such as mental health counseling or explaining the reasons an employee was not promoted. Pick information-rich channels with spoken words and facial expressions when you want to understand emotions and see the receiver's visual cues for immediate feedback. Managers and supervisors regularly use spoken communication to direct, instruct, motivate, train, lead, and control subordinates. This approach enables managers and supervisors to receive prompt feedback, answer questions, be visible, and develop closer working relationships with staff. Channels with low information richness may be used for simple, routine communications, such as reminders to order supplies. One-to-one communication is time-consuming and too costly for communicating with many people. Managers then use other channels, such as Twitter feeds, digital or print newsletters, mass e-mails, podcasts, blogs, Facebook pages, and speeches to groups of people. These channels are less information rich but also require less cost.

Many HCOs are using social media extensively as communication channels. To ensure these media are used effectively, managers often establish social media policies that provide guidelines for ownership of content, confidentiality, distribution, boundaries, and use during work hours. Examples may be found online, such as the "Healthcare Social Media Policy for Physicians and Staff" at www.symplur.com/healthcare-social-media-policy/.

Using multiple channels of communication can help ensure the correct message gets through. However, too much communication can be a problem. Communication overload causes "selective receiving," in which intended receivers select which messages to receive and which to ignore. Managers can ask stakeholders which channels and media they prefer and let people opt out of selected mass mailings.

Decoding Messages

For shared understanding to occur, receivers must receive messages and accurately decode (interpret) those messages. They must play back voicemail, read posts on a discussion board, observe coworkers' nonverbal cues, watch and listen to a webcast, read texts, and look at a PowerPoint presentation. Receivers have to assign meaning to words and symbols. They must interpret facial expressions and gestures. Senders can improve communication by encoding and transmitting messages in ways that make it easy for receivers to receive and accurately decode the messages.

Management and communication require effective listening to receive and decode messages, yet listening often is not done well. Perhaps this is because schools teach writing, reading, and speaking—but not listening. Here are useful tips to improve listening (Dunn 2016; Dye 2017; Griffin, Phillips, and Gully 2017):

◆   Realize that active listening is more than just passive hearing.

◆   Minimize distractions, noise, bias, and barriers.

◆   Pay attention and remain attentive.

◆   Listen for content (meaning of words) and for feeling (emotions of speaker).

◆   Avoid the urge to speak; do not interrupt.

◆   Be open-minded about content rather than quickly judging it.

◆   Show interest (verbally and nonverbally) in the speaker and what is said.

◆   Ask the speaker to clarify anything that is not clear.

◆   Occasionally sum up in your own words what you understand, and then ask if it is correct.

◆   Avoid judgment and negative reactions that will close off communication.

Decoding suffers when receivers too quickly skim through their messages. Rather than fully receive and decode the message, they may overlook content needed to correctly perform a medical procedure or a management project. To prevent this from happening, some senders may send messages via multiple channels over a period of time to increase understanding. Decoding also suffers when receivers try to "read between the lines" and infer extra content or hidden meanings. Receivers should ask senders about possible inferences (e.g., does this mean there will be layoffs?) rather than assume too much.

(→) TRY IT, APPLY IT

You can develop your listening ability to improve how well you receive and decode spoken messages. Doing so will make you a better manager. Consider the listening techniques previously stated. Which are typical of how you listen? Which are not? Identify the listening techniques you want to improve and then practice them. Make a reminder note for yourself. Ask friends to give you feedback on your listening skills. After talking with someone, think about how well you listened based on these guidelines. With practice, you can make these guidelines part of how you listen.

Communication Barriers

Barriers can interfere with all elements of the communication model and thereby thwart shared understanding. There are two types of barriers, environmental and personal. Environmental barriers arise from the environment in which communication takes place. Because the sender and receiver may be in different environments, both environments should be considered to avoid barriers and communication breakdowns. Personal barriers arise from the people who communicate—the sender and receiver. Here too, both must be considered to avoid problems.

Have you ever been talking with a friend while outside but suddenly could not hear because a loud vehicle passed by? Have you been unable to read in bad lighting? Have you missed a cell phone call because you were in a "dead zone"? These situations involve communication barriers created by the environment in which people try to communicate. HCO managers deal with (and even create) environmental communication barriers. A power failure occurs. Equipment and machines make distracting noises. A manager works behind a closed door. The organization structure and assigned work spaces separate workers. You cannot avoid all barriers, but you can anticipate and avoid some of them.

 USING CHAPTER 15 IN THE REAL WORLD

Tobacco use by young people was a serious problem in northeast Pennsylvania. Leaders from local units of the American Lung Association and the American Cancer Society invited representatives of HCOs, schools, churches, youth groups, and other organizations to form a coalition that would help middle school students avoid tobacco. The coalition members applied knowledge and tools about population health and determinants of health (that we studied in chapter 1). They used management theories, concepts, and tools (that we studied in chapter 2). The members applied the five management functions of planning, organizing, staffing, leading, and controlling (that we studied in chapters 3 through 12). Coalition members used tools and methods for decision making, problem solving, conflict resolution, and change management (that we studied in chapters 13 and 14). When doing all that, they used professionalism, emotional intelligence, cultural competency, and communication (that we studied in this final chapter). That helped the members to work well together and progress toward their goal. For example, when the coalition met for the first time, the representative of a small HCO did not know or feel at ease with the representative of a big, powerful HCO. Differences in job-related status of coalition members created barriers. However, professionalism, EI, cultural competency, and communication methods enabled the coalition members to work together, communicate well, and implement programs to help young people avoid tobacco use.

People create personal barriers to communication. Personalities, emotions, moods, beliefs, and biases impede communication. Personal barriers affect our willingness to even send or receive a message! Then they affect how we talk, write, hear, read, perceive, and interpret what others say and write. Bias may cause a person to listen to a webinar primarily from a financial perspective, for example. Emotions such as fear, anger, love, joy, and resentment affect how we send and receive communications. If we distrust a manager, we might filter what he says. Filtering may occur unconsciously and be hard to avoid. Many employees filter out bad news when communicating with their supervisor. Employees and others may be reluctant to communicate openly for personal reasons and because of others' perceptions of them. Busy executives may filter out and ignore e-mails that do not seem urgent. Cultural differences, studied earlier, lead to different attitudes and styles for speaking, listening, writing, and reading; preferred communication channels and languages; and many other aspects of communication. Limited vision, hearing, and dexterity also may interfere with communication. Excessive multitasking can create personal barriers for accurate communication. **Senders and receivers should intentionally assess communication situations for possible communication barriers.** Then they can adjust to avoid communication breakdowns.

TIPS FOR EFFECTIVE COMMUNICATION

As a manager, you can use the following suggestions to improve your communication at work (Dunn 2016; Griffin, Phillips, and Gully 2017; McConnell 2018):

◆ Help create an organization culture that values and rewards good communication.

◆ Be accessible and open to communication; visit employees' work areas; if you have an office, leave the door open when possible.

◆ Learn the communication preferences of various cultures.

◆ Pay attention to verbal and nonverbal feedback when communicating.

◆ Prepare to communicate by anticipating and removing barriers and by choosing how to encode and transmit your message so the receiver will understand it.

◆ When communicating with varied stakeholders, customize the communication content and process to fit specific receivers.

◆ Speak and write using clear, direct, and unambiguous language.

◆ Follow proper rules of writing, such as correct grammar, capitalization, and punctuation.

◆ Use EI when sending and receiving communications. Empathize by putting yourself in the receiver's situation.

◆ Use multiple channels and repetition when necessary.

◆ Read and listen for meaning and feeling (based on content and emotion).

◆ Practice communication skills, learn from role models, and obtain training if necessary.

Finally, to communicate effectively, use what you learned in this chapter about professionalism, emotional intelligence, and cultural competence.

ONE MORE TIME

To successfully perform the management work described in this book, managers at all levels of HCOs should use professionalism, emotional intelligence, cultural competency, and communication. These four competencies are interrelated. With practice and effort, a new manager can intentionally improve each of them.

Professionalism is the ability to align personal and organizational conduct with ethical and professional standards. Emotional intelligence is the ability to recognize and understand emotions in yourself and others and to use this awareness to manage your behavior and relationships. It includes self-awareness, self-management, social awareness, and relationship management. Cultural competence is the ability to interact effectively with people of different cultures. It involves consistently respecting and responding to beliefs, practices, cultures, and languages of diverse populations. With communication, managers transmit messages to other people to create shared understanding. Formal communication in an HCO is the official communication of the organization; informal communication (e.g., the grapevine) is outside the official organization structure. Although managers do not control informal communication, they should pay attention to it. Formal communication in an organization goes in all directions—mostly vertically and horizontally, but also diagonally.

Communication involves an idea, sender, message, channel, receiver, and barriers that interfere with communication. The sender encodes an idea (verbally or nonverbally) into a message and then transmits it through channels (media) to the receiver. The receiver decodes (interprets) the message by reading, listening, and observing. Environmental and personal barriers can distort, reduce, and even block communication at all stages of the process. After decoding a message, the receiver may provide feedback to the sender to ensure effective communication and shared understanding.

FOR DISCUSSION

1. What does professionalism mean to you? Why is it important for HCO managers?

2. In your own words, what is emotional intelligence? Why is it important for HCO managers?

3. In your own words, what is cultural competence? Why is it important for HCO managers?

4. Using the communication model in this chapter, discuss how communication occurs.

5. In your experience, which parts of the communication model have caused problems? How could you avoid those problems?

CASE STUDY QUESTIONS

These questions refer to the Integrative Case Studies at the back of this book.

1. Disparities in Care at Southern Regional Health System case: Explain how professionalism and cultural competence will be important for Mr. Hank as he tries to reduce disparities in care at Southern Regional.

2. Hospice Goes Hollywood case: Using all parts of the communication model presented in this chapter, describe how Ms. Thurmond could more effectively communicate with the clinicians. Explain how she could use EI to improve communication with them.

3. How Can an ACO Improve the Health of Its Population? case: Using all parts of the communication model presented in this chapter, explain how Ms. Dillow could communicate "to engage patients and community members in improving their health." Explain why cultural competence will be important for her.

4. "I Can't Do It All!" case: Using what you learned in this chapter, describe how professionalism and EI will be important for Mr. Brice as he works with the vice presidents.

5. The Rocky Road to Patient Satisfaction at Leonard-Griggs case: Using all parts of the communication model presented in this chapter, describe how Ms. Ratcliff could more effectively communicate with the office staff.

 RIVERBEND ORTHOPEDICS MINI CASE STUDY

Riverbend Orthopedics is a busy group practice with expanded services for orthopedic care. It has seven physicians and a podiatrist, plus about 70 other employees. At its big, new clinic building, Riverbend provides extensive orthopedic care. Several technicians provide diagnostic medical imaging, from basic X-rays to magnetic resonance images. The physicians perform surgery in their own outpatient surgery center with Riverbend's own operating nurses and technicians. Therapy is provided by three physical therapists and one part-time contracted occupational therapist. In addition to staff providing actual patient care, the clinic has staff for financial management, medical records, human resources, information systems/technology, building maintenance, and other administrative matters. Occasional marketing work is done by an advertising company. Legal work is outsourced to a law firm. Riverbend is managed by a new president, Ms. Garcia. She and Riverbend have set a goal of achieving "Excellent" ratings for patient experience from at least 90 percent of Riverbend's patients this year.

Dr. Chen told Ms. Garcia he feels that some employees do not have enough cultural competence. He gave specific examples pertaining to himself and some of his patients. One patient is upset about perceived lack of respect by Riverbend staff for her Chinese culture. Dr. Chen asked Ms. Garcia to talk with his patient, which she agreed to do.

MINI CASE STUDY QUESTIONS

1. Using information from this chapter about professionalism, EI, cultural competency, and communication, describe what Ms. Garcia should do when talking with Dr. Chen's patient.

2. Explain how Ms. Garcia could use professionalism, EI, cultural competency, and the communication model when managing Riverbend's efforts to achieve its patient experience goal.

REFERENCES

American College of Healthcare Executives (ACHE). 2018. "ACHE Healthcare Executive 2018 Competencies Assessment Tool." Accessed April 14. www.ache.org/-/media/ache/career-resource-center/competencies_booklet.pdf.

———. 2017. *ACHE Code of Ethics*. Amended November 13. www.ache.org/about-ache/our-story/our-commitments/ethics/ache-code-of-ethics.

Armstead, C. 2016. "Sharpen Your Inclusion Skills for Career Success." *Healthcare Executive* 31 (3): 76–79.

Benson, K., and C. Hummer. 2014. "Creating a Culture of Professionalism." In *New Leadership for Today's Health Care Professionals: Concepts and Cases*, edited by L. G. Rubino, S. J. Esparza, and Y. S. Reid Chassiakos, 77–88. Burlington, MA: Jones & Bartlett Learning.

Bjorseth, L. 2007. "Ten Principles of Communication." *Healthcare Executive* 22 (5): 52–55.

Bowen, D. J. 2016. "Cultivating Leadership Acumen Amidst Change." *Healthcare Executive* 31 (5): 8.

Cummings, T. G., and C. G. Worley. 2015. *Organization Development and Change*. Stamford, CT: Cengage Learning.

DeVito, J. A. 1986. *The Communication Handbook: A Dictionary*. New York: Harper & Row.

Dolan, T. C. 2013. "Aspirations of a Servant Leader." *Healthcare Executive* 28 (6): 30–38.

Drafke, M. W. 2009. *The Human Side of Organizations*, 10th ed. Upper Saddle River, NJ: Pearson Education.

Dunn, R. 2016. *Dunn and Haimann's Healthcare Management*, 10th ed. Chicago: Health Administration Press.

Dye, C. F. 2017. *Leadership in Healthcare*, 3rd ed. Chicago: Health Administration Press.

Forte, J. 2018. Interview with author, April 26.

Freshman, B., and L. Rubino. 2002. "Emotional Intelligence: A Core Competency for Healthcare Administrators." *Healthcare Manager* 20 (4): 1–9.

Goleman, D. 2015. "How to Be Emotionally Intelligent." *New York Times.* Published April 7. www.nytimes.com/2015/04/12/education/edlife/how-to-be-emotionally-intelligent.html.

———. 1998. *Working with Emotional Intelligence.* New York: Random House.

Griffin, R. W., J. M. Phillips, and S. M. Gully. 2017. *Organizational Behavior: Managing People and Organizations*, 12th ed. Boston: Cengage Learning.

Kivland, C. 2018. "Successfully Managing Emotions and Behavior." *Healthcare Executive* 33 (1): 68–71.

———. 2014. "Your Future Gets Brighter with Emotional Intelligence." *Healthcare Executive* 29 (1): 72–75.

Liebler, J. G., and C. R. McConnell. 2004. *Management Principles for Health Professionals*, 4th ed. Sudbury, MA: Jones & Bartlett.

McConnell, C. R. 2018. *Umiker's Management Skills for the New Health Care Supervisor*, 7th ed. Burlington, MA: Jones & Bartlett Learning.

Molinari, C., and L. Shanderson. 2014. "The Culturally Competent Leader." In *New Leadership for Today's Health Care Professionals: Concepts and Cases*, edited by L. G. Rubino, S. J. Esparza, and Y. S. Reid Chassiakos, 57–72. Burlington, MA: Jones & Bartlett Learning.

Substance Abuse and Mental Health Services Administration. 2016. "Cultural Competence." Updated November 10. www.samhsa.gov/capt/applying-strategic-prevention/cultural-competence.

US Department of Health and Human Services Office of Minority Health. 2018. "The National CLAS Standards." Modified May 22. https://minorityhealth.hhs.gov/omh/browse.aspx?lvl=2&lvlid=53.

A MANAGEMENT CASE STUDY: PARTNERS HEALTHCARE

Partners HealthCare: Connecting Heart Failure Patients to Providers Through Remote Monitoring

Andrew Broderick

Reprinted with permission from The Commonwealth Fund.

Case Studies in Telehealth Adoption, January 2013.

Overview

Partners HealthCare (Partners), an integrated health system in Boston, is undergoing a mission-driven, system-level transformation by aligning the organization with external forces shaping the future organization, financing, and delivery of healthcare. Its strategic initiatives center on making patient care more affordable and accountable through providing integrated, evidence-based, patient-centered care. Partners' strategy implementation group has been looking at performance improvement in a number of priority conditions. These initially included diabetes, acute myocardial infarction, coronary artery bypass graft surgery, stroke, and colorectal cancer, but other conditions will be added to the initial care redesign portfolio over time. Care redesign initiatives are working to move the organization from an episodic and specialty approach to a longitudinal, condition-based, and patient-focused orientation. These include determining how technology can contribute toward improving care quality and cost-effectiveness and identifying strategies for their successful introduction into practice.

A key strategic priority at Partners has been to reduce 30-day readmissions to improve quality of care and patient satisfaction, and to minimize Partners' financial risk for potential reductions in Medicare payments. Initiatives that work toward meeting those goals include: providing patients with critical information at discharge to promote safer transitions, using transitions teams and health coaches, participating in the Center for Medicare and Medicaid Services' care coordination pilot demonstrations, and programs that connect chronic care patients with specialized outpatient care services.[1] Health information technologies, including patient-centered telehealth technologies, serve as a strategic tool across many of these process improvement initiatives. In the future, widespread use of connected health solutions at Partners will be driven by structural changes like new reimbursement models and the introduction of patient-centered medical homes.

Partners' Center for Connected Health (CCH)[2] leads the development of patient-centered telehealth solutions and remote health services for a variety of chronic health conditions, potentially leading to reductions in preventable readmissions. The shared goal of these telehealth solutions is to improve outpatient care management. Partners' experience with the implementation of technology into workflow and care management practices indicates that the technology has a positive impact on patient activation and engagement in self-care and plays a critical role in realizing better clinical outcomes. This evidence is critical in demonstrating to providers that this new program supports behavior changes that lead to improved care and quality outcomes. However, Partners' experience indicates that organizations must be prepared for potential implementation delays imposed by the current fee-for-service environment's adverse impact on staff behavior. To overcome workforce resistance, organizations must demonstrate to clinicians and other staff that new programs will support care and quality outcomes.

BACKGROUND

Boston-based Partners HealthCare is an integrated health system. In addition to the two academic medical centers, Brigham and Women's Hospital and Massachusetts General Hospital, the Partners' system includes community and specialty hospitals, community health centers, a physician network, home health and long-term care services, and other health-related entities. The spectrum of care offered at Partners includes prevention and primary care, hospital and specialty care, rehabilitation, and home care services. As one of the nation's leading medical research organizations and a principal teaching affiliate of Harvard Medical School, the nonprofit organization employs more than 50,000 physicians, nurses, scientists, and caregivers.

Partners' mission includes a commitment to its community and the recognition that increasing value and continuously improving quality are essential to maintaining operational excellence. Partners is also dedicated to enhancing patient care, teaching, and research and to taking a leadership role as an integrated healthcare system. The organization also prizes technology adoption and innovation to drive improvements in operations, productivity, and patient care. Its success to date in the large-scale adoption of electronic health record (EHR) and computerized physician order entry (CPOE) systems attests to the organizational culture of openness, preparedness, and ability to adapt to change. Such attributes have helped to ensure that the rollout of new technologies is minimally disruptive and seamless to workflow.

Partners has launched efficient care redesign efforts for five conditions—diabetes, acute myocardial infarction, coronary artery bypass graft surgery, stroke, and colorectal cancer—that reflect its shift toward longitudinal, condition-, and patient-focused orientation in care. The care redesign initiative is being led by Partners Community HealthCare (PCH), the management services organization for the Partners' network of physicians and hospitals. PCH encompasses more than 5,500 employed and affiliated physicians and seven acute care hospitals within the system. If opportunities for using technology-enabled strategies to aid in redesigned care have been identified, Partners' Center for Connected Health will lead the design and development of patient-centered telehealth solutions and remote health services. PCH will help introduce them into practice across the Partners' network.

PERFORMANCE IMPROVEMENT INITIATIVES THAT REDUCE PREVENTABLE READMISSIONS

A top strategic priority at Partners is to reduce 30-day readmissions to improve the quality of patient care and patient satisfaction and minimize risk for reductions in Medicare payments. In a survey of Massachusetts hospitals, more than 10 percent of patients were reported to have been readmitted for the same or unrelated complaints within 30 days.[3] Processes that ensure seamless transitions from hospital to other care settings are essential. These include improvements in educating patients and caregivers, reconciling medications carefully before and after discharge, communicating with receiving clinicians, and ensuring prompt outpatient follow-up. Exhibit 1 illustrates 30-day readmission rates for heart failure, acute myocardial infarction, and pneumonia at selected Partners' hospitals.[4] Partners is currently pilot-testing several programs addressing patient safety,[5] experience,[6] and quality,[7] with a goal of reducing 30-day readmission rates for patients at high risk of readmission. These include programs that target critical failures in communication and information exchange during care transitions across settings and caregivers.

THE CENTER FOR CONNECTED HEALTH'S ROLE IN ADVANCING PATIENT-CENTERED TECHNOLOGY

In 1995, Partners established Partners Telemedicine to use consumer-ready technologies to enhance the patient–physician relationship and deliver remote care. This entity later evolved to become the Center for Connected Health. "Connected health" signifies new patient-centered technology strategies and care models that use information and communications

EXHIBIT 1.

30-Day
Readmission
Rates at Selected
Partners Hospitals
for Acute
Myocardial
Infarction, Heart
Failure, and
Pneumonia

	Brigham & Women's Hospital	Faulkner Hospital	Mass. General Hospital	Newton-Wellesley Hospital	North Shore Medical Center	U.S. National Rate
Acute myocardial infarction	21.1%	21.1%	22.1%	20.8%	18.6%	19.8%
Heart failure	23.7	27.0	23.7	23.8	22.8	24.8
Pneumonia	20.4	20.0	19.0	17.1	18.6	18.4

Partners HealthCare Data Period: July 1, 2007–June 30, 2010.

Partners HealthCare Source: Hospital Compare.

Reference Point Source: U.S. National Rate for Heart Failure, Acute Myocardial Infarction, and Pneumonia for Medicare Patients.

technology—cell phones, computers, networked devices, and simple remote monitoring tools—to support the healthcare needs of patients in community-based settings without disrupting their day-to-day lives. CCH solutions help providers and patients manage chronic conditions, maintain health and wellness, and improve adherence, engagement, and clinical outcomes. To date, CCH has generated more than 100 scholarly publications and helped more than 30,000 patients. In 2011, CCH collected its one-millionth vital life sign from program participants.[8]

CCH's programs use a combination of remote monitoring, social media, and data management applications to enhance patient adherence and engagement to realize improvements in care quality and cost outcomes. The center also supports mobile health initiatives, including a prenatal care text-messaging program for expectant mothers, and wellness programs, such as Step It Up and Virtual Coach, that emphasize activity and exercise among elementary school children and overweight people, respectively. The center offers video-based, real-time consultations and an online second-opinion service, Partners Online Specialty Consultations. CCH recently spun off a health service company, Healthrageous, to provide self-management tools that offer personalized support and motivation in health and lifestyle management.

CCH focuses on applying technologies to conditions that have standard clinical measures of success or offer a clear business case in terms of the potential cost savings or return on investment. For example, the Medicare payment reductions associated with 30-day readmissions provides the heart failure program with a clear business case in terms of the negative financial implications from poor care outcomes. For management of diabetes, HbA1c is a well-accepted clinical marker used to measure success. One program that has been successfully piloted and implemented at scale across Partners is the Connected

Cardiac Care Program (CCCP). It provides home telemonitoring and patient education over a four-month period to enable patients to collect frequent readings and become more engaged in their care.

Exhibit 2 outlines two connected models of care that are currently being deployed at Partners to address congestive heart failure, as well as diabetes and hypertension.

EXHIBIT 2.

Connected Health Models of Care at Partners

The Diabetes Connect and Blood Pressure Connect programs offer patients and their care providers a way to track their blood sugar or blood pressure readings and to collaborate on establishing a shared care plan between office visits. These programs differ from the Connected Cardiac Care Program (CCCP), which uses a centralized telemonitoring model. Diabetes Connect and Blood Pressure Connect operate on a distributed model where each practice comes up with its own structure and protocols for managing patients. Nurses, certified diabetes educators, pharmacists, or primary care physicians can monitor patients' data. The driver to adopt is greater provider efficiency and quality outcomes, and less focus on cost savings. The programs help manage patients by providing structured data frequently and engaging patients actively in their care management. Both programs are available at several primary care practices affiliated with Massachusetts General and Brigham and Women's Hospitals, and through the Partners Community HealthCare network of physicians and hospitals.

Connected Health Program	Summary Description
Connected Cardiac Care Program	A centralized telemonitoring and self-management and preventive care program for heart failure patients that combines telemonitoring capabilities with nurse intervention and care coordination, coaching, and education. The daily transmission of weight, heart rate, pulse, and blood pressure data by patients enables providers to more effectively assess patient status and provide "just-in-time" care and patient education. The program has led to an approximate 50 percent reduction in heart failure–related hospital readmissions for participants.
Diabetes Connect Blood Pressure Connect	Provide practices with tools for the self-management and monitoring of patients with diabetes and hypertension. A recent clinical study with 75 enrolled patients found that participants in Diabetes Connect achieved an average drop in HbA1c of 1.5 percent, while 22.3 percent of participants enrolled in Blood Pressure Connect achieved a 10mmHg or greater drop in systolic blood pressure, compared with 16.7 percent among nonparticipants.

Source: Center for Connected Health.

CARE OUTCOMES

Remote monitoring improves the health of ambulatory patients who have been recently hospitalized for heart failure and leads to reductions in hospital readmissions. A 2006 pilot study of CCCP with 150 heart failure patients, with an average age of 70, who had been admitted to Massachusetts General Hospital and received six months of follow-up care did not reach statistical significance. However, the results indicated a positive trend in reducing readmissions (Exhibit 3). Sixty-eight patients received usual care for heart failure; the remaining 82 patients were offered remote monitoring. Forty-two patients accepted and 40 declined to participate. The remote monitoring group had a lower rate of all-cause readmissions compared with usual-care patients and nonparticipants. Patients in the remote monitoring group also had fewer heart failure–related readmissions. However, all-cause emergency room (ER) visits were higher among the remote-monitoring group than for usual care and nonparticipating patients. This higher frequency of reporting to the ER may be a result of closer monitoring.

EXHIBIT 3.
Remote Monitoring CCCP Pilot Results at Six-Month Follow-Up

	Control (n=68) Mean rate (± standard deviation)	Intervention (n=42) Mean rate (± standard deviation)	Nonparticipant (n=40) Mean rate (± standard deviation)	P-value
Hospital readmissions				
• All-cause	0.73 (±1.51)	0.64 (±0.87)	0.75 (±1.05)	.75
• Heart failure–related	0.38 (±1.06)	0.19 (±0.45)	0.42 (±0.93)	.56
Emergency room visits				
• All-cause	0.57 (±1.43)	0.83 (±1.08)	0.65 (±1.0)	.10
• Heart failure–related	0.25 (±1.02)	0.26 (±0.49)	0.35 (±0.80)	.31
Length of stay				
• All-cause	10.64 (±9.7)	9.16 (±9.00)	13.2 (±13.4)	.85
• Heart failure–related	8.52 (±8.3)	10.57 (±12.5)	10.78 (±9.1)	.78

Source: A. Kulshreshtha, J. C. Kvedar, A. Goyal et al., "Use of Remote Monitoring to Improve Outcomes in Patients with Heart Failure: A Pilot Trial," *International Journal of Telemedicine and Applications*, published online May 19, 2010.

Process Efficiencies

Initial studies of CCCP that involved patients receiving skilled nursing care from a home care provider found that introducing telemonitoring not only affected care outcomes but also indicated a trend toward a decreasing need for nurse visits. The studies did not have a large enough sample to definitively demonstrate cost savings, nor did they indicate that telemonitoring would replace home visits. However, telemonitoring was seen as providing a critical adjunct to patient care and workload efficiency for nurses. The impact was significant enough to support adoption of telemonitoring as part of the care plan for heart failure patients. This led Partners in 2007 to fund the program's expansion systemwide for all heart failure patients that met the inclusion criteria. To date, more than 1,200 patients have been enrolled. Exhibit 4 shows that the proportion of enrollees in CCCP with one or more heart failure hospitalizations in the year following disenrollment was 13.3 percent compared with 39.8 percent one year prior to enrollment.

User Satisfaction

Eleven research studies were conducted at Partners-affiliated hospitals to measure patient perceptions of connected health technologies; namely, if patients feel empowered to better

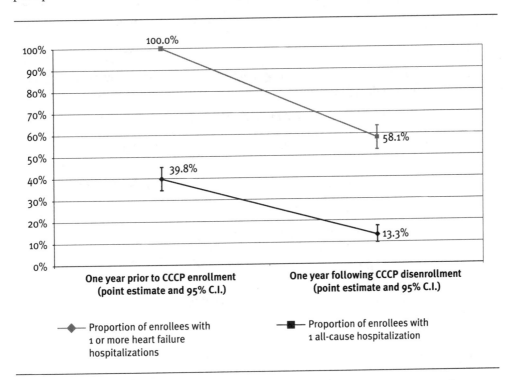

EXHIBIT 4.

Proportion of Connected Cardiac Care Program Enrollees with One or More Hospitalizations

Data include 332 CCCP enrollments among 301 unique patients discharged from the CCCP program prior to July 1, 2009. Results are similar within more recent cohorts of enrollees discharged from the program prior to October 1, 2009, and prior to January 1, 2010.

manage their care, if they have increased satisfaction with care, and if their overall health is improved.[9] Patients in CCCP reported the program increased their confidence and improved their understanding of heart failure and helped them avoid hospitalizations (Exhibit 5). Of the 20 participants in the pilot's remote monitoring group who returned the satisfaction survey, high levels of program satisfaction were recorded (93%). All patients reported that the equipment was easy to use, resulted in greater confidence to self-manage, and helped them stay out of the hospital. In general, once patients are enrolled in the program, less than 10 percent opt out of the program. Those that do drop out usually do so because of personal factors, such as preferences, and not as a result of problems with the technology. Diabetic patients report that blood sugar monitoring was most valuable when they were newly diagnosed or trying to regain control of their diabetes. Electronic communication between providers and patients outside of scheduled office visits was perceived as important in improving diabetes management.

THE CONNECTED CARDIAC CARE PROGRAM

CCCP is developing new ways to help patients at risk for hospitalization to manage their heart disease, by integrating technology into remote patient care and supporting self-monitoring. Contract changes to the Medicare payment structure for the home care industry—in which Medicare provided a prospective payment rate for up to 60 days of service—presented

EXHIBIT 5.

Results of Connected Cardiac Care Program Patient Satisfaction Survey

- 98% of patients reported learning more information about heart failure because of being enrolled in the CCCP

- 85% reported they felt in control of their health because of the program

- 85% reported they were able to gain control over their heart failure while in the program

- 82% reported they were able to stay out of the hospital because of the program

- 82% reported they were able to avoid the emergency room because of the program

- 77% reported they will continue to check their weight daily

- 64% reported they are confident that they can independently manage their heart failure

- 77% reported they would like their treatment providers to offer this program to other heart failure patients

Note: A subset of CCCP participants returned the satisfaction survey (n=93).
Source: Center for Connected Health.

an impetus to create CCCP. Partners HealthCare at Home (PCAH), one of the region's largest home care providers, partnered with the Center for Connected Health to develop CCCP, and provides all of the telemonitoring nurses and clinical support for the program. PCAH, which is recognized as a top-performing agency by the Centers for Medicare and Medicaid Services, offers medical, therapeutic, and supportive home-based services for patients who are recovering from a hospitalization, managing chronic illness, or those who need assistance to remain in their own homes.

CCCP's core components are care coordination, education, and development of self-management skills through telemonitoring. Patients use equipment—a home monitoring device with peripherals to collect weight, blood pressure, and heart rate measurements, and a touch-screen computer to answer questions about symptoms—on a daily basis for four months. Telemonitoring nurses monitor these vitals, respond to out-of-parameter alerts, and guide patients through structured biweekly heart failure education (Exhibit 6). This concentrated effort is effective in meeting the primary goal of reducing hospital readmissions.

PCAH was initially interested in using telehealth under the new Medicare reimbursement model to leverage staff across more patients. Heart failure was targeted as a priority condition because of the high costs involved in caring for heart failure patients and the potential savings from preventing unnecessary admissions to hospitals. The support of Partners' senior leadership was critical to the program's expansion. In particular, the leadership's interest in connected health solutions as a way to augment care delivery systemwide and its commitment of funds to support the development of the program have been critical to scaling CCCP across Partners' network.

CCCP allows patients to monitor their physiological health on a daily basis and provides a virtual link to their healthcare team from their home. Daily monitoring, "just-in-time" teaching—based on the immediacy of interventions in response to monitored patient data—and weekly structured education sessions help patients become aware of their daily behaviors. This impact leads to changes in behavior and the development of new self-management skills. The CCCP team provides the technology, support, and training. It also installs equipment in patients' homes and shows them how to use it. PCAH and other clinical partners provide the expertise for successfully designing and implementing the technology for use in care practices.

There is no cost to patients to enroll or for use of the equipment. The program is open to all patients with a Partners' affiliated primary care physician or cardiologist. Patients are referred by hospital case managers, nurse practitioners, primary care physicians, cardiologists, and other clinicians. Since the inception of CCCP in 2006, the program has included eligible patients from across the Partners HealthCare system on an opt-out basis.

Evaluations of CCCP have been limited to before and after evaluations rather than randomized controlled trials. Such assessments have shown a positive, sizable effect in reducing readmissions, which increased the comfort level among Partners senior leadership

Exhibit 6.

Key Features of the
Connected Cardiac
Care Program

√ Four-month home telemonitoring of congestive heart failure patients by a telemonitoring nurse

√ Intervention by telemonitoring nurse based on physician orders

√ Interactive patient education and lifestyle management

√ Reports posted in electronic health record with email alerts to physicians and nurse practitioners

√ No cost to the patient

√ Open to patients with a Partners' affiliated primary care physician or cardiologist

Who is eligible?	Who is *not* eligible?
• Patients age 18 and older with a diagnosis of heart failure	• Patients currently receiving skilled home care services***
• Patients considered to be at high risk for hospitalization	• Patients with end-stage renal disease on dialysis
• Patients who have a Partners' affiliated primary care physician or cardiologist	• Patients with organ transplant
	• Patients in hospice
• Patients covered by Medicare, Medicaid, or certain patients in the safety net*	• Patients with an active cancer diagnosis
	• Patients who reside in nursing homes
• Patients able to speak and read English**	• Patients who do not have a stable environment to conduct the monitoring
• Patients mentally competent and willing**	• Patients with any physical disability that precludes use of telemonitoring equipment
• Patients with a traditional phone line	

* Limited funding available for some patients with commercial insurance.

** Or those with a primary caregiver willing to assume responsibility for telemonitoring.

*** Exception: Partners' Health at Home skilled Medicaid and commercial patients.

Source: Partners HealthCare System, Connected Cardiac Care Program, http://www.connected-health.org/media/224132/cccp summary 6 2 11.doc.

with the intervention. There has also been ongoing iterative research using small groups of people to assess the intervention and identify the need for modifications. CCH has also been working with PCH to test effective adoption and the role of financial incentive mechanisms to facilitate spread. CCH's in-house analysis estimates that the program has generated total cost savings of more than $10 million since 2006 for the more than 1,200 enrolled patients (Exhibit 7).

Exhibit 7.
Reducing Hospital
Readmissions with
the Connected
Cardiac Care
Program

Program outcomes

√ 51% reduction in heart failure hospital readmissions*

√ 44% reduction in non–heart failure hospital readmissions*

√ Improved patient understanding of heart failure and self-management skills

√ High levels of clinician and patient acceptance and satisfaction

Savings**

A case study prepared by the Center for Connected Health outlines the following cost savings:

Cost of CCCP:	$1,500 per patient
Total savings from reduction in hospitalizations:	$9,655 per patient
Total net savings:	$8,155 per patient
Total savings:	$10,316,075 for 1,265 monitored patients since 2006

* N=332 patients

** This program targeted reductions in unplanned heart failure and non–heart failure related admissions. The savings realized factor involves the cost of running the program, including marketing, referral management, telemonitoring nurse support, and technology.

Source: Center for Connected Health.

LESSONS LEARNED IN TAKING CCCP FROM PILOT TO SCALE

Partners' experience with connected health technologies and with successfully implementing telehealth-enabled programs across the provider network highlights the significant potential value of transforming care delivery, improving care outcomes, and lowering costs. Social processes are as important in ensuring program success as are the technical factors. Key social factors include leadership support and the championing of technology, the integration of patient data into the workflow to enable providers to more effectively assess patient status and provide just-in-time care and education, and using personal health data to help educate and motivate patients to make necessary lifestyle changes. Even though it has not always been met with immediate success, the organization has persevered to introduce telehealth-enabled care management solutions, to generate evidence of impact, and to use that evidence to advocate for broader deployment across the provider network. This experience imparts important lessons for the successful planning, implementation, and deployment of telehealth-enabled care management programs at scale and for identifying future opportunities for continued program advances in patient care management.

PATIENT ACTIVATION AND ENGAGEMENT ARE CRITICAL TO PROGRAM SUCCESS

With the decision by PCAH to use telehealth to leverage staff across more patients in response to Medicare reimbursement changes, CCH became a strategic partner to PCAH. CCH and PCAH collaborated in the design of the technology-enabled clinical program, the selection of the technology, and the staffing of the operational model. Both parties market and perform outreach of CCCP to patient referral sources. There was a low level of adoption in the initial phase of the program. Nurses at first saw CCCP as driving a wedge between them and their patients. They resisted the introduction of the program and the replacement of the more traditional high-touch approach to care. An important factor in overcoming that initial pushback from staff—and an important lesson for the adoption of patient-centered technology in general—is the positive impact the technology has once it's placed in patients' hands. With CCCP, patients felt more connected and nurses learned to develop relationships with patients accordingly with the help of technology. Another important insight in terms of adoption is that patients need to be aware that the provider is engaged in order for them to regularly use the technology as a self-management tool.

AUTOMATIC ENROLLMENT OF PATIENTS IMPROVES CLINICIAN INVOLVEMENT AND SATISFACTION

As the program was extended beyond home care throughout the Partners system, pushback came from other sources, primarily primary care physicians and cardiologists, such that physician referrals and enrollment into the program were challenged. The program struggled initially but the key watershed point came with the decision to change patient enrollment to an opt-out process. Once a patient is identified for enrollment in CCCP, clinicians are responsible for notifying CCCP that they do not want the patient in the program. As a result, enrollment has increased, readmission rates have declined, and satisfaction levels among doctors have increased as benefits in patient care became evident. The refusal rate to participate among doctors went from 10 percent to less than 1 percent.

DATA CAN MOTIVATE AND EMPOWER CLINICIANS AND PATIENTS

Outcomes in controlled trials, as well as in before-and-after studies, have consistently demonstrated an approximate 50 percent drop in cardiac-related readmissions for patients enrolled in CCCP. One driver of that outcome is patients learning self-management skills and receiving constant feedback about how lifestyle factors affect health outcomes. Another is just-in-time care, whereby remote monitoring and intervention by nurses sends a strong message to patients that they are accountable. CCH's commitment to research allows the organization access to the data and studies to counter resistance and arguments from clinicians about the impact on quality and patient experience. CCH is also able to prepare the business case and concomitant cost-savings argument. But the traditional business case approach cannot convey the full impact that other factors, such as patient experience and staff satisfaction, have on improved health outcomes and higher quality of care.

NEW TECHNOLOGY-ENABLED SOLUTIONS DO NOT FIT OLD POLICY FRAMEWORKS

CCH faces challenges in optimizing the impact of connected health programs on care outcomes. The current fee-for-service environment can present a mental barrier for clinicians, and pilots involving financial incentives that reward provider engagement have not led to significant behavior change. Many doctors view the move toward a patient-centered medical home as requiring more staff, such as nurses and pharmacists, rather than an opportunity for leveraging technology in support of fewer staff. While the widespread use of connected health solutions will require structural changes in the form of reimbursement and new care models like the patient-centered medical home, a significant amount of work remains to be done in promoting the use of technology to leverage existing staff across more patients.

IMPLICATIONS FOR U.S. HEALTHCARE ORGANIZATIONS

Being in an integrated delivery network that owns a home care service business has allowed Partners to be ahead on the adoption curve with telehealth relative to other health systems. Organizations—particularly ones lower on the adoption curve—that are considering technology-enabled solutions will need to address the following issues: establishing acceptance that the technology can clinically make a difference, identifying the method by which the organization will implement and integrate the technology, determining whether a one-size-fits-all approach will be feasible across the network or system, and evaluating whether the prevailing financial system can support an economical approach to scaling.

From an organizational readiness perspective, it is critical to recognize the role of champions who understand workflow and also to understand the requirements for successfully integrating solutions into practice. To gain buy-in from staff, it is important to put the data in the hands of motivated individuals, like clinicians who want to help their patients. It is also important to aggregate external data, integrate it with clinical health information systems, and communicate it to patients and providers alike. Data cannot be maintained in separate data silos and must be placed in the EHR to be meaningful and useful in clinical decision support. Patients need access to the patient portal, with the ability to retrieve clinical information and perform administrative functions. CCH has invested significant resources in developing a platform to support the integration and management of data, which will also serve as a platform for the development and implementation of other applications.

However, recognizing that not all systems are equal in the U.S. healthcare delivery system, CCH's experience also points to common pitfalls to avoid rather than just best practices to adopt. A common mistake is attempting to shoehorn a connected health program into the traditional care model. Technologies such as telemonitoring can be disruptive to workflow and represent a change in the way care is delivered. Organizations often tend to view connected health solutions as simply requiring a technical interface to existing programs rather than a redesign of the care delivery model. Partners' experience indicates that connected health requires a different mind-set to program design and execution. Otherwise, there is a low likelihood that it will change practice and lead to desired outcomes. Looking forward, Partners is developing a predictive algorithm as a screening strategy of a hospitalized patient's risk for readmission. This will help contribute toward a more aggressive segmentation of the population and tiering of the program to meet the needs of more acute patients on discharge and to manage them so they can exit the program.

Dedicating staff members to the implementation and oversight of the program is more critical than the technology itself in understanding why programs sometimes fail. But often, many technology-enabled solutions in healthcare fail to recognize the need for solutions that are social in nature rather than solely technological. In the current fee-for-service environment, organizations have to also be prepared for the delays that payment systems can impose on staff behavior. Organizations must show clinicians that connected health programs will support care and quality outcomes, while planning workflow changes very carefully and taking the time and making the effort to work methodically and systematically through issues that may arise. Finally, it takes time to integrate technology into health delivery and to allow staff to adapt to the new work model. As a result, structure, coordination, planning, and setting goals, as well as expectations, for the program are critical preparatory steps for success.

Notes

1. Partners HealthCare System, Quality, Safety and Efficiency, http://qualityandsafety.partners.org/.

2. Partners HealthCare System, Center for Connected Health–Changing Healthcare Delivery, http://www.connected-health.org/.

3. Partners HealthCare System, Annual Report 2010, http://www.partners.org/Assets/Documents/AboutUs/PartnersHealthCare_2010AnnualReport.pdf.

4. Partners HealthCare System, Efficiency: 30-Day Readmission Rate to Discharging Hospital for AMI/HF/PNE, http://qualityandsafety.partners.org/measures/readmissionv2.aspx?id=93.

5. Partners HealthCare System, Report Card: Patient Safety Measures, http://qualityandsafety.partners.org/measures/overview.aspx?id=2.

6. Partners HealthCare System, Report Card: Patient Experience, http://qualityandsafety.partners.org/measures/overview.aspx?id=17.

7. Partners HealthCare System, Report Card: Quality Measures for Clinical Conditions, http://qualityandsafety.partners.org/measures/highquality.aspx?id=3.

8. "Center for Connected Health Reaches Milestone of One Million Vital Signs Collected from Patients via Remote Monitoring," Partners HealthCare press release, Oct. 20, 2011, http://www.connected-health.org/media-center/press-releases/center-for-connected-health-reaches-milestone-of-one-million-vital-signs-collected-from-patients-via-remote-monitoring.aspx.

9. "Center for Connected Health Presents Growing Evidence of the Benefits of Technology to Improve Patient Satisfaction and Empowerment," Partners HealthCare press release, April 8, 2008, http://www.connected-health.org/media-center/press-releases/center-for-connected-health-presents-growing-evidence-of-the-benefits-of-technology-to-improve-patient-satisfaction-and-empowerment.aspx.

INTEGRATIVE CASE STUDIES

These case studies enable you to apply and integrate what you have learned throughout the book. At the end of each chapter are questions for several cases. Multiple chapters are required to fully resolve the problems in each case, so each case has questions in multiple chapters. By answering questions in several chapters for a single case, you will develop your ability to use and combine management tools and methods described throughout the book. You may also make up more questions for these cases to strengthen your ability to apply management theories, methods, principles, models, and tools to current real-world healthcare organizations and situations.

Four cases—"Disparities in Care at Southern Regional Health System," "How Can an ACO Improve the Health of Its Population?," "Increasing the Focus on Patient Safety at First Medical Center," and "Managing the Patient Experience: Facing the Tension Between Quality Measures and Patient Satisfaction"—are reprinted, with permission, from *Health Services Management: A Case Study Approach*, 11th edition, by Ann Scheck McAlearney and Anthony R. Kovner (Health Administration Press 2018). Three cases—"Hospice Goes Hollywood," "I Can't Do It All!," and "The Rocky Road to Patient Satisfaction at Leonard-Griggs"—are reprinted, with permission, from *Managing Health Services: Cases in Organization Design and Decision Making* by Deborah E. Bender with Julie Curkendall and Heather Manning (Health Administration Press 2000).

CASE: DISPARITIES IN CARE AT SOUTHERN REGIONAL HEALTH SYSTEM

Theo Hank leaned back in his chair and closed his eyes. He had been afraid that the reports would contain bad news, and he now had to figure out what to do with this new information. Flipping through the first binder on his desk—reporting results of the recent Robert Wood Johnson Foundation–sponsored assessment of the cardiovascular care provided by his organization—he was increasingly concerned.

Southern Regional Health System was based in Jackson, Mississippi, an area known for its diverse population and high poverty rates. Poverty and unemployment in the area affected whites and nonwhites differently: Black and Hispanic residents were about three times more likely than white residents to live in poverty, black residents were two and a half times more likely than whites to be unemployed, and Hispanic residents were more than twice as likely as whites to be unemployed. Beyond poverty and unemployment concerns, however, was the issue of disparities in healthcare—that is, different care being given to different patients. Although such disparities had received increasing attention nationwide, Hank thought that the care provided at Southern Regional was "color-blind." Under the health system's mission of providing "excellent quality of care for all," he assumed that the care was equitably delivered across patients and patient populations.

Apparently, this was not the case. The first report presented heart care data that had been collected over the past year, and it showed significant disparities in the care provided by Southern Regional. For instance, using the four core measures for heart failure that the Centers for Medicare & Medicaid Services currently collects and reports, the data indicated that only 41 percent of Southern Regional's patients were receiving all recommended heart failure care and that the number was lower for nonwhite patients than it was for whites. Whereas 68 percent of whites received all recommended care, the comparable number among nonwhites was just 27 percent. Disparities were also apparent in the percentage of heart failure patients who received discharge instructions: Only 65 percent of Hispanic patients received the information, compared to 85 percent of non-Hispanic patients. Also troubling Hank was the fact none of the measures was close to 100 percent. The data clearly indicated that the care provided at Southern Regional was not the type of care Hank would want offered to his own family. He truly did not understand how his hospital could be providing such disparate care.

The second binder on his desk offered little information to ease his concerns. This report, the "Assessment of Organizational Readiness to Change" for Southern Regional, showed that few individuals in the hospital were aware of the nationwide problem of disparities in care and that even fewer were aware that such an issue might be problematic within their own hospital. The evaluation also showed a strong tendency among hospital employees and physicians to resist proposed changes and instead "go with the flow."

Hank now possessed data showing significant gaps in the care provided to African American and Hispanic patients relative to white patients, and he knew that he had to bring this issue to the forefront of hospital concerns. A meaningful reduction in these disparities would be a legacy he would love to leave. Yet he still was not sure how best to address this issue at Southern Regional.

CASE: HOSPICE GOES HOLLYWOOD

Hollywood Hospice is a not-for-profit, 85-bed hospice facility located in the small, but populous, town of Hollywood, California. Like all other hospices, its mission is to provide high-quality palliative care to the terminally ill. Because it is located in a competitive environment that receives much media coverage, Hollywood Hospice is extremely conscious of its image. Hollywood Hospice, therefore, maintains top clinicians and administrative staff, has an attractive facility, and recently attempted to make adjustments to apply for JCAHO (Joint Commission on Accreditation of Healthcare Organizations) accreditation. The administrative staff worked for several months revising policies and procedures and determining areas in which work practices should change to comply with JCAHO standards. The staff believed that improving standards for compliance would improve the quality of care and bring prestige to the facility, even though it already has approval from the National Hospice Organization.

The administration of Hollywood Hospice knew that the changes were vital to achieving accreditation and had to be made quickly. The director, Ms. Cynthia Thurmond, distributed to each clinical and administrative department two-inch binders that contain details about the implementation procedures for accreditation. Shortly after distributing the binders and sending a reminder e-mail to all staff about the urgency of the implementation, Ms. Thurmond began to receive complaints from the administrative staff; the staff complained that most of the changes were not being followed by the clinicians. Ms. Thurmond expressed her frustrations to her assistant Glenn: "I don't understand why the clinicians aren't following the new protocols we gave them. Without full compliance with the new protocols, we have no chance for accreditation or for increased quality care."

"I know, but some of the changes are proving harder to implement than others; I'm not sure which ones we should have them focus on," Glenn responded. "I don't believe the clinicians understand that all of the new protocols have to be followed strictly. They just don't seem to care! Maybe we should create an incentive system so they'll do what we want," he suggested.

Meanwhile, down the hall, the medical director, Dr. George Frank, became very aggravated after reading the documents. "I can't believe they want us to make changes this quickly without giving our staff adequate training, and without even asking for our input!" he complained to a nurse. The nurse agreed, "All of these new policies and procedures are just more useless bureaucracy; who needs accreditation when we know we provide good quality healthcare? We have enough work as it is and we don't need more non-clinicians telling us what to do or how to do it."

Hollywood Hospice's compliance efforts appear to have reached a stalemate. Although its administration is ready to implement new policies and procedures for accreditation, the implementation lacks clinician support.

CASE: HOW CAN AN ACO IMPROVE THE HEALTH OF ITS POPULATION?

Vandalia Care, an accountable care organization (ACO), had been successfully developed as part of Vandalia Medical Center (VMC), but the new ACO's leadership had become concerned. Specifically, they worried that their mission to reduce care costs while improving the health of the population was at risk. In the six months since Vandalia Care had been established, the number of patients served had increased, but VMC was having difficulty determining whether and how the ACO model was having an impact on the health of its population.

VMC had an electronic health record (EHR) that was operational in both inpatient and outpatient settings, but not all providers could access all elements of the EHR. Now that Vandalia Care had been implemented, a new problem arose with respect to data. Vandalia Care had associated hospitals and providers, but because of the way ACO contracts were written, patients attributed to the ACO were not required to use those facilities and clinicians. As a result, when patients attributed to Vandalia Care visited providers external to the ACO, data about those visits were virtually impossible to collect. Considering that Vandalia Care's goal is to improve the health of the entire ACO population, lack of access to the comprehensive health records of all attributed patients was problematic.

Lindsey Dillow, the new manager of care coordination for Vandalia Care, wanted to help solve this problem. Drawing from recent research on ACO development, Dillow believed that Vandalia Care patients, like other ACO patients, did not know they were actually part of the ACO. Patients might be loyal to their primary care physicians, but when they needed specialty care or hospitalization, they went wherever they wanted to go, regardless of whether the setting was part of Vandalia Care. As a result, Dillow did not know these patients had sought services outside the ACO until she received claims data several months after the admission or visit, thus significantly compromising her ability to coordinate care. Further, costs that could have been controlled via ACO contracts with specialists, hospitals, and even skilled nursing facilities were left unchecked.

Vandalia Care's launch had included a mass mailing to members of the community, but Dillow believed more needed to be done to engage patients and community members in improving their health. She knew that the ACO's leadership was open to supporting a major initiative to connect with the community, so she needed to carefully consider her strategy. Dillow recognized that a true focus on population health management had to be less about branding the ACO and more about engaging consumers and encouraging them to care about their health. In particular, she believed that an important element of this outreach had to focus on connecting physicians with community members. She wondered whether focusing on a particular segment of the population first—children, for instance—made sense, or whether staging her outreach plan by geographic area or community was a better alternative. Dillow had access to the Vandalia EHR to inform her plan, but she needed to figure out what to do first.

CASE: "I CAN'T DO IT ALL!"

Based in Walnut Creek, California, Healthdyne is a health maintenance organization (HMO) that provides healthcare to the northern California Bay Area. It serves approximately 1.2 million enrollees composed mainly of upper-class, white-collar professionals. Healthdyne occupies a relatively small corner of the market, but is quickly gaining prominence in the area and has developed a solid financial footing with bright prospects. It is located in a growing community, with a 15 to 20 percent annual growth rate projected for the next five years.

For the past 20 years, Healthdyne's former president, Amanda Huggins, has successfully carried out the organizational mission—to provide more affordable and better quality healthcare for its members by setting the statewide standard for excellence and responsiveness. As one of the key players in the organization since its inception, Ms. Huggins is a recognized expert in the managed care industry. Corporate legend has it that her motto was "It doesn't happen without my signature!" Upon Ms. Huggins's retirement, Arnold Brice was recruited to take her place.

When Mr. Brice, who is the former CEO of Atlantic Healthcare, was brought in as president, he inherited an executive staff composed of the vice presidents of the marketing, finance, and professional services departments as well as a medical director, all of whom were capable of fulfilling their managerial responsibilities. However, within a few weeks of joining Healthdyne, Mr. Brice perceived a serious flaw with his staff—none of the vice presidents would make a decision, not even on routine matters such as personnel questions, choice of marketing media, or changing suppliers. The vice presidents frequently presented him with issues in their areas of responsibility and requested that he make the decision. This troubled Mr. Brice. Before long, the situation seriously impeded his efforts to engage in strategic planning for the HMO.

At a regular staff meeting, when every member of his staff had an issue that required his attention, Mr. Brice finally blew up. The catalyst to this incident was this question from the Finance vice president: "What font do you want this in?"

Waving his arms in exasperation, Mr. Brice shouted, which is very uncharacteristic of him, "I cannot do it all! You are going to have to make these decisions yourselves."

The meeting broke up with the staff looking very puzzled and Mr. Brice realizing that he had to make serious changes.

CASE: INCREASING THE FOCUS ON PATIENT SAFETY AT FIRST MEDICAL CENTER

At First Medical Center (FMC), the goal for the past decade has been to simultaneously improve quality and patient safety by implementing projects, initiatives, and programs either focused on an organizationwide intervention or targeted at one department, unit, or floor within the organization. This effort has resulted in a piecemeal approach to quality improvement, with one intervention layered on top of another. FMC's newly appointed chief quality and patient safety officer, Dr. Emily Frame, believes they can do better.

Emily sees a major opportunity to centralize and standardize quality initiatives through a systemwide initiative focused on both cultural change and quality improvement. Specifically, she wants to implement the Crew Resource Management (CRM) program across all units of FMC. CRM is a systematic approach to training leadership, staff, and physicians, and it incorporates customizable safety tools aimed at generating permanent culture change around patient safety. Emily is aware that adopting a unified approach to safety and quality improvement will require significant organizational change, but she believes the long-term results will justify the expected difficulty.

Given the circumstances at FMC, Emily believes that the first challenge will be to get the leaders of the institution to understand that a gap exists in patient safety and to recognize the opportunity for improvement. She is well aware that cultural transformation needs engaged leadership, and she knows that only through shared vision and purpose can such widespread programs succeed. If leaders are not engaged and supportive, the program will struggle to get off the ground, making the desired transformation virtually impossible.

Another major challenge related to executive leadership buy-in involves the financial resources necessary for implementation. Healthcare organizations have a large number of competing financial priorities, not the least of which are training and education. Training for CRM requires dedicated time away from patient care (between two and four hours), so the organization will have to backfill that nursing and physician care time. Once put into practice, however, CRM has the potential to save money by averting patient safety events. The research literature provides some evidence for these savings, particularly in critical care and surgery specialties, though systemwide implementation has never been studied. CRM has to be seen as value added and a top priority for the organization and the care of its patients.

An additional area of concern for Emily involves how she will be able to measure success. If CRM aims to improve teamwork and promote a culture of safety, how can one prove that it works? What metrics would FMC leaders, providers, and patients regard as indicators of success? As Emily well knows, cultural transformation is hard enough to define, let alone measure.

CASE: MANAGING THE PATIENT EXPERIENCE: FACING THE TENSION BETWEEN QUALITY MEASURES AND PATIENT SATISFACTION

Bryce Jackson has recently been appointed chief experience officer for Academic Medical Center (AMC), a large tertiary-care health system consisting of six hospitals with a total of 1,500 inpatient beds and an annual average of 60,000 discharges. In this role, he will oversee the Department of Patient Experience, which has responsibility for patient satisfaction data, patient family complaints/grievances, patient advocacy, volunteer services, information desks, and employee engagement. Bryce will report directly to the chief quality and patient safety officer, who is responsible for quality and performance improvement across the system.

Bryce has a decade of experience working in various middle management roles within AMC's Department of Patient Experience. During this time, he has noted a growing tension between patient satisfaction and quality measures. At AMC, although all health system leaders are tasked with improving satisfaction and quality measures, fragmentation and tension result from the involvement of different leaders tasked with improving specific metrics. Bryce recently completed a master's in healthcare administration (MHA) program through a school of public health affiliated with AMC, and he found during his studies that he is not the only one to notice the growing tension.

Prominent health administrators and researchers have noted that the current structure of the Centers for Medicare & Medicaid Services (CMS) Hospital Value-Based Purchasing (HVBP) program has contributed to, and perpetuates, this tension. One specific issue is that the CMS HVBP program now reimburses for an ever-increasing number of metrics. The pie charts in exhibits 1 and 2 illustrate the changes in the HVBP program at AMC. The proportion of the reimbursement pie that is derived from patient satisfaction scores (the Hospital Consumer Assessment of Healthcare Providers and Systems, or HCAHPS, survey) has remained relatively steady, but the other segments of this pie are continually shifting. In 2013, clinical process measures filled out the rest of the pie, but for the coming fiscal year, outcomes and efficiency will be added, incorporating a variety of metrics related to quality and patient safety.

Bryce feels that use of this reimbursement pie at AMC has resulted in fragmentation of the concept of patient experience, as well as tension among organizational leaders challenged with maximizing performance for the individual metrics in each leader's piece of the pie. Discussions with peers at other institutions have convinced Bryce that this problem is not isolated to AMC; in fact, these tensions are felt in health systems across the country.

The competing priorities are most evident at the point of patient care, with the patient often becoming the victim of the tension. For instance, steps taken to meet a goal in patient fall prevention—a key quality and safety metric—may be in direct conflict with a goal of improving the patient's experience as reflected in patient satisfaction scores. During his time in middle management, Bryce has been in several staff meetings where frontline nursing staff have discussed this problem. Staff are concerned that use of bed alarms will lead to hospitalized patients feeling restrained, thereby worsening their experience of care and lowering the resulting patient satisfaction scores.

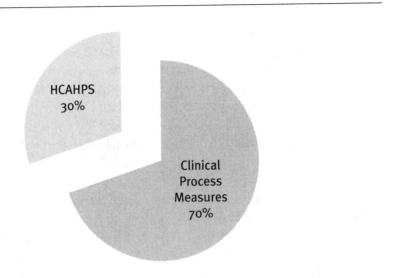

Exhibit 1
Breakdown of CMS
Hospital Value-
Based Purchasing
Categories, 2013

Note: HCAHPS = Hospital Consumer Assessment of Healthcare Providers and Systems.

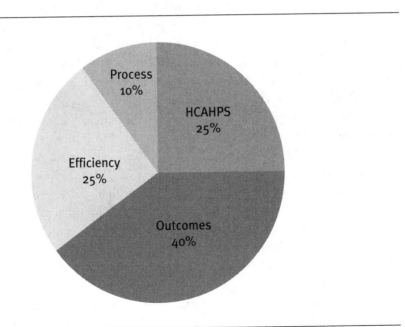

Exhibit 2
Breakdown of CMS
Hospital Value-
Based Purchasing
Categories,
Upcoming Fiscal
Year

Note: HCAHPS = Hospital Consumer Assessment of Healthcare Providers and Systems.

Just a few months ago, a patient had been injured in a fall, triggering a patient safety event review process that highlighted this type of tension. After the fall was reported, the nurses on the care team and the physician lead reviewed the incident, and because the case was of high severity, it was discussed at the weekly significant event meeting. The administration present at the meeting called for a root-cause analysis, which took 45 days and involved speaking with every party in the case. Discussions with the nurse assigned to the patient at the time of the fall noted that the patient had a bed alarm and that the alarm had gone off twice in the 24 hours preceding the fall when the patient had tried to get out of bed unassisted. Members of the staff had had a discussion about placing the patient in arm restraints, but they were concerned about infringing on the patient's rights. They knew the patient would be distraught by the use of physical restraints, but they were under great time pressure and did not know if they would be able to have a prolonged discussion with the patient about the need to have both a safe and positive experience. Staff debate about the next course of action was ongoing when the patient suffered the injury fall.

Based on this incident, and a variety of other prior experiences, Bryce has formed the opinion that much of the tension could be resolved through the development of a program to establish patient expectations. A recent large-scale survey research study, which had been included on the reading list for his capstone MHA class, indicated that patients' "met" expectations were associated with their postvisit satisfaction scores—thus supporting Bryce's idea that managing expectations may be key to solving the problem. Bryce feels that, in the ambulatory setting, patients could be provided with information about what to expect as inpatients, including the needs of the hospital and its staff, to balance safety and satisfaction. This approach would be similar to airlines' efforts to emphasize flight attendants' roles in flight safety rather than just their roles in providing passenger service on board.

Specifically, Bryce envisions appointing a multidisciplinary working group comprising all stakeholders to develop a Patient Expectation of Inpatient Care curriculum. The working group could develop an educational video to play on the hospital channel on the television in each inpatient bedroom. The video would directly present to patients the tension between satisfaction and safety and specifically highlight the recent patient fall case in which the debate over arm restraints was a factor. Each admitted patient could be directed to this video when they were assigned to a room. Bryce is confident that this approach could address the problem without involving the staff nurses directly in the education effort; nurses' direct involvement could be viewed as self-serving and would also add to their significant workload.

Bryce views his new appointment as an opportunity to address tensions, build bridges, and knock down silos. Specifically, he feels that this new role, chief experience officer, is the ideal platform from which to implement his program of patient expectation management. However, despite his enthusiasm, Bryce realizes that he must prioritize his agenda and develop a long-term plan.

CASE: THE ROCKY ROAD TO PATIENT SATISFACTION AT LEONARD-GRIGGS

Leonard-Griggs Primary Care System is a network of physician practices located in rural South Carolina. The network presently includes five sites. Three of the sites, including the parent site and the two larger satellite clinics, are located in Haycock County. These sites are well established and have positive relationships with the community. The other two satellite clinics, located in separate adjoining counties, have been recently acquired by Leonard-Griggs. Neither county has any major metropolitan areas. The communities of these counties are traditionally underserved, change comes less easily for them, and their satellite clinics have had some difficulty establishing themselves and marketing their services among this very dispersed population. The satellite clinics are no more than 20 miles from the main clinic and administrative office.

Leonard-Griggs's mission is to provide comprehensive, quality primary and preventative healthcare services to all citizens of the region, regardless of the patient's financial or insurance status. Leonard-Griggs is important to the community because it is committed to serving everyone regardless of one's ability to pay. By providing primary healthcare services to the "unassigned" or underinsured patients in the area, Leonard-Griggs supports the medical staff, enhances physician retention and recruitment efforts, and reduces the overall healthcare costs for the community. To maintain the current patient base and attract new patients to sustain revenue, Leonard-Griggs must continue to perfect its patient focus and service per requests of the patients.

Leonard-Griggs employs 12 providers and a support staff of approximately 60 individuals including nurses, certified nursing assistants, clerical support staff, and billing personnel. The majority of the employees, particularly those who assist in the individual physician offices, have worked for Leonard-Griggs since its opening. The responsibilities of these employees, as well as various other staff members, generally do not differ greatly from day to day.

To try to better serve patients, Sadie Ratcliff, the executive director, decided to implement a patient satisfaction effort at each of the five physician practices. Key to the effort would be the ongoing collection of data using a survey instrument. The surveys would reveal patient opinions of services, office staff, nursing staff, providers, and geographic location of the site. Ms. Ratcliff informed each of the administrative managers of her intentions at the weekly meeting and enlisted the assistance of the summer intern, Jessie Hartley, in starting the project. The manager of Human Resources was especially supportive of the surveys: "These surveys will reveal any possible changes in personnel I should make and will show just where our system's focus should be." Jessie was assigned to deliver the surveys, along with incentives for patients to complete the surveys, to all five sites. The incentive is that each patient would receive a gift—a notepad with the network logo and site-specific information—at checkout for agreeing to complete the survey there or take it home.

On Monday morning, Jessie walked into Shady Bluff Medical Clinic, the first site to receive the surveys. She began to explain the plan of action to Ms. Robin, the employee responsible for checkout procedures—collecting payments at the time of patient departure and scheduling return appointments. Ms. Robin has worked for Shady Bluff since it opened 17 years ago, so she has established a particular way to perform every aspect of her job and perform them quite naturally. Although the people she has met since Leonard-Griggs purchased Shady Bluff seemed like good people, she still was not sure about their new methods, including distributing the patient satisfaction survey.

"I'm not sure I can remember to give out the surveys as patients come to my window to check out," Ms. Robin explained to Jessie. "Why should I have to take the time to explain the survey format to patients, especially those who are ill, and give out notepads? I just can't do all of my work and this work, too!"

"Ms. Robin, please do the best you can," Jessie cautiously replied. "If you miss a few patients, no big deal. Just try to hand the surveys to patients as often as you can and stress the importance of responses. Management feels patient satisfaction surveys are tools that can lead to a more efficient, patient-friendly organization and I'm sure your efforts will be appreciated."

As Jessie walked out the front door of the office, Ms. Robin placed the boxes of surveys and notepads under the counter. "Well, it appears that Ms. Ratcliff does not feel obligated to personally speak with office staff about the issue," Ms. Robin thought. "The instructions Jessie gave me are so vague, so I see no reason to go out of my way to tell patients to complete them. Besides, I'm tired of handling duties that are not included in my job description. These additional tasks involve just enough work to make my day even more hectic."

Jessie continued to deliver the surveys and gift notepads to the remaining four sites. At each clinic, office personnel were surprised at the new procedure that took effect right away. Mrs. Lorene, an employee at the Oak Grove site, offered her concerns: "Many of our regular patients cannot read and some can't write. Can relatives or friends complete the surveys? What about children who come in for check-ups and are too young to speak for themselves? These things are more trouble than they are worth."

While driving back to the administrative office, Jessie was confused and discouraged. She wondered why Ms. Ratcliff had not mentioned the survey implementation process to employees at last month's staff meeting. Certainly, Jessie thought to herself, patients could sense tension in the attitudes and actions of the support staff, which could create a negative perception of the office visit and, therefore, result in negative responses on the survey.

Jessie and Ms. Ratcliff met for an hour the same afternoon. Jessie relayed the responses of the office employees and her own concerns: "I feel caught in the middle, and the employees are not willing to listen to me. I think an administrator probably needs to provide guidance. I don't want to be thought of as a know-it-all."

Ms. Ratcliff gave her a few suggestions for responding to the complaints and promised to send a memo to "get everyone on board with this endeavor." Jessie was somewhat encouraged, but still feared overstepping her boundaries. She wanted to tell Ms. Ratcliff that confusion and low employee morale seemed to be two deterrents to the success of the implementation, but she was not sure whether or not she should share her opinions because she was only an intern.

Many procedural questions were left unanswered, including what to do with the surveys as they came back to the clinics and whether patients could receive more than one survey given that most of them returned for rechecks. Jessie realized that making employees feel like team players would help them accept increased job responsibility with enthusiasm. A plan for turning the patient satisfaction survey crisis around needed prompt consideration.

REAL-WORLD APPLIED
INTEGRATIVE PROJECTS

Healthcare organizations (HCOs) have to implement big projects and accomplish important goals. For example, many of them must become more eco-friendly, improve population health, integrate clinical services, strengthen diversity and inclusion, create more joy in work, implement mobile health, reduce costs, enhance patient experience, prevent medical errors, or merge with another HCO. You can probably think of other big projects and goals.

There are plenty of ways to become more eco-friendly, such as reducing energy use, recycling waste, and carpooling to work. But how do managers get their HCOs to save energy, recycle, and carpool? Costs can be reduced in many ways, such as by doing procedures right the first time and not wasting supplies. But how do managers make their organizations and employees do it right the first time and not waste supplies? Patient experience may be enhanced by more compassionate employees and reduced wait times. So how do managers make employees more compassionate to enhance patient experience? We can think of good ideas to help an HCO be eco-friendly, reduce costs, and so on. But how can managers bring those good ideas to life and actually make them happen in their HCOs?

Managers cannot just wave a magic wand and expect employees to do these things. Instead, managers can apply management theories, principles, models, techniques, and tools from this book. For example, managers can use principles from chapters 2 and 4 to assign responsibility to specific jobs for reducing energy. Managers can use the information in chapter 3 to revise the organization's mission to state that the HCO will be green and eco-friendly. To help an HCO become eco-friendly, a student might say, "Let's have a green team." OK, good idea. Let's use the material in chapter 6 to form an *effective* green team. And let's use motivation theories and methods from chapter 10 to influence workers so they actually do carpool and reduce energy usage. Chapter 14 presents useful methods for managing change so that an HCO can become greener and more eco-friendly. You can identify, apply, and integrate many management theories, principles, models, techniques, and tools from this book (listed at the end of chapters and in the Your Management Toolbox appendix) to help an HCO achieve a major goal and implement a major project.

Listed below are ten real-world projects that many HCOs are involved in. Later, when you become a manager, you probably will be involved in many of these projects.

1. Manage an HCO to become greener and more eco-friendly.

2. Manage an HCO to improve population health.

3. Manage an HCO to integrate clinical services.

4. Manage an HCO to strengthen diversity and inclusion.

5. Manage an HCO to create more joy in work.

6. Manage an HCO to implement mobile health.

7. Manage an HCO to reduce costs.

8. Manage an HCO to enhance patient experience.

9. Manage an HCO to prevent medical errors.

10. Manage an HCO to merge with another HCO.

The instructor may vary assignments using some of these suggestions:

◆ Students work alone or in groups.

◆ Students are required to use at least 10 different chapters or 20 different management tools.

◆ Students work on a project week-by-week, chapter-by-chapter during class as a learning activity, or as a semester-long, integrative cumulative assignment due late in the semester.

◆ Students make presentations in class, write reports, or produce videos.

◆ Students explain how to implement these projects for various types of HCOs, such as a medical group practice, nursing home, health insurance company, hospital, medical supply company, outpatient diagnostic test center, or primary care clinic.

YOUR MANAGEMENT
TOOLBOX

These management tools, methods, theories, models, and concepts will be especially useful to you in your healthcare management career. The chapter from which the tool is drawn is indicated in parentheses.

GLOSSARY

administrative theory. An integrated set of ideas to organize work, positions, departments, supervisor–subordinate relationships, hierarchy, and span of control to design an organization.

appraising performance. Evaluating workers' job performance and discussing those evaluations with them.

authority. Power formally given to a job position to make decisions, take actions, and direct and expect obedience from subordinates.

balanced scorecard. Report with performance measures typically for finances, customer service, internal business processes, and growth and learning; other kinds of measures may also be used.

bounded rationality. Limits to human rational decision making.

cause-and-effect diagram. A tool that visually identifies which factors might affect performance.

centralization. How high or low in an organization the authority exists to make a decision.

channels. Methods and media that transmit a message from sender to receiver.

collaborative leadership. Leadership used to form alliances, partnerships, and other forms of interorganization relationships.

committee. A formal group with an official purpose and official relationships with other parts of the organization.

communication. Transmitting a message to someone else to develop shared understanding.

compensating staff. Determining and giving wages, salaries, incentives, and benefits to workers.

conflict of interest. A situation in which a person's self-interest interferes with that person's obligation to another person, organization, profession, or purpose.

contingency theory. Theory that there is no single best way to organize; the best way depends on factors that differ from one situation to another.

contingent. Dependent on something.

continuum of care. A range of services needed to care for a person or population.

control. To monitor performance and take corrective action if performance does not meet expected standards.

controlling. Comparing actual performance to preset standards and making corrective adjustments if needed to meet the standards.

coordination. Connecting individual tasks, activities, jobs, departments, and people to work together toward a common purpose.

cultural competence. The ability to interact effectively with people of different cultures.

culture. The values, norms, guiding beliefs, and understandings shared by members of an organization and taught to new members as the correct way to think, feel, and behave.

decision making. The process of choosing from among alternatives to determine and implement a course of action.

delegate authority. Give authority to a subordinate position to make decisions and take actions.

departmentalization. Organization of jobs and work into departments, bureaus, divisions, sections, offices, and other formal groups.

designing jobs and work. Determining work tasks to be done by a job, along with the job's qualifications, supervision, working conditions, rules, and schedules.

developing staff. Helping employees acquire new knowledge, skills, attitudes, behaviors, and competencies for current and future jobs.

diagonal communication. Communication to someone at a higher or lower level of an organization and outside of one's own vertical chain of command or hierarchy.

differentiation. Differences in departments' structures and how their workers think and feel.

directing. Assigning work to workers and motivating them to do the work.

diversity. The range of human differences that include the primary (internal) dimension such as age, gender, race, ethnicity, physical and mental ability, and sexual orientation and the secondary (external) dimension such as thought styles, religion, nationality, socio-economic status, belief systems, military experience, and education.

division of work. How work is separated into smaller, more specialized tasks and activities.

divisional structure. An organization structure that organizes departments and positions to focus on particular groups of customers or services.

downward communication. Communication to someone at a lower level in one's own vertical chain of command or hierarchy.

emotional intelligence. Ability to recognize and understand emotions in yourself and others, and then to use this awareness to manage your behavior and relationships.

ethical climate. The shared perceptions of how ethical issues should be addressed and what is ethically correct behavior for an organization.

ethical dilemma. A situation in which any decision or course of action will have an undesirable ethical outcome.

ethics. Values and moral principles regarding what is right and wrong.

evidence-based management. An approach to making decisions through the conscientious, explicit, and judicious use of the best available evidence from multiple sources.

external equity. Fairness in compensation for a job compared to compensation for other similar jobs outside the organization.

force field analysis. Graphical technique that shows and evaluates the strength of various forces that are *for* and *against* a change.

formal organization. The official organization as approved by managers and stated in written documents.

functional structure. An organization structure that organizes departments and positions according to the functions workers perform and the workers' abilities.

Gantt chart. Graphic arrangement of tasks needed to complete a project, in sequence and with start and end dates for each task; may include other information, such as the person responsible and resources needed for each task.

garbage can decision making. Seemingly random organizational decision making resulting from evolving streams of problems, solutions, participants, and decision-making opportunities.

goal. A specific, measurable outcome that will help achieve the mission and vision.

group. Two or more people who interact with each other and share a common purpose.

groupthink. A process in which group members quickly agree without considering diverse ideas and thoughtful analysis, usually to maintain group harmony.

health. A state of complete physical, mental, and social well-being; not merely the absence of disease or infirmity.

healthcare. The maintaining and restoration of health by the treatment and prevention of disease and injury, especially by trained and licensed professionals.

health disparity. A health difference that is closely linked with social, economic, or environmental disadvantage.

hiring staff. Recruiting and selecting people for jobs, which may include reassigning existing workers by promotion or transfer.

horizontal communication. Communication to someone at the same level of an organization and outside of one's own vertical chain of command or hierarchy.

horizontal structure. An organization structure that organizes work into core processes that are performed by self-managed, multidisciplinary teams of workers.

human relations. A type of management based on psychology and sociology that considers employees' feelings and behaviors, especially in groups.

inclusion. The active, intentional, and ongoing engagement of diversity, where each person is valued, respected, and supported for his or her distinctive skills, experiences, and perspectives, to create a working and learning environment where everyone has an opportunity to experience personal fulfillment and participate fully.

incremental decision making. The process by which a big, complex decision is gradually made from a series of small decisions during a lengthy time period that may involve backing up to further diagnose problems, rethink ideas, and revise prior choices.

informal organization. Workers' own unofficial and unwritten work rules, procedures, expectations, agreements, and communication networks (e.g., the grapevine), which coexist and may conflict with the official ones of the formal organization.

integrator. A person who works full-time coordinating the work of multiple departments toward a common purpose.

internal equity. Fairness in compensation for a job compared to compensation for other jobs inside the organization.

intuition. The process of knowing, believing, or deciding based on experience, hunches, or unconscious processes rather than on logical conscious thinking and reasoning.

job. A group of activities and duties that entail natural units of work that are similar and related; may be performed by more than one person.

job description. A statement that indicates the job title and work to be done; often includes minimum qualifications and describes the job's authority, reporting relationships, equipment and materials used, working conditions, work schedule, mental and physical demands, interactions with others, and salary range. Also called *position description*.

key performance indicator. A metric linked to a target or standard of performance.

knowledge management. A system for finding, organizing, and making available an organization's knowledge, including its experience, understanding, expertise, methods, judgment, lessons learned, and know-how.

leading. A process by which a person tries to influence someone else to voluntarily accomplish a task, goal, or vision.

Lean production. Design of work processes to reduce waste, increase efficiency and speed, and thereby produce more value for customers.

line jobs. Jobs that contribute directly to achieving an organization's purpose and main goals.

line of authority. The vertical chain of command, authority, and formal communication up and down an organization.

management. The process of getting things done through and with people.

managerial ethics. Ethics that guide right and wrong in the practice of management.

matrix structure. An organization structure that organizes work by combining functional and divisional structures; uses vertical and horizontal authority to manage workers.

mechanistic. Emphasizing specialized, rigid tasks; centralized decisions; strict hierarchy, control, and rules; and vertical communication and interaction.

medical ethics. Ethics that guide right and wrong in the practice of medicine.

mission. The purpose of an organization; why the organization exists.

moral distress. A situation in which an organization's constraints prevent someone from doing what the person thinks is ethically right.

motivation. The set of forces that leads people to behave in particular ways.

network structure. An organization structure that organizes work by outsourcing much of it to a network of other organizations connected by interpersonal relationships, contracts, and information systems.

nonprogrammed decisions. Decisions that are new, unusual, hard to define, and hard to diagnose; they present fuzzy alternatives with uncertain cause and effect relationships and without existing decision rules to follow.

nonverbal encoding. Representing ideas without using words, such as with icons, diagrams, attire, objects, body language, touch, behavior, and actions.

norms. Behaviors and attitudes expected of people in a group, organization, or society.

onboarding. The process of helping new hires adjust to social and performance aspects of their new jobs.

organic. Emphasizing shared flexible tasks; teamwork; decentralized decisions; loose hierarchy, control, and rules; and horizontal communication and interaction.

organization chart. Visual portrayal of vertical hierarchy, departments, span of control, reporting relationships, and flow of authority.

organization development. A process that applies behavioral science knowledge and practices to help organizations build their capability to change and achieve greater effectiveness.

organization learning. A process that enhances an organization's capability to acquire and develop new knowledge.

organization structure. The reporting relationships, vertical hierarchy, spans of control, groupings of jobs into departments and an entire organization, and systems for coordination and communication.

organizational socialization. The process by which employees learn (and share with others) their organization's culture, including what is and is not acceptable behavior.

organizations. Social entities that are goal-directed, designed as deliberately structured and coordinated activity systems, and linked to the external environment.

organizing. Arranging work into jobs, teams, departments, and other work units; arranging supervisor–subordinate relationships; assigning responsibility, authority, and other resources.

outcome measures. Measures of results and effects.

patient experience. All that a patient experiences and perceives while interacting with the healthcare system, healthcare organizations, and healthcare workers.

personal power. Power based on a person.

planning. Deciding what to do and how to do it.

planning for staff. Forecasting the staff (workforce) the organization will require in the future and planning how to effectively obtain and retain that future staff.

point-factor system. A system for determining a job's value, in which points are assigned to each job based on how each job rates on a common set of factors used to evaluate all jobs; total points for a job determine pay for that job.

politics. The use of power to influence decisions.

population health. The health outcomes of a group of individuals, including the distribution of outcomes within the group.

position. A group of activities and duties that are performed by only one person.

positional power. Power based on a position in an organization.

power. The ability to influence others to achieve outcomes.

process. A set of tasks, activities, and steps performed sequentially to transform resource inputs into outputs and thereby accomplish a specific outcome.

process map. A tool that identifies and shows in sequence the flow of tasks, activities, and steps required to complete a process.

process measures. Measures of the work that is done, how it is done, and the activities performed.

professional ethics. Ethics that guide right and wrong for a profession, such as the nursing profession.

professionalism. The ability to align personal and organizational conduct with ethical and professional standards.

programmed decisions. Decisions that are well defined, routine, easily diagnosed, and easily solved with existing decision rules, formulas, algorithms, and procedures.

project. A temporary endeavor undertaken to create a unique product, service, or result.

project management. The application of knowledge, skills, tools, and techniques to project activities to meet the project requirements.

protecting staff. Ensuring that workers have proper and safe work conditions, their rights are protected, and their opinions are considered by managers.

rational decision making. The process of making a decision based on logical reasoning and deliberate analysis.

refreeze. Lock in the new way and make it the correct way of doing something.

root-cause analysis. A structured problem-solving technique to find and fix the ultimate cause of a problem rather than the visible symptoms of the problem.

satisfice. To decide on a satisfactory (rather than the best) solution that will suffice.

scientific management. A type of management that uses standardization, specialization, and scientific experiments to design jobs for greater efficiency and production.

servant leadership. Leadership style that emphasizes that a leader should serve the followers by respecting, empowering, hearing, teaching, and supporting workers and helping them succeed.

Six Sigma. A performance improvement program that aims to reduce variation and defects in work processes and outputs to meet customers' quality requirements.

social responsibility. Ethics that guide right and wrong for the good of society.

span of control. How many subordinate workers a manager is directly responsible for; how many workers report directly to that manager (sometimes called *span of supervision* or *span of management*).

specialization. The width of the range of tasks and work done by an employee or department.

staff jobs. Jobs that use specialized skills, abilities, and expertise to support line jobs and thereby indirectly contribute to the organization's main goals.

staffing. Obtaining and retaining people to fill jobs and do work.

stakeholders. For a designated organization, people and other organizations who have a stake (interest) in what the organization does.

strategic planning. A decision-making activity that defines where an organization is going, sets its future direction, and guides its future efforts to move the organization toward its intended future.

strategy. An idea that guides an organization's decisions, actions, and behaviors in a consistent way to gain competitive advantage.

structural inertia. Resistance to change created by organization structures and systems.

structure measures. Measures of resources, staff, equipment, competencies, inputs, facilities, and characteristics of the organization; how the organization is set up.

subculture. Culture of a distinct part of an organization (e.g., a team or department) that exists within the organization's overall culture.

SWOTs. Strengths, weaknesses, opportunities, and threats.

system. A set of interrelated parts that function as a whole to achieve a common purpose.

team. A special kind of group whose members share a common goal and accountability for outcomes and coordinate tasks, skills, and resources interdependently.

Theory X. Leader assumes people dislike work, are lazy and stupid, are motivated by rewards from others, lack self-discipline, want security, and do not want responsibility.

Theory Y. Leader assumes people like meaningful work, are creative and capable, are motivated by rewards from within themselves, have self-control, can direct themselves, and want responsibility.

Theory Z. Leader emphasizes concern for workers, develops long-term cooperative relationships, provides slow yet steady long-term growth opportunities for workers, and promotes individual and collective responsibility.

transactional leadership. Leadership based on transactions; workers perform tasks to achieve goals and then the leader gives workers pay and other rewards.

transformational leadership. Leadership that uses a compelling vision, inspiration, charisma, intelligence, and attention to employees' individual needs to revitalize an organization with change for the greater good of all.

unfreeze. Create dissatisfaction with the current way and motivate people to want change.

unity of command. Arrangement in which a worker takes commands from and is responsible to only one boss.

upward communication. Communication to someone at a higher level in one's own vertical chain of command or hierarchy.

value stream mapping. A visual diagram of all steps in a process used to transform inputs into outputs when creating a product or service for customers.

values. Deeply held beliefs, ideals, and standards of behavior.

verbal encoding. Using written or spoken words to represent ideas.

vision. What the organization wants to be in the long-term future; what it aspires to become.

INDEX

ABOUT THE AUTHOR

Peter C. Olden, PhD, MHA, LFACHE, earned a BS in business from Miami University and an MHA from Duke University. For 14 years, he held executive positions at a community hospital, teaching hospital, and regional medical center. Initiating a career change, he completed a PhD in health services organization and research at Virginia Commonwealth University, then joined the faculty at the University of Scranton (Pennsylvania). There he became a full professor and also served as a program director and a department chair. He taught undergraduate and graduate healthcare management courses for many years, including the undergraduate and graduate capstone courses. His teaching included healthcare management lectures and workshops abroad.

Dr. Olden's scholarship focused on healthcare organizations and management, preventive health, the US healthcare system, and health administration education. He authored chapters for healthcare management textbooks and published articles in *Health Services Research*, *Journal of Healthcare Management*, *Health Care Management Review*, *The Milbank Quarterly*, *Health Care Manager*, *Journal of Health Administration Education*, and other journals. He presented at conferences of the Academy of Management, Association of University Programs in Health Administration, AcademyHealth, American Public Health Association, and other organizations. Dr. Olden reviewed proposals and abstracts for national conferences, reviewed manuscripts for peer-reviewed journals, and served on editorial boards. As a volunteer, he contributed to health organizations, especially the American Cancer Society, which he served at the local, state, and national levels. During his hospital management career, he was a Fellow of the American College of Healthcare Executives (ACHE). He is a Life Fellow of ACHE, which honored him with its Service Award in 2008. Dr. Olden retired in 2018 from being a full-time professor and is now professor emeritus.